Better Homes and Gardens®

FOOD FOR HEALTH & HEALING

Medical Reviewer:
George Blackburn, M.D., Ph.D.
Associate Director of Nutrition
Division of Nutrition
Harvard Medical School

Better Homes and Gardens® Books
Des Moines, Iowa

Better Homes and Gardens® Books
An imprint of Meredith® Books

Better Homes and Gardens® Food for Health & Healing
Food Editor: Kristi M. Fuller, R.D.
Associate Art Director: Lynda Haupert
Copy Chief: Catherine Hamrick
Copy and Production Editor: Terri Fredrickson
Contributing Editor and Recipe Development: Marcia K. Stanley, R.D.
Contributing Copy Editor: Angela K. Renkoski
Contributing Proofreaders: Susie Kling, Debra Morris Smith, JoEllyn Witke
Illustrator: Eric Grotenhuis
Indexer: Sharon Duffy
Electronic Production Coordinator: Paula Forest
Editorial and Design Assistants: Kaye Chabot, Judy Bailey, Treesa Landry, Karen Schirm
Test Kitchen Director: Sharon Stilwell
Test Kitchen Product Supervisor: Marilyn Cornelius
Production Director: Douglas M. Johnston
Production Manager: Pam Kvitne
Assistant Prepress Manager: Marjorie J. Schenkelberg

Meredith® Books
Editor in Chief: James D. Blume
Design Director: Matt Strelecki
Managing Editor: Gregory H. Kayko
Executive Health Editor: Alice Feinstein

Director, Sales & Marketing, Retail: Michael A. Peterson
Director, Sales & Marketing, Special Markets: Rita McMullen
Director, Sales & Marketing, Home & Garden Center Channel: Ray Wolf
Director, Operations: George A. Susral

Vice President, General Manager: Jamie L. Martin

Better Homes and Gardens® Magazine
Editor in Chief: Jean LemMon

Meredith Publishing Group
President, Publishing Group: Christopher M. Little
Vice President, Consumer Marketing & Development: Hal Oringer

Meredith Corporation
Chairman and Chief Executive Officer: William T. Kerr

Chairman of the Executive Committee: E. T. Meredith III

All of us at Better Homes and Gardens® Books are dedicated to providing you with information and ideas to ensure your family's health. We welcome your comments and suggestions. Write to us at: Better Homes and Gardens® Books, Health Editorial Department, 1716 Locust St, LN 116, Des Moines, IA 50309-3023. If you would like to purchase any of our books, check wherever books are sold.

Our seal assures you that every recipe in Better Homes and Gardens® *Food for Health & Healing* has been tested in the Better Homes and Gardens® Test Kitchen. This means that each recipe is practical and reliable, and meets our high standards of taste appeal. We guarantee your satisfaction with this book for as long as you own it.

Contributing Writers

Jan Bresnick has written and edited for a number of national health magazines. Her special areas of interest and expertise include men's health, women's health, and weight control. She was a contributing writer for the book *Energy Forever*.

Susan A. Fiske is a writer for numerous national health and popular women's magazines.

Sara J. Henry has authored a number of popular health books, including *Arthritis: What Works*. Fitness is her area of special interest and expertise. She has also edited several health and fitness books on such topics as diabetes, surgery, running, carpal tunnel syndrome, and sports massage.

Mark Ingebretsen of Des Moines, Iowa, is a former senior editor of *Better Homes and Gardens*® magazine. He is currently a freelance writer, whose works have been published in the nation's top magazines.

Claire Kowalchik is the author of *The Complete Book of Running for Women*.

Judith Lin is a certified personal trainer whose work has appeared in several magazines and health books.

Diane Quagliani, R.D., is a national media spokesperson for the American Dietetic Association. Her health and nutrition articles have appeared in several of the nation's top magazines. She is a contributing writer to a number of Better Homes and Gardens® books, including *New Dieter's Cookbook* and *Eating Well with the Food Guide Pyramid*.

Maureen P. Sangiorgio has written for many health and popular magazines and has contributed to numerous health books, including *The Doctor's Book of Home Remedies for Women*.

Porter Shimer is the author of *Fitness Through Pleasure, More Fat-Burning Foods*, and *Native American Healing Secrets*. He also has contributed to numerous health books and written for a number of health magazines.

Elizabeth Somer, R.D., is the author of *Food & Mood, The Nutritional Desk Reference, The Essential Guide to Vitamins and Minerals*, and *Nutrition for Women: The Complete Guide*.

Selene Yeager, a certified personal trainer, is the co-author of *New Foods for Healing* and *Alternative Healing Secrets*. She also has contributed to several books, including *The Complete Book of Alternative Nutrition* and *Healing with Vitamins*.

Contents

Foreword

How would you like to extend your life by a quarter of a century? You can!

"Good eating can add an extra 25 years of life," says the medical reviewer of this book, George Blackburn, M.D., Ph.D., Associate Director of Nutrition in the Division of Nutrition at Harvard Medical School. He's not alone in his opinion, either. Experts at the American Cancer Society, for example, estimate that each year approximately one-third of America's 500,000 cancer deaths are due to this nation's unhealthy eating habits.

In fact, a mountain of medical research—done in the top research institutions in this country by the top nutritional researchers—bears witness to this simple message: Eating the right way can help keep you healthy. And if you're sick, eating the right way can very often help you heal. So, what exactly is the right way?

Better Homes and Gardens® Food for Health & Healing makes it simple for you. It shows you how a diet of wonderfully delicious foods—whole grains, vegetables, and luscious fruits—can help you prevent cancer, heart disease, diabetes, and high blood pressure. It shows you how eating the healthy way can help you lose weight,

look younger, and give you more energy. None of this is difficult.

Chapter 1, "The 7 Keys to Healthy Eating" contains seven simple concepts that are the basic keys to healthy eating. You can continue to use these simple keys to make healthy food choices for you and your family for the rest of your lives.

It would be great if all you had to do these days was concentrate on selecting and preparing healthy foods. Unfortunately, there are some new microbes in the world that you need to defend yourself against. Clean, safe food preparation has never been more important than it is today. **Chapter 2, "The 6 Rules for Food Safety"** can save your life—literally.

Chapter 3, "Conditions and Diseases," builds on the important foundation laid in the opening chapters. Here you will find lots of information about healing a specific disease or condition by eating healthy food. But remember this critical point: It would be unwise to rely *only* on food to prevent disease and help you heal. And although research may point to certain foods as helpful, it has involved a limited number of participants. Every individual is different, every body is different, including yours.

So when you move beyond the basic rules of good, healthy eating and consider specific healing foods or even supplements, talk to your doctor. He or she, usually working in concert with a registered dietitian or other health care professional, can help you put together a customized eating plan that's just right for you.

One more thing needs to be said: *Enjoy* your food! **Chapter 4, "Healing Recipes,"** a section of luscious recipes, all tested in the Better Homes and Gardens® Test Kitchen should help you with that mission. The need for high fiber foods comes up again and again in this book. High fiber foods include beans, which are not exactly on everyone's list as a pleasure food. But with recipes like Three-Bean Salad, Caribbean Beans and Rice, and North African Bean Stew to get you started, plain old beans can take on a whole new meaning.

We hear again and again that soy foods are good for you and especially helpful in preventing many women's health problems. Soybean Pilaf and Fruity Tofu Shakes make it easy to increase your soybean intake. Stymied about how to get more whole grains into your diet? Try Roasted Vegetables and Quinoa, Millet-Stuffed Squash, or Nutty Brown Rice Patties. And for sheer pleasure, you can't beat desserts like Apple-Plum Crostata or Mango Mousse.

Besides tasting good, all the easy, innovative recipes in this book were designed with a specific health mission in mind. But they all taste so good, you can forget about the nutrients and concentrate on enjoyment. Healthy eating is such a pleasure. Isn't it wonderful that it's also good for you?

Alice Feinstein
Executive Health Editor
Meredith® Books

good eating

YOUR INSURANCE POLICY FOR GOOD HEALTH

❮❮ You are what you eat.
— Dr. Henry Lindlahr ❯❯

When you take stock of the riches in your life, where does good health appear on the list? Like many people, you likely count it as your single most precious asset. After all, being healthy allows you to fully enjoy the many other treasures that life offers.

You have your health today. But will you have it tomorrow? Does good health sometimes seem like an unpredictable blessing that can vanish without warning?

It's true that some factors that influence your health are beyond your control—getting older, for example, or a family history of a particular disease.

But many factors are well within your control. Among them are whether you smoke, how much alcohol you drink, how physically active you are, and—the focus of this book— the food you eat.

Healthful Eating: What's in It for You?

Just how important is a healthful diet in the mix of factors that paint your total health picture?

"What you eat is very important to good health," explains Tim Byers, M.D., M.P.H., professor in the Department of Preventive Medicine and Biometrics at the University of Colorado School of Medicine in Boulder. "In fact, in terms of health benefits, eating well is a two-for-one deal that's hard to beat. It pays off now by helping you feel good today and pays off later by helping prevent many chronic diseases that may occur as you get older."

Today, healthful eating habits power you with energy to tackle that long "to do" list, contribute to good looks and maintaining a healthful weight, and help prevent annoying problems such as irregularity that can slow you down.

A lifetime of good eating helps prevent or delay a number of illnesses that can rob you of your zest for life or result in premature death. Need convincing? Scan this list of relationships between diet and

health claims

that enhance your health

Scientific research has uncovered several solid relationships between what we eat and our health. To guide us in making healthful food choices, the Food and Drug Administration (FDA) permits health claims about these relationships to appear on some food packages. Only foods meeting strict criteria may use a health claim on their package, but not all foods meeting the criteria opt to list this information. The following are 11 relationships between diet and disease prevention you may read about on food packages:

● A calcium-rich diet helps maintain bone health and may reduce risk of osteoporosis.

● Limiting the amount of sodium you eat may reduce risk for high blood pressure.

● Limiting the total amount of fat in your diet may help reduce your long-term risk for some types of cancer.

● Diets low in saturated fat and cholesterol may help reduce risk of heart disease.

● Diets rich in fiber-containing grain products, fruits, and vegetables may reduce risk for some types of cancer.

● Eating fruits, vegetables, and grain products that contain soluble fiber may reduce risk of heart disease.

● Eating fruits and vegetables that contain dietary fiber, vitamin A, or vitamin C may reduce risk of some types of cancer.

● Consuming adequate folate may reduce a woman's risk of having a child with a brain or spinal cord defect.

● Sugar alcohols (such as xylitol, sorbitol, or mannitol) do not promote tooth decay.

● Soluble fiber from whole oats may reduce risk of heart disease.

● Soluble fiber from psyllium may reduce risk of heart disease.

disease, established by years of scientific research. It's an eye-opener:

Poor eating habits contribute to contracting heart disease, cancer, stroke, and diabetes—four of the 10 leading causes of death in the United States.

Being overweight increases risk for a bevy of illnesses, including heart disease, stroke, high blood pressure, diabetes, and several types of cancer. An alarming one in three Americans is overweight, a jump up from one in four just two decades ago. One in five children and adolescents is overweight as well.

Eating too much fat increases risk for heart disease and cancers of the colon, rectum, prostate, and endometrium.

The saturated fat found in meats, dairy products, and coconut and palm oils is the biggest dietary culprit for high blood cholesterol, a major risk factor for heart

the 9 red flags of junk science

The next time you read a confusing or conflicting nutrition report, see if it raises one of these red flags. If so, beat a hasty retreat.

1. Recommendations that promise a quick fix.
2. Dire warnings of danger from a single product or regimen.
3. Claims that sound too good to be true.
4. Simplistic conclusions drawn from a single study.
5. Dramatic statements that are refuted by reputable scientific organizations.
6. Lists of "good" and "bad" foods.

7. Recommendations made to help sell a product.
8. Recommendations based on studies published without peer review.
9. Recommendations from studies that ignore differences among individuals or groups.

(Source: Food and Nutrition Science Alliance, September 1995.)

attack. One in five Americans has high blood cholesterol.

More than one in three (35 percent) of all cancer deaths are related to what we eat. Up to 90 percent of colon and rectal cancers are caused by diet. The links to increased risk? Eating too much fat and too little fiber.

Eating too much sodium drives up blood pressure in up to 30 percent of Americans.

Low calcium intake can lead to osteoporosis, the crippling, bone-thinning disease that results in 1.5 million bone fractures each year. More than 28 million Americans, mostly women, are at high risk of developing osteoporosis.

Drinking too much alcohol may increase risk for breast cancer.

But, enough dietary gloom and doom! A healthful eating plan chock-full of whole grains, vegetables, and fruits, and light on

saturated fat from sources such as meat and dairy products does wonders for staying healthy and preventing disease, according to Byers. "National nutrition surveys show that the American diet is slowly improving," he says. "Since the 1960s, we've gradually been eating more fruits and vegetables and less saturated fat. At the same time, average blood cholesterol levels have declined."

While other factors such as advances in medical treatment and a decline in smoking also contributed to this improvement, diet is surely an essential part of the mix.

What does all this mean to you? It's really good news. With the sure knowledge that medical science backs you up, you can now count healthful eating as your powerful ally for maintaining vibrant good health. And in this fast-paced, ever-changing world, isn't it nice to know that making good food choices is one important way you can take charge of your health?

Barriers to Better Eating

Okay, you're convinced. You know that a healthful diet positively impacts your health both today and years from now. But, if you're like many Americans, knowing isn't necessarily doing. Do you see yourself in these statistics?

A whopping eight in 10 Americans believe nutrition impacts their health, but only half (four in 10) are doing all they can to eat right, according to a recent survey by The American Dietetic Association.

What's causing this short circuit between believing and doing?

People who participated in the survey reported that their top three barriers to eating better are:

1. Confusion over conflicting media reports about nutrition.
2. Fear of having to give up their favorite foods.
3. Believing that healthful eating takes too much time.

Don't let these barriers trip up your good intentions to eat right! Let's knock them down right now with help from registered dietitian Cindy Moore, a spokesperson for The American Dietetic Association and director of Nutrition Therapy at the Cleveland Clinic Foundation in Cleveland, Ohio.

Barrier Number 1:
Confusion over Mixed Media Messages

You know the drill:
● *Butter's bad and margarine's good.* Then butter's back and margarine's on the back burner.
● *Oat bran is fabulous, then it fizzles.* Now it's back again with its very own health claim on food labels.

Why do we continually see these frustrating nutrition flip-flops in the news? And what's the best advice to follow?

Moore explains it this way: "Credible nutrition advice is based on hundreds of research studies conducted over many years until a pattern emerges. During this process, results from different studies will sometimes contradict each other. Scientific research has worked this way for years. But

call for help

A registered dietitian (RD) is a specially trained nutrition professional who can answer your nutrition questions or create a customized eating plan that's right for you.

For a free referral to an RD near you, call The American Dietetic Association's Consumer Nutrition Hot Line toll-free at 800/366-1655.

To speak directly with an RD who will answer your specific food and nutrition questions, call 900/CALL-AN-RD (900/225-5267).

today, people are so hungry for nutrition information that the media reports on many studies before researchers reach a consensus."

"That's why you shouldn't change your eating habits based on only a study or two," advises Moore. "Instead, wait for agreement from respected health authorities such as The American Dietetic Association, the American Heart Association, and the American Cancer Society." Or, ask your doctor. You might also consult a respected nutrition professional such as a registered dietitian. (See "Call for Help," on page 12 to find a registered dietitian who can answer your questions.)

Barrier Number 2:
Fear of Forgoing Favorite Foods

Mmmm, juicy, sizzling steak; crispy, golden french fries; devilishly dense chocolate cake… You'd hate to give up your favorite dishes forever, wouldn't you?

Unfortunately, many people envision eating right as a dreary regimen devoid of taste. They see ho-hum, boring foods and (yawn) a lifetime of boring, boring, boring meals stretching out into a dull, gray infinity. Fortunately, nothing could be further from the truth.

"Any food you like can fit into a healthful meal plan," says Moore. The trick is to keep the portion size reasonable and

---

a word about the word "diet"

The word "diet" gets a bad rap. That's because it's often associated with strict, unsafe, or downright silly weight-loss schemes. Rest assured, when you see the word "diet" throughout these pages, it's meant as it should be: the foods and beverages that make up the sum total of what you eat— your eating style, if you will.

---

watch how often you indulge in yummy goodies. In other words, you can have your cake and eat it, too—just not the whole cake and not every day!

Moore's favorite portion control strategy is to freeze brownies or cookies in individual packets. Then, when the urge hits, she takes out a single serving and savors it.

What if you occasionally throw portion control to the wind and scarf down half a pizza loaded with pepperoni and extra cheese? Don't fret, says Moore. Over the next day or so, simply balance out your indulgence by choosing more lower-fat foods such as whole grains, vegetables, and fruits and by upping your physical activity regimen a bit.

Barrier Number 3:
You Can't Eat Healthy in a Hurry

Nonsense! People crave convenience, says Moore, so the food industry now provides a tremendous number of options that are both fast and healthful. Just one example is the

good nutrition advice
in a nutshell

Be realistic. Make small changes over time in what you eat and the level of activity you do. After all, small steps work better than giant leaps.

Be adventurous. Expand your tastes to enjoy a variety of foods.

Be flexible. Go ahead; balance what you eat and the physical activity you do over several days. There's no need to agonize about just one meal or even one day.

Be sensible. Enjoy all foods; just don't overdo it.

Be active. Walk the dog; don't just watch the dog walk.

(Source: The Dietary Guidelines Alliance)

explosion of ready-to-use fresh vegetables such as salads, baby carrots, cut-up broccoli and cauliflower, slaw, and stir-fry mixes.

As a busy professional who works long hours, Moore is a fan of the "big batch" method of convenience. "I make a huge batch of oatmeal and store it in the fridge. In the morning, I microwave a portion with some milk and sweetener. My breakfast is ready in less than a minute." Moore also makes large portions of long-cooking dishes such as soups and brown rice to freeze in small containers. "It's a snap to defrost them in the microwave," she says.

And what could be faster than fresh fruit? Moore keeps a bowl of her favorite apples, bananas, pears, and grapes right in her office, ready for speed snacking.

The Best Barrier Busters

Consider Chapter One your game plan for breaking down all your personal barriers to better eating.

For starters, you'll learn about the best nutrition advice around—the Dietary Guidelines for Americans—seven simple, scientifically sound keys to eating for good health. You'll find easy strategies for putting the Guidelines into practice, including "how-tos" on using the Food Guide Pyramid and the Nutrition Facts food label.

And because we couldn't agree more that food must taste great and be convenient, too, you'll find lots of ideas for selecting healthful, great-tasting food fast. The recipes in this book, which begin on page 289, will go a long way toward helping you enjoy healthy eating. They're easy, kitchen-tested in the Better Homes and Gardens® Test Kitchen, and healthy. What's more, they taste good.

Let's start busting those barriers right now!

chapter 1

the 7 TO keys healthy eating

{ He who has health has hope, and he who has hope, has everything. — Arabian Proverb }

Every year you make thousands and thousands of decisions that have an impact on your health. And, if you shop and cook for your family, you make thousands of little decisions that, taken together, have an impact on your family members' health.

Although keeping up with all the latest nutrition research can be overwhelming—a full-time job for a dietitian, as a matter of fact—the good news is that you don't have to. You can unlock the secrets to healthy eating with just seven simple keys. Taken together, these seven keys are known as the Dietary Guidelines for Americans.

The Guidelines provide nutrition advice for healthy Americans age two years and older. To develop these Guidelines, the U.S. Department of Agriculture (USDA) and U.S. Department of Health and Human Services assembled the country's top health and nutrition authorities to create easy-to-follow nutrition advice for eating right. The question is, do these government guidelines really work?

"You can be sure these nutrition guidelines are scientifically sound," says Sachiko T. St. Jeor, Ph.D., R.D., a member of the 1995 Dietary Guidelines Advisory Committee and professor and director of the Nutrition Education and Research Program at the University of Nevada School of Medicine in Reno. "The committee evaluated the enormous and ever-changing body of nutrition research to provide consumers with the best nutrition advice available today."

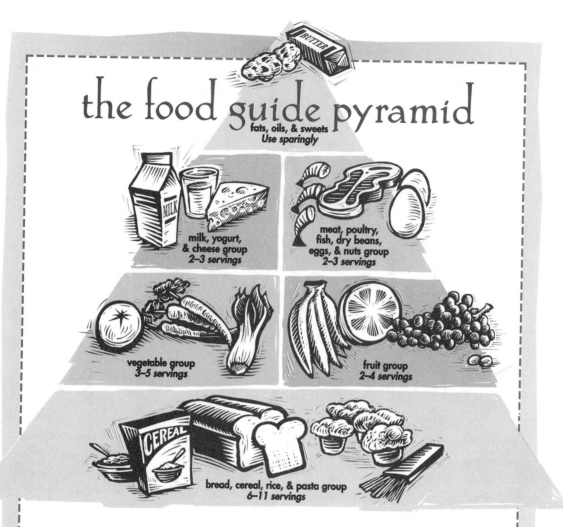

the food guide pyramid

fats, oils, & sweets
Use sparingly

milk, yogurt,
& cheese group
2–3 servings

meat, poultry,
fish, dry beans,
eggs, & nuts group
2–3 servings

vegetable group
3–5 servings

fruit group
2–4 servings

bread, cereal, rice, & pasta group
6–11 servings

The USDA's Food Guide Pyramid is a reliable road map for translating the seven keys into the food choices that end up on your plate. The pyramid helps you select foods that meet your calorie and nutrition needs without getting too much fat, saturated fat, cholesterol, sugar, and sodium.

Can you spot the Pyramid's biggest clue to a healthful eating plan?

Compare the sizes of each food group. The biggest groups at the Pyramid base (grains, vegetables, and fruits) should make up the biggest part of your diet. The meat and dairy groups, though also important for good health, are smaller and should be enjoyed in moderation. The Pyramid tip is not an official food group but includes "extras" such as butter, margarine, oils, and sweets. The tip is smaller because these foods supply calories, but few, if any, vitamins or minerals. Most of us can afford to eat only small amounts.

Look for the Pyramid Pointers throughout this chapter to learn more about using the Pyramid as a tool to help you eat for health.

The Nutrition Facts Label

The Nutrition Facts label, *right*, found on almost all packaged foods in the grocery store, helps you create an eating plan that meets the Dietary Guidelines. You can use Nutrition Facts to learn about the nutrition value of foods, make comparisons between products, and plan your and your family's meals and snacks. **The nutrition numbers and percentages** you see on the Nutrition Facts label are based on current health recommendations for a 2,000-calorie diet.

The % Daily Value column shows you how much total fat, saturated fat, cholesterol, total carbohydrate, and dietary fiber one serving of a food contributes to a healthful 2,000-calorie diet. The % Daily Values for sodium, vitamins, and minerals apply to all calorie levels. In the example shown, one serving of the food provides 5 percent of the daily total fat budget and contributes 4 percent of needed calcium.

To stay within healthful guidelines for total fat, saturated fat, cholesterol, and sodium, make sure the % Daily Values for your daily food choices don't add up to more than 100 percent. For nutrients we sometimes fall short on—total carbohydrate, dietary fiber, vitamins, and minerals—shoot to reach the 100 percent level each day.

Some labels show Daily Values for 2,000- and 2,500-calorie diets. Use these numbers as a quick reference for how much total fat, saturated fat, cholesterol, sodium, total carbohydrate, and dietary fiber are recommended each day for these two calorie levels.

What about foods without labels? The Nutrition Facts label only appears on packaged foods, but that doesn't mean you're in the dark when purchasing fresh meat, poultry, seafood, vegetables, and fruits. Most stores display nutrition information for fresh foods on posters or in brochures right in the department.

Nutrition Facts

Serving Size 1 cup (228g)
Servings Per Container 2

Amount Per Serving

Calories 90   Calories from Fat 30

	% Daily Value*
Total Fat 3g	5%
Saturated Fat 0g	0%
Cholesterol 0mg	0%
Sodium 300mg	13%
Total Carbohydrate 13g	4%
Dietary Fiber 3g	12%
Sugars 3g	
Protein 3g	

Vitamin A 80%	•	Vitamin C 60%
Calcium 4%	•	Iron 4%

*Percent Daily Values are based on a 2,000-calorie diet. Your daily values may be higher or lower depending on your calorie needs:

		Calories:	2,000	2,500
Total Fat	Less than		65g	80g
Sat. Fat	Less than		20g	25g
Cholesterol	Less than		300mg	300mg
Sodium	Less than		2,400mg	2,400mg
Total Carbohydrate			300g	375g
Dietary Fiber			25g	30g

Calories per gram:

Fat 9 • Carbohydrate 4 • Protein 4

the 7 keys

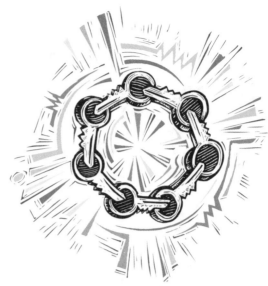

On the following pages, you'll learn why each of the seven keys is important for safeguarding your and your family's health. And you'll find dozens of quick and easy tips, techniques, and tactics to help you make each guideline a part of your life.

1: variety

Eat a Variety of Foods

You know variety is the spice of life, but do you know it's also a key to good health?

Your body needs more than 40 different nutrients to stay in top shape, but you can't get them all from one food. Oranges are loaded with the vitamin C you need for healthy body tissues and to fight infections, for example. But you can't eat an orange to get the vitamin B12 you need for healthy red blood cells. Cheese contains vitamin B12 and calcium. But you won't get any vitamin C from a piece of cheese. All of these foods are good, healthful foods. But none of them provides everything. So, you see, one food simply can't do it all. And it's a good thing, too. Eating lots of different foods is an endless source of pleasure.

First Aid for the Variety Averse

A staggering 15,000 new food products appear in supermarkets each year, yet the majority of many Americans' weekly food choices include the same eight or 10 foods. With so many choices available, why are we so averse to variety? Why is trying something new such a big challenge for so many people?

"I see many adults who are in food ruts," says registered dietitian Elizabeth M. Ward, a nutritionist at Harvard Vanguard Medical Associates in Boston and spokesperson for The American Dietetic Association. "They eat chicken or pasta five nights a week because they can get it on the table fast." But, she says, adding some variety to your daily menu can be fast and fun. Here's how to do it:

🍎 **Rev up your culinary repertoire.**
"There's a big wide world of foods out there," says Ward, "and plenty of quick, tasty recipes to help you and your family enjoy them." Earmark interesting recipes, then invest some weekend time to try them out. Make a big batch so you'll have extra for a quick meal during the week. You can start

pyramid pointer

Let the Pyramid serve as your variety guide. Each day, choose the right number of servings from all five Pyramid food groups and eat many different foods from within each group. This chart will help you determine the number of servings you and your family need from each food group based on how many calories you eat. For many people, eating with the Pyramid guidelines means consuming a lot less meat and more whole grains, fruits, and vegetables.

Sample Daily Diets for Three Calorie Levels

1,600 calories is about right for many sedentary women and some older adults.

2,200 calories is about right for most children, teenage girls, active women, and many sedentary men. Women who are pregnant or breast-feeding may need somewhat more.

2,800 calories is about right for teenage boys, many active men, and some very active women.

	Lower (about 1,600)	Moderate (about 2,200)	Higher (about 2,800)
Bread group servings	6	9	11
Vegetable group servings	3	4	5
Fruit group servings	2	3	4
Milk group servings	2-3*	2-3*	2-3*
Meat group (ounces)	5	6	7
Total fat (grams)	53	73	93
Total added sugars (teaspoons)	6	12	18

*Women who are pregnant or breast-feeding, teenagers, and young adults to age 24 need 3 servings.
Meat group amounts are listed here in total ounces.
Reprinted from USDA Home and Garden Bulletin Number 252

with the easy-to-make healthy recipes at the back of this book.

🍎 **Turn the day upside down.** "Have breakfast for dinner or dinner for breakfast," suggests Ward. "Fruit-topped French toast and a glass of milk make a speedy, nutritious supper. For breakfast, try a cheese sandwich or a slice of leftover pizza with a glass of juice." Kids will love these topsy-turvy meals, too.

🍎 **Add color to your cart.** Eating many different-colored fruits and vegetables helps you get the variety of nutrients you need. And stocking a cart brimming with color adds little time to your shopping trip. Simply grab a red, yellow, and green pepper instead of all one color. Mix a few sweet potatoes in with the whites. Choose a bunch of bananas, a few shiny red apples, a couple of oranges, and a cluster of purple grapes instead of a big bag containing one single type of fruit.

🍎 **Custom-make a morning taste treat.** Mix together two or three different breakfast cereals for a unique flavor. Bananas have appeal, but try a new topper such as blueberries, nectarines, or kiwi.

🍎 **Supercharge your soup and sandwich.** At lunch, swap the same old chicken noodle soup for lentil or mushroom-barley. "These soups satisfy and boost your fiber intake, too," says Ward. Build your usual turkey and Swiss sandwich on a new bread such as focaccia, seven-grain, or pita. Try a new topping such as arugula, roasted red peppers, and honey mustard.

🍎 **Go exotic with ethnic cuisine.** Break free of your dining-out routine—try a brand-new cuisine! Thai, Japanese, Middle Eastern, Indian, and Greek are just a few tantalizing choices. Many ethnic cuisines feature low-fat dishes heaping with grains and vegetables—just what the Pyramid ordered. Many large supermarkets also offer a wide selection of ready-made ethnic dishes or quick-to-fix staples.

Why Not Just Pop a Pill?

There's no dispute that getting enough vitamins and minerals is essential to good health. So, why not simply rely on a supplement to get what you need?

"A supplement is just that—it's a supplement, not a substitute for a healthful diet," explains Ward. "A vitamin and mineral tablet can't provide all the nutrients you need for good health. Only food can. Besides, foods offer benefits we don't even fully understand yet." For example, Ward cites research into the disease-fighting potential of phytochemicals found in grains, fruits, and vegetables. In addition, taking large amounts of some single supplements can be harmful or interfere with the delicate balance of other important nutrients.

variety:
unexpected benefits?

A steady stream of scientific research is focusing on phytochemicals—plant compounds found in grains, vegetables, and fruits that protect against cancer and heart disease. Registered dietitian Elizabeth Ward says the phytochemicals in broccoli, berries, legumes, cooked tomatoes, and soy products such as tofu are just a few that show promise as disease fighters. "It pays to eat a wide variety of foods because you never know which food will show a benefit next," she advises.

Supplements are a good idea for some people. For instance, strict vegetarians who don't eat meat, poultry, fish, eggs, or milk products may need a vitamin B12 supplement because this vitamin is found naturally only in animal products.

But, for most of us, eating a wide variety of foods is the best nutrition strategy. If you opt for a supplement as an "insurance policy," Ward says, stick with a multivitamin and mineral tablet containing no more than 100 percent of the U.S. Recommended Daily Allowance for each nutrient.

In some cases, extra amounts of a particular nutrient may be appropriate for preventing or fighting a particular disease. If you fall into this category, you should discuss supplements with your doctor rather than trying to prescribe for yourself.

2: activity

Balance Food You Eat with Physical Activity—Maintain or Improve Your Weight

The formula seems so simple: To maintain a healthful weight, the number of calories you eat must equal the number of calories you burn.

Yet, in recent years, the number of overweight American adults has jumped to one in three. At the same time, Americans spend $30 billion each year on diet plans, products, and potions.

Clearly, as a nation, our ability to achieve and maintain a healthful weight is out of whack. If you need to lose weight,

walk the talk

What's the best activity for most people? The hands-down winner is walking, says exercise expert Steve Farrell, Ph.D. "You can walk almost anytime, anywhere. Walking doesn't require expensive equipment, has a low risk of injury, and suits people at a variety of fitness levels."

How do you know you're exercising at the right intensity—not too high and not too low? "Take the talk test," suggests Dr. Farrell. "You should be able to talk comfortably during your workout. If you can't talk, you're working too hard. If you can sing, you're not working hard enough."

you'll find specific advice in "Overweight," which begins on page 256.

This section will help you determine whether your current weight is healthful. You'll also learn the importance of physical activity for either maintaining or improving your weight and for its great health-enhancing benefits.

Benefits of Staying in Balance

Sure, you want to achieve a healthful weight to look good. But, keeping extra pounds at bay throughout your life positively impacts your health, too. Weight gain increases risk for several serious conditions such as heart disease, high blood pressure, diabetes, gallstones, osteoarthritis, and some cancers.

Because of these risks, a good philosophy is "don't gain ... maintain," says obesity expert Dr. St. Jeor.

If you are already overweight, there's good news. Losing just 5 to 10 percent of your body weight—or about 12 pounds for someone who weighs 165 pounds—can help reduce your risk or improve your condition for health problems such as high blood cholesterol, high blood pressure, and diabetes, says Dr. St. Jeor.

Rating Your Weight

So, how do you know whether your weight is healthful? Perhaps you've tried comparing the number on the scale to a numerical range on a weight chart. Scales and charts provide general guidelines. They don't provide a complete picture of whether or not you're at a healthful weight. The scale, for example, does not tell you how much of your weight is from unhealthy amounts of fat versus muscle, bone, or fluid.

rate your weight

Use this formula to calculate your Body Mass Index (BMI):

Multiply your weight by 700, then divide by your height (in inches). Divide that number by your height again. For example, a 145-pound woman who stands 5'6" tall has a BMI of 23:

$$145 \text{ pounds} \times 700 = 101{,}500 \div 66 \ (5'6'') \div 66 = 23$$

Now compare your BMI to the chart below:

Body Mass Index (BMI)	
18.5 to 24.9	Healthful weight
25 to 29.9	Moderate overweight
30+	Severe overweight

The Dietary Guidelines say your weight is healthful if your BMI is between 19 and 25, you've gained less than 10 pounds since reaching your adult height, and you are otherwise healthy.

You need to lose weight if your BMI indicates you are overweight and you carry extra fat on your abdomen, have a weight-related medical problem, or have a family history of such a problem.

A BMI below 19 is healthful for some people, but for others can signal an eating disorder or other serious health problem.

If you have questions about your weight, consult your physician or a registered dietitian.

moderate amounts of activity
that burn 150 calories

Each of the following activities burns approximately 150 calories in the time indicated. Note that a more strenuous activity, such as running, requires less time than a moderate activity such as walking. (Also note that moderate activity may take longer, but it gets the job done.)

- Washing and waxing a car for 45 to 60 minutes
- Washing windows or floors for 45 to 60 minutes
- Playing basketball for 45 minutes
- Playing volleyball for 45 minutes
- Playing touch football for 30 to 45 minutes
- Gardening for 30 to 45 minutes
- Walking 1¾ miles in 35 minutes (20 minutes a mile)
- Bicycling 5 miles in 30 minutes
- Dancing fast for 30 minutes
- Pushing a stroller 1½ miles in 30 minutes
- Raking leaves for 30 minutes
- Shooting baskets (basketball) for 30 minutes

- Walking 2 miles in 30 minutes (15 minutes a mile)
- Water aerobics for 30 minutes
- Swimming laps for 20 minutes
- Bicycling 4 miles in 15 minutes
- Jumping rope for 15 minutes
- Running 1½ miles in 15 minutes (10 minutes a mile)
- Shoveling snow for 15 minutes
- Climbing stairs for 15 minutes

Note: If you have health problems or are a man older than 40 or a woman older than 50, consult your doctor before you begin a new physical activity program.

Source: U.S. Department of Health and Human Services

And most charts don't account for individual characteristics such as your age, gender, and frame size. Like the scale, charts simply can't tell you whether you are carrying an undesirable amount of body fat.

One method for determining whether your weight puts you at risk for health problems is the Body Mass Index (BMI). "A BMI between 19 and 25 indicates you're at a healthy weight," says Dr. St. Jeor. "The higher your BMI is above 25, the greater your risk for weight-related illnesses."

See the "Rate Your Weight" work box on page 22 to determine whether your weight is putting you at risk for health problems.

The Activity Factor

Physical activity helps keep your weight in balance by burning calories and revving up your metabolism so you continue to burn extra calories for up to several hours. Being

what's the big deal about one-fifty?

Can 150 calories really make much difference in your weight? You bet it can! Consuming a calorie excess of just 150 calories each day—the amount of calories in one can of soda or a small bag of chips—can add up to a 15-pound weight gain in a year! On the flip side, achieving a daily deficit of 150 calories through extra physical activity or cutting back a bit on what you eat could mean you'll be 15 pounds lighter this time next year!

active also promises an impressive array of health benefits, says Steve Farrell, Ph.D., associate director of the Cooper Institute for Aerobics Research in Dallas, Texas. These benefits include strong bones, muscles, and joints, and reduced risk of heart disease, high blood pressure, diabetes, colon cancer, and osteoporosis. And if that's not enough, activity just plain makes you feel good by reducing feelings of depression and anxiety, and by promoting a sense of well-being.

With all that activity has to offer, you'd think we'd all be bounding out the door for a daily workout. Not so. The fact is, more than 60 percent of American adults aren't physically active on a regular basis, and one in four adults isn't active at all. What gives?

For starters, cars, computers, and remote controls. "We're a sedentary society," says Dr. Farrell. "We drive instead of walking, work at a computer or surf the Internet after school, and transform into TV couch potatoes by night."

Many people avoid exercise because they still believe the old "no pain, no gain" exercise cry from the 1980s. Forget all that

nonsense, says Dr. Farrell. A 1996 report from the U.S. Surgeon General says you can reap health benefits and burn extra calories from just a moderate amount of physical activity each day. And meeting this goal is easier than you may think.

Moderate activity is defined as any activity that burns about 150 calories a day, or 1,000 calories per week. "Moderate Amounts of Activity That Burn 150 Calories" on page 23 shows several options for fitting moderate physical activity into your day. For best results, choose a variety of activities that you enjoy and that fit easily into your lifestyle. (And hallelujah! Household chores such as raking leaves and washing windows count toward your total.)

3: veggies
Eat Lots of Grains, Vegetables, and Fruits

A bounty of benefits awaits when you load your plate with grains, vegetables, and fruits. These foods supply important nutrients and fiber and, when eaten as part of a balanced, low-fat diet, may reduce your risk for heart disease and some types of cancer.

The Dietary Guidelines say these foods should make up the biggest proportion of what we eat. That's why the breads, cereals, rice, and pasta group and the vegetables and fruits groups are the biggest Pyramid food groups. Let's find out more about what makes grains, vegetables, and fruits so great— and how you can get plenty on your plate.

Enjoy the Goodness of Grains

Breads, cereals, rice, pasta, breadsticks, pizza crust, crackers, pretzels, popcorn, pancakes, and bagels are only a few of the foods made from grains. They're great for us because they're naturally low in fat and high in energy-giving complex carbohydrates, says registered dietitian Elizabeth Ward. Plus, grains provide B vitamins, vitamin E, iron, zinc, calcium, magnesium, and copper. Whole grains, such as whole wheat bread, bran flakes, and brown rice, also supply valuable fiber.

With all that grains have going for them, it's no wonder the Food Guide Pyramid recommends we get six to 11 daily servings of them. Yet Americans average only four to five daily servings, at best a full serving short of even the minimum number recommended. If you're falling short on grains, try these tips:

🍎 **Double up in the morning.** Ward gets a jump on her grain servings each day by breakfasting on a double serving of whole grain cereal. To double your health benefits, too, she says, choose a cereal with at least 7 grams of fiber per serving. (Choosing your breakfast cereals is a good place to exercise your label-reading smarts.)

🍎 **Sneak in some extra cereal.** Mix your favorite into yogurt or pudding or sprinkle it on ice cream.

🍎 **Snack smart.** Stash pretzels, air-popped popcorn, fun-flavored rice cakes, and baked bagel chips in your desk, car, or backpack to munch on during your mid-afternoon break.

🍎 **Explore new side-dish options.** Try an intriguing, quick-cooking grain such as Middle Eastern bulgur, Indian basmati rice,

nutrition facts focus

spotlight on
serving size and calories

The nutrition numbers listed on the Nutrition Facts label are based on one serving in the **Serving Size** shown. If your serving size differs, adjust the nutrition numbers up or down. Look carefully at the number of **Servings Per Container.** Sometimes a small package that looks like a convenient single serving actually contains more than one serving. (This is a little trick that food manufacturers use to keep those calorie counts down; don't let yourself be fooled.)

To keep your weight in balance, look carefully at the number of **Calories** in each serving. The number of **Calories from Fat** are already included in the total **Calories.**

North African couscous, or South American quinoa—all as close as your supermarket shelf.

Make a speed-scratch spaghetti supper. A mere half-cup of cooked pasta is one grain serving—and who eats just half a cup? (Timesaving tip: Registered dietitian Cindy Moore says you can have a meal of spaghetti with already prepared tomato sauce, a microwaved vegetable, and Italian bread on the table in 15 minutes flat.)

Say good night with a grain. Savor a bran muffin or a few graham crackers with a cup of tea.

Ways to Get Your "Five a Day"

Fewer than one in three American adults gets the minimum five daily servings of vegetables and fruits recommended by the Food Guide Pyramid. And it's a shame because produce provides a cornucopia of good nutrition.

Almost all vegetables are low in calories and fat and provide beta-carotene (which the body turns into vitamin A), vitamin C, folic acid, iron, magnesium, and fiber. Fruits are fat-free and supply beta-carotene, vitamin C, potassium, and fiber.

Beta-carotene and vitamin C, along with vitamin E and selenium, are antioxidants—nutrients that may help slow the aging process and protect against some cancers, heart disease, strokes, and cataracts. In addition, plant foods offer a wealth of disease-fighting phytochemicals.

Enjoy these fun and fast ways to get your five a day:

Start the day the "high C" way. An orange, a cantaloupe half, a cup of strawberries, or a kiwi all provide 100 percent of your daily vitamin C requirements. (Tip: To eat a kiwi quickly, cut it in half and scoop out the fruit with a spoon.)

Make it easy to snack on fruit. Keep a bowl of grab-and-go fruits on the kitchen counter. Apples, bananas, pears, and plums are tasty options.

Think Middle Eastern. Make a quick lunch of hummus (chickpea spread). Dig in with whole wheat pita triangles, red pepper strips, baby carrots, and zucchini rounds.

Get juiced. Six ounces of fruit juice (not fruit "drink") is a refreshing pick-me-up that counts as one fruit serving.

Try a little sweet and dry. Tote mini-boxes of raisins in your bag or briefcase for a fast snack.

Love those sweet potatoes. These wonderful tubers are rich in beta-carotene. Microwave, dot with butter, and dust with cinnamon for a yummy snack or side dish.

Don't let a busy day sabotage your dinner. Zip by the supermarket salad bar to pick up ingredients for a fast veggie stir-fry.

Sneak in extra veggies. Add carrots, corn, peas, peppers, green beans, onions, and garlic to soups, stews, casseroles, chili, and pasta dishes.

Dress up your usual salad. Grab a bag of prewashed lettuce (dark green varieties such as romaine are most nutritious). Toss in some chopped dates, apples, and nuts.

Pile your pizza with a variety of veggies. Try red and green peppers, mushrooms, sliced tomatoes, artichokes, onions, and garlic.

Have a fast fruit dessert. Top frozen yogurt or low-fat ice cream with a mix of sliced strawberries and bananas (or your own favorites). For a taste of the tropics, squeeze fresh lime juice on prepared pineapple chunks (fresh or canned).

Stock up on frozen and canned vegetables and fruits. They're high in quality and nutrients—and you'll never be caught shorthanded.

Fantastic Fiber

Yet another reason that fruits, grains, and vegetables are so important to your diet is fiber. Fiber is found naturally only in plant foods such as whole grains, beans, peas,

---

nutrition facts focus

spotlight on

carbohydrates

Health experts recommend that carbohydrates—plentiful in grains, vegetables, and fruits—make up 60 percent of your daily calories. The % Daily Value shown on the Nutrition Facts label for **Total Carbohydrate** is based on this target for a 2,000-calorie daily diet. The % Daily Value for **Dietary Fiber** is based on 25 grams of fiber.

Vegetables and fruits are excellent sources of vitamins A (as beta-carotene) and C. The % Daily Values for these vitamins are required on the label. The % Daily Value for **vitamin A** is based on 5,000 international units (IUs) and for **vitamin C** on 60 milligrams.

---

vegetables, and fruits. Fiber comes in two forms: insoluble and soluble.

● *Insoluble fiber* moves through your digestive tract without dissolving, so it helps keep you regular and may protect against colon cancer. Some good sources of insoluble fiber are whole wheat bread, bran cereals, and vegetables and fruits with edible skins (such as potatoes) and seeds (such as kiwi).

● *Soluble fiber* dissolves to a gummy texture as you digest it. Eating foods containing soluble fiber as part of a low-fat diet may help reduce risk of heart disease and control blood sugar in people with diabetes. Good sources of soluble fiber include oatmeal, dried beans and peas, lentils, barley, carrots, and apples.

The National Cancer Institute recommends we get 20 to 35 grams of fiber each day, but government surveys say we average only about 15 grams. Use the

Nutrition Facts label and the Fiber Foods chart on page 108 to make sure you get enough fiber. To avoid digestive discomfort, increase your fiber intake gradually and drink plenty of fluids.

Get your fiber from whole grains, vegetables, and fruits instead of fiber pills or powders. Foods provide a mix of both insoluble and soluble fiber, plus vitamins, minerals, and phytochemicals, with benefits a fiber supplement can't deliver. (Of course, if your doctor recommends a fiber supplement, you should take it.)

4: low fat

Choose a Diet Low in Fat, Saturated Fat, and Cholesterol

First the good news: Americans are getting the message that eating too much fat, saturated fat, and cholesterol can increase risk for heart disease by driving up blood cholesterol levels. In fact, our average intake of fat, saturated fat, and cholesterol are declining and heart disease rates are down. (For details on getting your cholesterol levels down, see "High Cholesterol," which starts on page 193.)

Now the not-so-good news: We still eat amounts of fat, saturated fat, and cholesterol that are above recommended levels for good health, and heart disease remains our number one killer. Eating too much fat also increases risk for several types of cancer, and, because of fat's calorie-rich nature, can contribute to being overweight.

For good health, the Dietary Guidelines recommend following an eating plan that averages no more than 30 percent of calories from fat, less than 10 percent of calories from saturated fat, and no more than 300 milligrams of cholesterol. If you eat a lot of processed foods—things like lunch meats, frozen dinners, baked goods— it can be challenging to keep your fat intake this low. That's all the more reason to get used to eating with the Pyramid in mind and to pay attention to food labels.

A Healthy Heart's Biggest Food Foe

The saturated fat in foods raises your blood cholesterol—and so your risk for heart disease—more than anything else you eat. (Saturated fat is the kind that tends to be hard at room temperature. This includes fats such as those found in butter and shortening. See "Fat & Cholesterol Primer" on page 29 for a good look at the different kinds of fat and how they act in your body.)

"The more saturated fat you eat, the more cholesterol your body makes," explains registered dietitian Connie Diekman, a spokesperson for The American Dietetic Association, who is based in St. Louis, Missouri.

What about the cholesterol in food, once thought to be your heart's worst dietary enemy? Health experts now believe that dietary cholesterol plays a lesser role in increasing blood cholesterol levels than does saturated fat. However, says Diekman, concern about the cholesterol in food is still important. It's especially important if you

fat & cholesterol primer

Saturated fat raises blood cholesterol levels. Often solid at room temperature, it's plentiful in animal products such as whole milk, cheese, butter, lard, fatty meats, and in some vegetable oils such as coconut, palm, and palm kernel oils. Poultry, fish, and shellfish also contain some saturated fat, though generally less than meat.

Monounsaturated fat can help lower blood cholesterol if substituted for saturated fat in your diet. This type of fat seems to work by lowering "bad" LDL cholesterol while preserving the level of "good" HDL cholesterol. Olive, canola, and peanut oils are mostly made up of monounsaturated fat.

Polyunsaturated fat can also help lower blood cholesterol provided it replaces saturated fat. Corn, soybean, sesame, sunflower, and safflower oils are mostly made up of polyunsaturated fat. Fish oils, or omega-3 fatty acids, are also polyunsaturated and found abundantly in such cold-water fish as herring, tuna, salmon, mackerel, and sardines.

Cholesterol is not a type of fat, but it can raise your blood cholesterol levels. Dietary cholesterol is only found in foods that come from animals, such as meat, poultry, fish, and dairy products.

have heart disease or it runs in your family. But, in general, saturated fat is by far the bigger concern.

"Most of the saturated fat we eat comes from animal foods such as meats and dairy products," says Diekman, "so keep an eye on portion sizes and choose tasty, lower-fat versions of these foods when you can." A simple and effective dietary strategy, she says, is to cut back on the total amount of fat you eat because your intake of saturated fat and cholesterol will automatically fall, too.

Cut the fat with these shopping tips and cooking tricks:

🍎 **Get lean and mean at the red meat counter.** The leanest cuts contain the words "loin" or "round" in the name. Examples include beef round steak, ground round, and pork tenderloin.

🍎 **Try ground turkey in burgers, tacos, and spaghetti sauce.** Make sure the fatty turkey skin is not included. Ask for breast meat ground without the skin or look for the words "ground turkey meat" on packages.

🍎 **Eat more fish and seafood meals.** They're naturally low in fat (unless you have them deep fried, of course). Fish such as salmon, mackerel, and sardines contain more fat, but it's mostly unsaturated. Those fish varieties are rich in omega-3 fatty acids, a polyunsaturated fat that appears to protect against heart attacks.

nutrition facts focus

spotlight on

fat, calcium, and iron

Health experts recommend limiting your total fat intake to no more than 30 percent of daily calories and your saturated fat intake to no more than 10 percent of daily calories. The % Daily Values shown on the Nutrition Facts label for **Total Fat** and **Saturated Fat** are based on these targets for a 2,000-calorie daily diet. The % Daily Value for **Cholesterol** is based on 300 milligrams. You should be aware that it's perfectly okay to get less of both these substances.

Meats are excellent sources of iron, and dairy products are rich in calcium. The % Daily Values for these minerals are required on the label. The % Daily Value for **Iron** is based on 18 milligrams and for **Calcium** on 1,000 milligrams.

🍎 **Don't chew the fat.** Cutting away any visible fat reduces the fat in meats by about 40 percent. Remove skin from chicken to trim fat by 60 percent. (It's okay to remove chicken skin after cooking because the meat doesn't absorb much of the fat.)

🍎 **Lighten up on milk fat.** Choose from the wide variety of delicious reduced-fat and low-fat dairy products such as cheese, sour cream, and yogurt. Low-fat or fat-free milk is your best choice.

🍎 **Think "lite."** You can gain big fat savings by substituting reduced-fat or fat-free mayo, salad dressing, or tartar sauce for regular versions. But let flavor serve as your guide, advises Diekman. "If you don't like the taste of the lower-fat products," she advises, "use the 'real thing.' Just make sure to measure the amount."

🍎 **Don't abandon eggs.** Eggs have gotten a bad cholesterol rap in recent years. But the American Heart Association says it's okay for healthy people to enjoy up to four egg yolks each week (all the cholesterol is found in the yolk).

Once you reach your limit, you can substitute two egg whites for each whole egg or try an egg substitute.

🍎 **Get an oil change.** Cook and bake with a monounsaturated oil such as olive, canola, or peanut oil, or a polyunsaturated oil such as corn, safflower, or sunflower oil. Just remember that all oils contain 120 calories per tablespoon.

🍎 **Use fat-trimming cooking techniques.** Roast, broil, grill, steam, or microwave. Sauté foods in broth or use a nonstick cooking spray.

🍎 **Flaunt the rules.** When preparing rice, pasta, and other grains, don't add the butter, margarine, or oil called for in package directions. They'll taste just fine without the extra fat.

🍎 **Make a few strategic substitutions.** Use evaporated skim milk in place of light or heavy cream in soups, sauces—even pumpkin pie filling. In cake, quick bread, and muffin recipes, replace part of the fat with applesauce or a fruit puree.

fiber for small fry

Kids need fiber, too. The right amount of fiber helps fight childhood obesity and the development of heart disease, cancer, and diabetes. But how much do they need?

The American Health Foundation provides this easy-to-use formula to calculate daily fiber needs for kids ages 3 through 18: Just add 5 to your child's age to get the number of total grams of daily fiber your child needs. For example, a 10-year-old needs about 15 grams (10 + 5 = 15). As you slowly increase fiber-containing foods in your child's diet, increase fluids such as water and juice, too.

5: low sugar

Choose a Diet Moderate in Sugars

Let's begin with a quick quiz. Answer true or false:

1. Sugar causes diabetes.
2. Sugar causes tooth decay.
3. Sugar makes kids hyperactive.

Over the years, sugar has been blamed for causing diabetes and hyperactive behavior. But these allegations just aren't true. Sugar does play a role in tooth decay, but so do starchy foods such as bread and crackers. (To learn more about the causes of diabetes and tooth decay, turn to pages 123 and 113.) And sugar does not make kids hyperactive. We'll go into more detail in just a minute.

The sweet truth is, no convincing evidence shows that eating moderate amounts of sugar is harmful to health. But just how much is a moderate amount?

There aren't specific guidelines for healthful sugar consumption like there are for fat or fiber. But, because sugar and many sugary foods contain calories but few nutrients, you can overdo sugar. You are eating too much of the sweet stuff if:

● Your sugar habit dulls your appetite for eating your recommended servings from the Food Guide Pyramid food groups.
● You are overweight because a steady stream of candy, cookies, soft drinks, and other sweets pushes your daily calorie total over the limit.

Otherwise, it's fine to include some sweets as part of a healthful, balanced diet.

Don't Get Hyper over Kids and Sugar

Many people believe that sugar causes hyperactive behavior in children. But according to a review of 16 research studies published in the *Journal of the American Medical Association*, it just isn't so. The results showed that sugar does not

spotlight on sugars

The Nutrition Facts label lists in grams the amount of **Sugars** in one serving of a food. This number includes both sugars found naturally in foods such as milk and fruit, as well as sugars added to foods during processing. Sugars don't have a % Daily Value because there is no evidence that a certain amount of sugars in the diet is appropriate or inappropriate.

To calculate how many teaspoons of sugar are in a serving of a food, divide the number of grams in one serving by 4 (1 teaspoon of sugar weighs 4 grams). For example, a serving of food with 8 grams of sugar contains 2 teaspoons of sugar ($8 \div 4 = 2$).

affect either children's behavior or their cognitive performance.

But tell this to any parent who has a little one bouncing off the walls after a dose of sugar and you're bound to encounter skepticism. For some possible explanations, we turned to registered dietitian Julie H. Burns, owner of SportFuel in Western Springs, Illinois, and mother of five-year-old triplets:

The element of excitement. A child may get "hyper" from being in an unusual and exciting situation, rather than from eating sugar. "Think of a birthday party," says Burns. "Sure, kids are eating lots of cake and ice cream. But they're also wound up from running around, laughing, and playing with a large group of children." But, sugar takes the blame for their high-spirited high jinks.

The caffeine factor. Sugar and caffeine pair up in some of kids' favorite foods—soft drinks and chocolate, for instance. Burns says it's the caffeine, not the sugar, that revs up her tiny trio: "Even small amounts of caffeine from the chocolate in pudding, chocolate chip cookies, or a couple of chocolate kisses really affect their behavior."

Great expectations. Children are masters at sensing their parents' moods. So, if you expect your child to act extra lively after a dose of sugar, he or she will be only too happy to oblige you. Though sugar is cleared of causing hyperactivity, a steady stream of candy, cookies, and cupcakes is obviously not okay. Too many sugary treats can dull a little one's appetite for nutritious grains, vegetables, fruits, lean meats, and dairy products from the Food Guide Pyramid— what Burns and her brood call "big and strong" foods. "My kids know they have to eat their 'big and strong' foods first," she says. "Then they can have a little dessert." Good advice for adults and kids alike.

The Many Faces of Sugar

When you think "sugar," do you automatically picture a heaping spoonful of the granulated white stuff? Well, there are a lot more sugars than meet the eye.

Sugars are carbohydrates, which the body converts to glucose (blood sugar) to use for its main source of fuel. Sugars are found naturally in fruits, vegetables, grains, legumes, and milk, but sugar's claim to fame is the pleasing sweetness it provides when added to goodies such as cakes, cookies, and candies. You may be surprised to learn that sugars are also added to many not-so-sweet foods such as salad dressings and tomato sauce.

The names below are all types of sugars. The ingredients listed on food packages are shown in descending order by weight, from most to least. A food may be high in sugar if one of these names is the first or second ingredient, or if several types appear on the list:

- brown sugar
- corn sweetener
- corn syrup
- fructose
- fruit juice concentrate
- glucose (dextrose)
- high-fructose corn syrup
- honey
- invert sugar
- lactose
- maltose
- molasses
- raw sugar
- sugar (sucrose)
- syrup

6: low salt

Choose a Diet Moderate in Salt and Sodium

Your body needs sodium to maintain proper fluid balance, blood pressure, and normal heart action. But if a little sodium is a good thing, isn't a lot more even better? Not really. All it takes is 500 milligrams of

pyramid pointer

The Pyramid Tip. Sugary foods such as table sugar, jam, jelly, soft drinks, candy, and most sweet desserts are found in the Pyramid Tip. These foods supply calories, but few or no nutrients. Serving-size suggestions aren't provided for foods in the tip. Use them sparingly.

sodium each day to perform these vital functions, but many Americans consume 10 times that amount.

Eating too much sodium increases blood pressure in about 30 percent of people, who are termed "salt sensitive." At this time medical experts can't predict just who is or isn't salt sensitive. Eating large amounts of sodium also has another effect: When the kidneys work to excrete excess sodium, valuable calcium may be excreted right along with the sodium.

For these reasons, the Dietary Guidelines recommend a moderate sodium intake for the general, healthy public. A healthful guideline is 2,400 milligrams of sodium per day. (That's the amount used on the Nutrition Facts label to calculate the % Daily Value for sodium.)

are salt and sodium the same?

No, but sodium is one of two minerals that make up salt.

The chemical name for table salt is sodium chloride, and it's built from four parts sodium and six parts chloride. According to the International Food Information Council, about 95 percent of the sodium we eat comes from sodium chloride. The remaining sodium comes from a variety of sodium-containing ingredients such as baking soda (sodium bicarbonate) or monosodium glutamate (MSG).

Sodium Surprise

Do you think you consume too much salt or sodium?

If you answered "no," you're not alone. According to government surveys, only one in four adults thinks his or her diet is too high in salt or sodium.

But, surprise! Americans generally eat significantly more sodium than the 2,400 milligrams recommended by many health experts. Men average about 4,000 milligrams and women 3,000 milligrams daily from food alone, not even counting the extra we shake on at the table.

Health experts recommend limiting your sodium intake to 2,400 milligrams per day. The % Daily Value shown on the Nutrition Facts label is based on this level.

If you decide to cut back on salt and sodium, try these tips from The American Dietetic Association's Connie Diekman:

🍎 **Be a sodium sleuth at the supermarket.** Seventy-five percent of the sodium we consume comes from what's added to foods during processing. "Check the Nutrition Facts label to see how much sodium is in the food you buy," advises Diekman. "Use the label to compare brands so you can make lower-sodium choices." Take advantage of reduced-sodium products such as canned broth, soups, bouillon cubes, luncheon meats, and bacon.

🍎 **Cook without salt.** You can reduce or omit the salt in any recipe that doesn't call for yeast. Remember, you can always add a little salt at the table if you really need to, but you won't be able to take it out.

🍎 **Intensify flavor with herbs.** Fresh and dried herbs such as basil, oregano, rosemary, and parsley add zest to foods without salt. Diekman's kitchen tip: Add dried herbs at the beginning of cooking so their flavor can intensify. Add fresh herbs at the end so their flavor won't fade. The smaller you snip fresh herbs, the more of their flavor you'll enjoy.

🍎 **Follow the three sodium rules.** Always taste food before salting to make sure it needs it, says Diekman. If necessary, add salt to food during cooking or at the table, not both, and, when you do add salt, measure the amount.

🍎 **Go slow.** "Cut back gradually to allow your taste buds to adjust," says Diekman. "It takes about six to eight weeks to lose your taste for salt and start to appreciate the natural flavors of food."

7 : alcohol

If You Drink Alcoholic Beverages, Do So in Moderation

Enjoying a glass of mellow wine at dinner or an icy cold beer with friends after work is a pleasurable experience. But moderate drinking doesn't just enhance your enjoyment of food or good company. Research suggests it may also protect against heart disease.

Results are not yet conclusive, so, if you don't already drink, don't start for this reason. And, experts caution, drinking alcohol does not take the place of essential heart-healthy habits such as eating a low-fat, fiber-rich diet, being physically active, and not smoking.

Why Moderation Is Key

Moderation—no more than a drink or two a day—is the real key to using alcohol to enhance your enjoyment and health.

Drinking too much alcohol can increase your risk for a host of health problems, including high blood pressure, stroke, heart disease, certain cancers, birth defects, and accidents. Heavy drinkers are at risk for liver and pancreatic disease, and brain and heart

moderation
one drink or two

Health experts define moderate drinking as no more than one daily drink for women or two daily drinks for men. Count as one drink:

12 ounces of regular beer
5 ounces of wine
1.5 ounces of 80-proof distilled spirits

damage. They are malnourished, too, because empty calories from alcohol replace nutrient-packed calories from food.

Some people who should keep alcohol strictly off-limits include:

● Children and adolescents. Not only is under-age drinking illegal, but alcohol puts developing youngsters at risk for the same health problems as adults.
● Women who are pregnant or trying to become pregnant. Heavy drinking during pregnancy causes serious birth defects such as fetal alcohol syndrome.
● People, such as recovering alcoholics, who can't consume alcohol in moderation.
● People taking prescription and over-the-counter medications. Alcohol can interfere with the way medications work by making them more potent or less effective.
● Anyone who is driving or performing activities that require attention and skill, such as operating complicated machinery.

alcohol calories count

Alcohol contains 7 calories per gram, compared to 4 per gram in carbohydrates and protein, and 9 per gram in fat. If you drink alcohol, make sure to count the calories in your daily calorie total. Here are average calorie counts for several popular beverages:

80-proof distilled spirits (1.5 ounces)	100
Wine (5 ounces)	100
Light beer (12 ounces)	100
Regular beer (12 ounces)	150
Gin & tonic (8 ounces)	180
Bloody Mary (8 ounces)	185
Screwdriver (8 ounces)	200
Piña colada (8 ounces)	465

What's a Woman to Do?

To drink or not to drink? For women, the answer is not crystal clear. While moderate drinking appears to reduce risk of heart disease—the number one killer of women—alcohol may also increase risk of breast cancer. Given these mixed messages about alcohol and health, what's the best advice?

"Having even one alcoholic drink a day may slightly increase a woman's breast cancer risk," explains Michael Thun, M.D., of the American Cancer Society. "Before menopause, women receive few cardiovascular benefits from drinking because premenopausal women are already at low risk for heart disease. After menopause, a woman's heart disease risk rises sharply and having that daily drink may reduce that risk. At that point, the benefits drinking provides for your heart may outweigh an increased breast cancer risk."

The bottom line: Each woman must assess her own benefits and risks for drinking alcohol. Before you drink, it's wise to discuss your personal health history and family predisposition for heart disease and breast cancer with your physician. And remember, moderation is key.

master key
Enjoy Eating!

Nutrition scientists created the Dietary Guidelines for Americans. Think of these guidelines as the seven keys to healthful eating. But—and this is a big but—these seven keys won't work if you don't put them to use.

You can get the keys to work—or get them to work better—if you also use the master key: remember to enjoy your food! It's simple and will help you stick with all the other guidelines over the long term.

fitting in higher-fat favorites

Do you put goodies like chocolate cake and french fries on the "Forbidden Foods" list because you fear their calories and fat?

Immediately refer back to our "Master Key Enjoy Eating!" on page 36 and remind yourself that any food can fit into a healthful eating plan.

Let's say a scoop of ice cream provides 250 calories and 20 percent of your Daily Value for Total Fat. While these numbers are high, it doesn't mean that you have to forgo the pleasure. Just use the Food Guide Pyramid and Nutrition Facts labels to help you balance the rest of your daily food choices so calories and fat stay within healthful limits.

And, for goodness sake, don't worry if you exceed your targets now and then. A healthful eating plan is built from what you eat over several days, not by any one food, one meal, or one day of eating. The best advice: Follow the Food Guide Pyramid, select mostly lower-fat choices from each group on most days, and go ahead and enjoy that ice cream now and then.

In survey after survey, people say that nutrition is important when making food choices. But by far and away, taste is given as the number one reason for choosing a particular food. After all, enjoying food is one of life's great pleasures. Putting foods you like on the "off-limits" list in the name of good health is unnecessary, and may even make you give up on healthful eating altogether. Fortunately, you don't have to sacrifice flavor for good nutrition. Here are several tips for putting the Master Key to work in your life.

🍎 **Plan to indulge.** Are you dreaming of a hot fudge sundae loaded with whipped cream and nuts? Go ahead! Savor that sundae. You can fit an occasional treat into a healthful eating plan by trimming portions just a bit throughout the day and by working in some extra physical activity.

🍎 **Name your non-negotiables.** An enormous number of low-fat and fat-free foods are available, but not all of them measure up in the taste department. If only "real" fudge brownies or creamy Roquefort dressing will do, enjoy them in sensible portions. Use fat-reduced foods with tastes you like to cut back on fat.

🍎 **Savor Mother Nature.** Juicy, just-picked peaches; sweet, crunchy corn on the cob; crispy, garden-fresh green beans; red, ripe tomatoes still warm from the sun. All these mouthwatering wonders of nature are naturally low in calories and fat, yet hard to beat in terms of taste.

🍎 **Give your taste buds time.** It takes several weeks—and sometimes months—to adjust to eating less fat or sodium. Make changes slowly but surely.

Quiz: Do You Know Your Nutrients?

The foods you eat and drink supply nutrients—substances your body needs to produce energy and to grow, maintain, and repair itself. Test your nutrient know-how. See if you can match each nutrient listed below with its correct definition.

A. Carbohydrate B. Protein C. Fat D. Fiber E. Water F. Vitamins G. Minerals

1. This nutrient supplies your body with amino acids—building blocks needed for growth and for tissue maintenance and repair. Foods from animals, such as meat, poultry, fish, milk, yogurt, and eggs are "complete" sources of this nutrient because they contain all nine essential amino acids your body can't make. Foods from plants, such as nuts, seeds, grains, and vegetables are missing one or more essential amino acids, but can combine with the amino acids in other foods to become complete. This nutrient contains 4 calories per gram.

2. Don't let this nutrient group's reputation for building strong bones, teeth, and nails fool you: Its members also work hard to regulate the body's fluid balance, muscle contractions, and nerve impulses.

3. This substance is not really a nutrient because your body can't digest or absorb it. Instead, it passes through your digestive tract without adding calories or nutrients to your diet. Yet, most of us could use more of it because it keeps us regular and helps protect against heart disease and some cancers. It's plentiful in whole wheat bread, bran cereals, oatmeal, kidney beans, lentils, peas, broccoli, oranges, and apples.

4. Clearly, this nutrient is a big part of us. It makes up 10 to 12 gallons of our body weight, but we lose about 10 cups each day from perspiring, eliminating, and breathing. In the body, it shuttles other nutrients and oxygen where they're needed, regulates body temperature, protects and cushions vital organs, lubricates joints, and helps eliminate waste. All that and calorie-free.

5. This nutrient is often considered a dietary villain, but it does good deeds, too. Your body needs it to absorb vitamins A, D, E, and K, and it supplies linoleic acid and linolenic acid, which children need to grow properly and adults need for healthy skin. The most calorie-rich nutrient of all, it contains 9 calories per gram. You'll find it in vegetable oils, butter, margarine, meats, dairy products, olives, and avocados.

6. This nutrient can be simple or complex, but, either way, your body converts it into glucose (blood sugar) to use for energy. Health experts recommend you get 55 to 60 percent of your daily calories from this nutrient, which contains 4 calories per gram. You'll find it in bread, cereal, rice, pasta, potatoes, dried beans, and fruits.

7. Though the body needs only minuscule amounts of these nutrients, they're in charge of regulating many body processes. Their jobs include regulating energy production in the body's cells; keeping bones, muscles, and other tissues healthy; fighting infections; and functioning as antioxidants to protect body cells against damaging free radicals. Members of this nutrient group are either fat-soluble or water-soluble.

Answers: 1-B; 2-G; 3-D; 4-E; 5-C; 6-A; 7-F.

chapter 2

the 6 rules FOR food safety

{{ A man too busy to take care of his health is like a mechanic too busy to take care of his tools. —Spanish Proverb }}

The night started out so right. You threw a juicy steak on the grill. Or popped last night's yummy leftovers into the microwave. Or picked up pasta at that new place on the corner.

Delicious! But now, a few hours later, you're in bed with an explosive stomach. Could it be something you ate? Yes, it could be.

Even if you haven't had a personal taste of food poisoning, you can't have helped hearing in the news about some of the more serious outbreaks. Hundreds of children contract hepatitis A virus from a school treat of strawberry shortcake. More than 1,000 people are taken ill with *Clyospora* after eating raspberries imported from Guatemala. Four children die from *E. coli* bacteria in undercooked hamburgers at a fast-food chain. Then there are worries about mad cow disease, pesticides, and additives.

It's enough to make anyone worry. The question is: Should you be worried?

America's food supply is among the safest in the world. Nevertheless, an estimated 6.5 to 81 million cases of foodborne illness occur each year, according to the Centers for Disease Control (CDC).

There's obviously a pretty big range between those figures. What gives? The exact figures aren't certain because many victims mistake food poisoning symptoms for the flu and don't report them. The CDC is more precise on the number of deaths from foodborne illness. They estimate that number at 9,000 each year.

Foodborne illness occurs when we consume small quantities of pathogens—disease-causing infectious microorganisms that thrive in everything from water to animal feces. These microorganisms can multiply in our bodies and make us sick. Pesticides and other substances in our food sometimes cause problems, too, but most experts agree that microbes are the greater part of the problem.

Something as innocuous as milk spoiling in your refrigerator or bird droppings contaminating apples can end up in illness. Man-made hazards like assembly line food processing add to the risk: Bacteria from one animal can sweep their way through an entire meat warehouse.

Our fast-paced American lifestyle increases food safety risks. We consume more meals away from home, which means less quality control over the food we eat. And our increasingly global food system brings us fruits and vegetables from underdeveloped countries, food that may have been grown under less than sanitary conditions.

If all that weren't challenge enough, increasingly dangerous pathogens keep popping up.

"What is growing as a problem in this country is the increasing virulence of certain bacterial and viral strains," says Caroline Smith DaWaal, director of food safety for the Center for Science in the Public Interest (CSPI). "While most food poisoning is still like having the flu, the newer bugs can put you in the hospital or even kill you."

For example, milder forms of *E. coli* have been around for decades. It's the more recently evolved *E. coli* O157:H7 strain that caused kidney disease and death in kids who ate undercooked burgers. *Salmonella* DT 104, the latest form of a bacteria found in meat, poultry, and eggs, is resistant to antibiotics, so it is very difficult to treat.

We are all at risk, some of us more than others.

"We eat pathogenic microorganisms in every meal," says O. Peter Snyder, Ph.D., a food scientist and president of the Hospitality Institute of Technology and Management, an organization that oversees food safety practices at restaurants and other food service operations. "Whether or not you become ill depends on the type of pathogen, how much you've eaten, and the state of your immune system."

Especially vulnerable are young children and the elderly: kids because their immune systems aren't fully developed, and older people because our immune response slows down with age. Being pregnant or having conditions such as diabetes or AIDS also puts one at greater risk.

recognizing & treating
foodborne illness

Many intestinal illnesses thought to be stomach flu are actually food poisoning, according to the Centers for Disease Control.

Symptoms:
Abdominal discomfort, vomiting, diarrhea, fatigue, and fever are the most common. Symptoms usually appear and pass within 4 to 48 hours after eating contaminated food. They can, however, appear anywhere from 20 minutes to two weeks after eating.

Treatment:
Your best bet is to rest and drink plenty of fluids to prevent dehydration. Don't use antidiarrheal medications because they may slow elimination of the bacteria from your system.

See a doctor if:
● Symptoms persist more than three days.
● Diarrhea or vomiting is excessive, which could lead to dehydration if fluid isn't replaced quickly. If you haven't urinated for 12 hours, you're probably dehydrated.
● Diarrhea is bloody. This could be a symptom of *E. coli* 0157:H7 infection, which could lead to kidney failure and death.
● You get a stiff neck, severe headache, and fever all at once. This could signal meningitis, inflammation of the brain's lining, which can be caused by *Listeria* bacteria.
● You're at high risk. Young children, elderly people, anyone whose immune system is compromised (persons undergoing treatment for cancer or people with AIDS, for example), and pregnant women are more vulnerable to serious illness.

the 6 rules

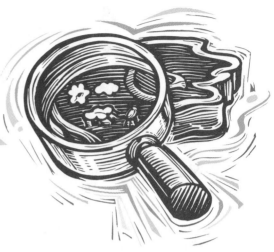

On the following pages, you'll learn 6 simple rules that are vitally important for safeguarding your and your family's health. These tips and techniques for shopping, food preparation, and food storage can help protect you from serious illness.

1: toxins

Know Your Enemy

At least 30 pathogens are commonly associated with foodborne illness. Along with bacteria and viruses, there are a number of other troublesome culprits. Here's a look at the main problems.

Bacteria

More than a dozen types of bacteria do their dirty work in one of two ways. Some, like *Salmonella*, multiply and cause irritation inside the intestinal tract. Others, such as *Staphylococcus aureus*, produce poisonous toxins in your intestines. The CDC has targeted four bacteria as the most worrisome:

E. coli O157:H7, found in everything from ground beef to unpasteurized milk and apple juice, causes some 21,000 illnesses and several deaths every year.

Salmonella, lurking in meat, poultry, milk, eggs, and even chocolate, sickens between two and four million Americans every year with abdominal pain and diarrhea; some people have died from its more virulent DT 104 strain.

Listeria monocytogenes, found in soft cheese, unpasteurized milk, and imported seafood products, makes an estimated 1,850 persons seriously ill every year and causes about 425 deaths.

Campylobacter, common in meat, poultry, unpasteurized milk, and untreated water, causes up to 6 million diarrhea cases a year.

Viruses

Microscopic forms of protein that multiply inside you, viruses can give you a cold or something a lot more serious, like the hepatitis A outbreak that resulted from contaminated strawberries. Raw shellfish and oysters from waters polluted by untreated sewage are a major viral hazard.

Parasites

Microorganisms that draw sustenance from other life forms, parasites are found in plants, animals, and water. Tainted water in Guatemala contaminated raspberries with *Clyospora* parasites and led to outbreak in the United States.

eating out safely

Eating out can be a great pleasure, but certainly not if the food ends up making you sick. Here's what experts say about assuring food safety:

● **Check cleanliness.** "Ask to visit the kitchen before you eat," advises food scientist Peter Snyder, Ph.D., who helped inspect restaurant kitchens in Los Angeles after a crackdown by that city's health department. "If it's well lit, if food isn't lying around on countertops, if the cooks and their uniforms are clean, and nobody's yelling at anybody, that's a well-disciplined kitchen, and chances are good that you'll get safe food."

A look at the restroom also helps, Dr. Snyder says. A dirty restroom probably signals a dirty kitchen.

"I personally look at the appearance of the waitstaff or counter staff," says food and nutrition specialist Angela Fraser, Ph.D. "If their hair is hanging loose, their uniform is dirty, they have long nails or lots of jewelry on their fingers, this means to me that food safety is not a priority of the management."

● **Choose food wisely.** If you have allergies or sensitivities to substances like MSG, be sure to inquire about ingredients used. To protect yourself from E. coli, when ordering a hamburger, don't ask that it be cooked "rare" or even "medium." In selecting food from a salad bar, check the temperature: Hot items should be hot, not lukewarm, and cold food should be chilled on ice. All food bars should be covered with a sneeze guard.

● **Inspect your food.** A hot entrée should be served piping hot, not lukewarm, which encourages the reproduction of bacterial toxins. Check meat with a fork to make sure it's cooked all the way through.

● **Be careful with leftovers or takeout.** If you're taking leftovers home in a doggie bag—or taking food out—make sure the food is already cool before it's put into the storage container. Then eat it within two hours or get it into your refrigerator as quickly as possible.

Natural Toxins

Lima beans contain low levels of cyanide, a deadly poison. There's no need to worry, however. It's present in such tiny amounts that it can't hurt you. Many herbs and spices contain a variety of toxic compounds as well. Again, these natural toxins are present in extremely low, harmless quantities. But some food toxins, such as the aflatoxins produced by molds that grow on peanuts, are poisonous and can pose a threat. The people who produce and process peanuts, for example, have to take steps to make sure their product is free of this toxin.

Pesticides

Farmers use pesticides to combat the abundance of insects, bacteria, viruses, fungi, and weeds that threaten their fields. Without pesticides, the U.S. Department of Agriculture (USDA) estimates, up to half of crops could be destroyed by pests. Nonetheless, pesticides can pose risks. In high doses, they've been linked to cancer and other illnesses. To be certain that non-toxic amounts of pesticide residue make it to our tables, the Environmental Protection Agency (EPA) closely regulates pesticide use.

Additives and Chemicals

Additives, most common among them sugar and salt, are used to preserve food; improve its taste, consistency, and appearance; and increase its nutrient content, says Angela M. Fraser, Ph.D., a food and nutrition specialist at North Carolina State University at Raleigh. Additives are strictly regulated by the U.S. Food and Drug Administration (FDA), which requires that the manufacturer submit scientific data proving that the chemical is harmless.

Some people have adverse reactions to some additives, Dr. Fraser says. This is a problem not of food safety but food sensitivity. (For a detailed treatment of this problem, see "Food Allergies," which begins on page 152.) Additives that have caused problems in some people include:

Monosodium glutamate (MSG). This flavor enhancer is commonly used in Asian food. Some people report reactions like flushing, dizziness, a headache, or nausea after consuming MSG.

Sulfites. These prevent browning of foods such as light-colored fruits and vegetables and baked goods. Sulfites are also used in wine-making because they inhibit bacterial growth but do not interfere with the desired development of yeast. Some people who have asthma report severe allergy-like reactions to sulfites, Dr. Fraser says.

Nitrites. Used to cure meats like hot dogs and lunch meat, nitrites have caused some concern because in large quantities they have been linked to the formation in the body of cancer-producing compounds called nitrosamines. However, meat processing today uses fewer nitrites, and the chemicals ascorbate or erythorbate are added to inhibit the nitrosamine reaction. Nitrites are not a significant cause of cancer, says the American Cancer Society.

Aspartame. Marketed as Equal and NutraSweet, aspartame has been reported by some users to cause adverse reactions like headaches, but studies by the FDA have concluded that there's not really a problem. The FDA also finds no evidence that aspartame causes cancer.

Olestra. This fake fat, used in potato chips, crackers, and other food products, can cause gastrointestinal problems, according to the Center for Science in the Public Interest. But so far, the FDA says olestra passes safe food muster.

Additives from Animals

Even when additives aren't put directly into the food you eat, they sometimes come to you via a more circuitous route: your meat counter. Here are a few additional items that cause concern in some food experts:

Antibiotics. Farmers often give livestock antibiotics to prevent illness. These can leave a residue in meat, says CSPI's Smith DaWaal. "But even more serious is that antibiotics kill off weak bacteria and leave the more virulent strains to survive," she says. "That's how, we believe, *Salmonella* DT 401 came into being."

Hormones. These can promote growth and other biological processes in animals. For instance, bovine somatotropin (BST), a hormone naturally produced by cows, is used as a supplement to increase cows' milk production. This probably isn't a risk to the consumer but is a risk to the cow, says Smith DaWaal. Higher milk production encourages infections of the udder, she says.

Mad cow disease. No cases of mad cow disease have been documented in the United States, but in England several people appear to have contracted this rare, degenerative disease of the brain and nervous system from eating meat infected with bovine spongiform encephalopathy (BSE). In the States, surveillance and prevention programs are in place to assure consumers that American beef and other foods derived from cattle are BSE-free.

2: shopping
Be on the Alert

Although food hazards are omnipresent, there's plenty you can do to protect yourself.

"Most food safety risks can be controlled by proper food handling," says Karen Penner, Ph.D., professor of food science at Kansas State University in Manhattan. "Every one of us must take the responsibility for assuring that our food is safe."

Proper selection, storage, cooking, and serving practices help assure that eating remains a delicious experience rather than a dangerous one.

You can take the first steps in protecting you and your family while shopping. "The consumer must be vigilant in choosing food," says Dr. Snyder. "Long-distance shipping, handling, and lots more can result in contamination of food before it even reaches the store."

Smart shopping gives you a head start on food safety, says Bessie Berry, director of the USDA's Meat and Poultry Hotline. For starters, she advises, shop for the least perishable items first and work your way toward the meat counter and frozen foods. Carrying perishable foods around the store in your cart for long periods invites pathogens to reproduce more quickly.

Here's an easy guide to shopping with safety in mind:

Dry and Canned Goods
🍎 **Use those labels.** Foods like pasta, dry beans, and just about anything in a can safely sit on a shelf for extended periods. Still, be sure to note the "use by" date on the label to make sure you'll be consuming the food before the date. Just because spaghetti sauce is on sale doesn't mean you should buy enough to last through the next two decades. Also check labels for ingredients you may be sensitive to, such as sulfites or MSG.

safe gifts by mail

These recommendations from food science professor Karen Penner help assure that mail-order food gifts are handled safely.

When you order a food gift:

● **Check on the cold source.** Ask how perishable food will be kept cold and how long the package will be in transit. The cold source must last long enough so that food arrives still frozen or firm and cold. Canned or processed foods labeled "keep refrigerated" should also be shipped with a cold source.

● **Make sure the message gets across.** Check that the package will be labeled as perishable food on the outside.

● **Set a workable delivery date.** Once you know how long the mailing takes, call your friends to find a date someone can be home to receive the gift. Mention that this "surprise" should go straight into the refrigerator.

When you receive a food gift:

● **Give it a feel.** Fresh or cooked meat, poultry, or fish should arrive frozen or still hard in the middle. If it was never frozen, it should at least be cold to the touch. With the exception of dry-cured country hams, baked hams and most canned hams need refrigeration and should arrive cold. Some hard, dry sausages like pepperoni and hard salami don't need refrigeration, while summer sausage and Thuringer do. If the label says "refrigerate," the sausage should arrive cold. Cheesecake, perishable because of its ingredients, should arrive fully frozen.

● **Inspect for mold.** There should be no mold on cheese except what is part of its nature, such as blue mold in blue cheese.

🍎 **Reject defects.** Inspect all cans to make sure they're not bulging or dented along any of the seams, advises Connie Diekman, R.D., a nutrition consultant in St. Louis and a spokesperson for the American Dietetic Association. A dent may signal the presence of clostridium botulinum, the toxin that causes botulism, a frequently fatal form of food poisoning.

🍎 **Allow for new forms of packaging.** You may notice foods like milk and tofu on the shelf along with the dry goods. These aseptically packaged items, sterilized and vacuum-packed, are perfectly safe for shelf storage for extended periods, says Snyder.

The Produce Aisles

🍎 **Be attracted to beauty.** Choose fruits and vegetables at their freshest: firm and healthy, not bruised, shriveled, or slimy, advises Diekman. This isn't simply a matter of aesthetics. Damaged or old produce is more likely to harbor bacteria inside and out, she says.

🍎 **Be conservative.** Purchase only the amount of produce you need in the next four days, says Diekman, because fruits and vegetables lose a big part of their nutritional value after that and also start spoiling.

🍎 **Go for difference.** Buy a variety of fruits and vegetables, advises CSPI's Smith DaWaal. This is not just good nutrition but lessens the risk of consuming high levels of pesticide residues. Different types of pesticides are sprayed on different crops, so your risk of getting a high dose of any one of them is lowered with a varied diet.

🍎 **Think domestic.** You may do well to limit your consumption of imported fruits and vegetables, suggests Dr. Snyder. Imports carry more risk of pathogens and also tend to have higher levels of pesticide residues, he says.

🍎 **Enjoy organic produce.** Buying organic (pesticide-free) produce also cuts pesticide risk, but eating organic foods is no assurance of safety from pathogens, says Smith DaWaal. Organic foods are exposed to exactly the same sorts of pathogens in nature and processing.

Dairy Products

🍎 **Chill out.** A proper storage temperature of 45° or less for dairy products is the single most important factor in maintaining their safety, says Dr. Snyder.

🍎 **Never buy warm milk or eggs,** advises the USDA's Berry. "Some may contain *Salmonella enteritidis* bacteria, which grow quickly if stored at room temperature."

🍎 **Buy only clean, pretty eggs.** Choose Grade A or AA eggs with clean, uncracked shells, Berry advises. Check for broken, cracked, or dirty eggs, which can carry a high number of pathogens.

🍎 **Check the dates and seals on all dairy products.** "Use by" dates are generally very accurate, says Diekman. If the product shows a "sell by" or "purchase by" date, you have about a week to use it. Be sure that all containers and wrappers are firmly sealed.

🍎 **Check for mold on cheese.** Although the kind of mold that grows on cheese isn't actually harmful, says Diekman, it's certainly not very tasty.

🍎 **Don't ever buy unpasteurized milk or milk products.** These can harbor deadly *Campylobacter jejuni*, *E. coli* 0157:H7, or other bacteria. (Don't buy unpasteurized juice either. Unpasteurized juice was linked to a big *E. coli* outbreak.)

Deli Items

"One of the biggest risks with deli foods is that they are being handled by yet another person," says Diekman.

🍎 **Check out the people.** Make sure that the person behind the counter looks clean and puts on a clean pair of plastic gloves to serve you. Also make sure he or she is not switching between raw meat and cooked deli items, which could cross-contaminate cooked food with pathogens.

🍎 **Use all your senses.** If any deli item looks or smells funny, don't buy it. Foods like chicken salad should be eaten within 48 hours of preparation, so ask the deli person when it was made.

🍎 **Don't reject mayo.** Salads made with mayonnaise pose no special risk, says Diekman, because mayonnaise is acid-based, which prohibits the growth of bacteria. The problem is with the perishable eggs, chicken, or other animal protein in the salad, she says.

🍎 **Make sure that hot deli items have been kept hot.** Lukewarm just doesn't do it. Temperatures below 150° allow bacteria to grow and produce toxins.

Meat

Proper cool storage of meat items is crucial to food safety, says Dr. Snyder.

🍎 **Check for coldness.** Find the meat department thermometer. It should read less than 35°. And do the touch test. When you pick up the item, it should be evenly cold to the touch.

🍎 **Check those vital signs.** Select meat that looks red and juicy, which indicates freshness, rather than flat or dull, advises Diekman. Chicken skin should be plump, not dehydrated, and fish should look clear and bright. Because of the risk of cross-contamination, don't buy cooked seafood if it's displayed in the same case as raw fish. (Never eat raw oysters or raw or undercooked mussels, clams, or whole scallops. These may be infected with *Vibrio vulnificus*, a killer bacteria.)

🍎 **Inspect the package.** Check the "purchase by" dates. All packaging should be completely sealed. If you notice ice crystals inside, this could mean that the item has been thawed and refrozen, a danger sign.

🍎 **Isolate any problems.** If a package of fresh meat or poultry is leaky, wrap it in another plastic bag to prevent the juices from cross-contaminating other food in your shopping cart. (And wipe your hands with soap and water or a paper towel to rid them of pathogens.) Place meat, poultry, and fish on the bottom of your shopping cart to avoid cross-contamination of other foods.

🍎 **Focus on frozen foods.** Do the touch test to be sure items are frozen all the way through, and check packages for holes that could allow bacteria in.

Heading Home

After shopping, you need to get perishable items into your refrigerator promptly, says the USDA's Berry. "You cannot go run errands or see friends and expect your food to be as wholesome and safe as it would have been if you'd gone straight home."

Refrigerated and frozen food items, plus hot deli items that you plan to refrigerate and eat later, have an absolute two-hour safety time limit. Milk spoils even faster. In hot weather, when your car temperature soars, even a half-hour out of the fridge can be too long. If you can't get home quickly, pack your perishables in an ice chest to give yourself a couple of extra hours.

3 : storage
Keep Foods Safe

Quick and careful storage helps assure that food stays safer longer.

Refrigerated Foods

The cooler your refrigerator, the longer food remains safe and tasty, says Dr. Snyder.

🍎 **Make sure your cold is really cold.** Set your refrigerator temperature no higher than 40°, the point at which most bacteria stop multiplying.

🍎 **Protect other foods from contamination.** Store meat and poultry in their original store wrappers on the bottom shelf, where

when to toss it

"If in doubt, throw it out," the saying goes. Going on a combination of observation and instinct may not seem like the most scientific approach to figuring out whether food in your refrigerator or cupboard is past its prime, but the saying reflects the fact that pathogenic bacteria usually can't be detected by sight or smell. "The best-tasting food you've ever had may be crawling with microbes and make you very ill," says food scientist Peter Snyder. These guidelines can help:

● **Refrigerated meat and poultry.** Steaks, roasts, and hamburger last one or two days in your fridge, three to four months in your freezer. Chicken is also fine one or two days in the refrigerator and up to a year frozen. Be sure to label and date everything.

● **Lunch meat and hot dogs.** They'll last two weeks unopened, one week opened.

● **Cheese.** Can be refrigerated for three to four weeks. If mold does develop, cut off the mold itself, plus about an inch of cheese around the mold.

● **Yogurt.** Good a week or two past the "use by" date, but if you spot reddish mold, toss it.

● **Eggs.** Raw, shelled eggs are good for three to five weeks. Hard-boiled eggs last only one week.

● **Milk.** Use by the "use by" date.

● **Fruits and vegetables.** Use within three to five days at the height of freshness and nutritional value.

● **Frozen vegetables, frozen dinners.** Can be frozen for up to a year.

● **Leftovers in general.** Use within five days for best quality, within 10 days for food safety.

● **Condiments.** Once opened and refrigerated, mayonnaise lasts two months; mustard and ketchup, six months; salad dressing, one to two months; barbecue sauce, three to six months; jam or jelly, one year.

● **Canned and dry goods.** Use by "use by" date for highest quality. Never, ever open a can that's swollen or dented near the top, bottom, or side seams. It could contain deadly *Clostridium botulinum* and could squirt up into your face. And never eat moldy peanuts, which can contain poisonous aflatoxins.

juices can't drip down to contaminate other food. Push it toward the back, too; the temperature in the back of your fridge is 10° to 15° cooler. Store milk and eggs on refrigerator shelves, not on the door where the temperature is highest.

🍎 **Save damaged goods.** If any eggs cracked on the way home, break them into a clean container, cover them tightly and keep them refrigerated. They must be used within two days.

🍎 **Leave a little breathing room.** Avoid packing food tightly, which interferes with cool air circulation, says Dr. Snyder.

🍎 **Use your crisper.** Store produce like lettuce and apples in the humidity-controlled crisper to keep them fresher longer, advises nutritionist Diekman. Fresher means less bacteria plus more nutrition.

🍎 **Wait to wash.** Don't wash fruits and vegetables until you are ready to eat them, because dampness encourages the growth of bacteria and mold.

🍎 **Pay special attention to frozen foods.** Frozen foods should be placed in your freezer in the original wrapper to avoid further handling, says Diekman. If you plan to use them in smaller quantities, rewrap them tightly in moisture-proof freezer paper, foil, or plastic. Write dates on all packages and containers, and move older items up front so they'll be used first.

🍎 **Clean out your "fossil" collection.** Food in your refrigerator or freezer won't last forever. One form of bacteria or another is still multiplying in your fridge, just more slowly. So use your food promptly.

🍎 **Refreeze.** Studies have shown that you can thaw frozen food to 40° (the temperature of your refrigerator), refreeze it as many times as desired, then cook it with no safety problems. If a frozen food has stayed outside of your refrigerator, you may safely refreeze it as long as it still contains ice crystals.

Canned and Dry Goods

Although canned and dry goods do last longer than foods that need refrigeration, they are not immortal.

🍎 **Aim for even temperature.** Store canned goods at room temperature—your pantry, not your back porch—because repeated heating and cooling brings quality down, says Dr. Snyder.

🍎 **Protect opened goods.** Put foods like flour, cereal, and pasta in tightly closed glass, plastic, or metal containers to keep them fresh and insect-free. Move older items to the front to be used sooner.

🍎 **Keep 'em dry.** Potatoes, carrots, and other root vegetables should be stored in a cool, dark place. But not under the kitchen sink, where leakage from pipes can damage food, or on the floor where insects or rodents can reach them.

4: be clean
Stop Germs Up Front

"The first cardinal rule of safe food preparation in the home is to keep everything clean," says Dr. Snyder. "This applies to the cook as well as the kitchen."

🍎 **Wash your hands.** "We all need to get into the habit of washing our hands," says Dr. Penner. "All day we've been touching dirty things, from going to the bathroom to petting the dog. Don't just head to the kitchen and grab something to eat or start fixing a meal. Wash your hands."

Hand-washing may sound awfully basic, but the Centers for Disease Control and Prevention report that one-third of the outbreaks of deadly foodborne illness caused by *E.coli* 0157:H7 could have been prevented by proper hand-washing.

🍎 **Use a little elbow grease.** Dr. Penner recommends a 20-second scrub, long enough to work up a soapy lather all the way up to your elbows. To be extra-thorough, scrub under your fingernails with a fingernail brush. Then dry with a paper towel or clean cloth towel.

👆 **Clean your work area.** Start out with everything in your kitchen clean, from your kitchen sink to your countertops, to assure that you're not contaminating food with germs from your kitchen. Then keep cleaning up to avoid cross-contamination as you work with foods containing pathogens.

Soap and water do just fine for cleaning your sink, countertops, and other work surfaces, says Dr. Penner. Antibacterial products are also good, especially if they contain bleach, which sanitizes. Or prepare your own sanitizer, using 1 teaspoon of bleach to 1 quart of water.

👆 **Soak those sponges.** If you use a sponge or scrub pad, soak in soapy water and rinse if the sponge has been sitting overnight, during which microorganisms were multiplying on it.

Or soak in a bleach-and-water solution for one minute followed by a rinse. Or if you have a dishwasher, throw the sponge into it once a day.

👆 **Clean your cans.** When using canned foods, clean the top of the can before you open to avoid getting dirt and infectious microbes inside. Also be sure to clean your can opener blade after each use.

Food Preparation

Pathogens like *Campylobacter jejuni*, *E. coli*, and more than 2,000 strains of *Salmonella* in your food are just waiting to break out and breed. Practicing caution every step of the way in preparing food can keep them under control.

👆 **Thaw meat, chicken, and fish in the refrigerator or microwave.** Forget thawing that package of ground beef or chicken on your kitchen counter all day, says Dr. Penner. Pathogens start multiplying the instant they're out of your fridge. Instead, thaw frozen foods overnight by placing them on the bottom shelf of your refrigerator where they won't drip on other food. If you're in a hurry, put the frozen item in your microwave on the defrost cycle or seal it in a plastic bag and immerse in cold water for about an hour.

👆 **Don't thaw frozen vegetables.** If you are cooking frozen vegetables, don't let them thaw before cooking. It's simply not necessary, and spoilage microorganisms multiply during thawing.

👆 **Wash raw poultry, fish, or meat carefully or not at all.** "Washing just removes any surface debris or juices," says the USDA's Berry. "It does not in any way render that product safe."

The big risk with washing these items is that you may spread pathogenic microorganisms around your kitchen, which can cross-contaminate other food. If you choose to rinse meat, poultry, or fish, do it in your sink under running water, pat dry with a clean paper towel, and dispose of the towel, Berry advises.

👆 **Prepare small amounts of food at a time.** Keep perishable food refrigerated as much as possible, says Dr. Penner.

Remove only those foods that you're immediately working on, and once you've finished preparing a piece of meat or assembling a casserole, start cooking or return it to the refrigerator right away. "Leaving the food on your counter invites bacterial growth," she says.

packing a safe school lunch

It's a scene played out all across America: children sent off to school with a homemade lunch in tow. But at least one in seven such lunches is a food poisoning risk, one survey shows. To keep your child safe, here's what nutritionists at Washington State University Cooperative Extension and the USDA suggest:

● **Choose foods that can be safely kept at room temperature.** Bacteria don't grow in foods that are high in acid or low in moisture. These include bread, peanut butter and jam (your basic peanut-butter-and-jelly sandwich), dry or hard cheeses, butter and margarine, raw vegetables, yogurt, pickles, mustard, and catsup, canned foods (until opened), and cookies. Cured meats such as salami and bologna are slow to spoil, too.

● **Prepare perishable foods with extra care.** Sandwiches and salads that contain cooked or processed meat, fish, or poultry, cooked vegetables, rice, beans, custards, puddings, and milk are all risky. Make sure you chop ingredients and assemble sandwiches and salads with sanitary and safe preparation practices in mind. (See "Be Clean," which begins on page 50.)

● **Take extra precautions with meat, chicken, and poultry.** These foods when cooked must be cooled quickly and thoroughly to slow toxin growth before they're made into a sandwich or salad. Even when cooled, these foods are risky. To increase sandwich safety, make the night before, pack in a thin plastic sandwich bag, and freeze it. Packed the next day in your child's lunch, the sandwich will thaw in time for lunch while also keeping the rest of the lunch cool. Other freezable fillings include cheese and peanut butter.

Reusable ice packs and insulated lunch carriers help keep food cool, as does a frozen can of juice.

● **Send cold milk to school in a thermos bottle.** Wash and rinse the bottle in boiling water after each use. Pack soup or stew in a thermos as well, only after bringing them to a full boil to keep the food hot for four to six hours.

● **Don't include custards, puddings, and cream pies in your child's lunch.** These are extremely vulnerable to bacterial growth. Individual servings of commercially prepared puddings are fine, however, as they don't require refrigeration.

Do all your marinating in the refrigerator and throw out the marinade when you're finished because it contains raw juices that may contain bacteria.

🍎 **Clean as you go.** Constantly clean up after yourself to prevent pathogens like *Salmonella* from spreading from one food to another. Wash your hands and wipe them with a paper towel you dispose of. Don't get into the habit of wiping your hands on your shirt or jeans. And don't use a dish towel that gets used for other things later.

Clean your countertops, your sink, and, perhaps most importantly, your cutting board and knives. Food processors and other equipment should also be cleaned thoroughly to avoid cross-contamination.

🍎 **Pay special attention to your cutting board.** One of the biggest cross-contamination hazards is using a cutting board and knives for several food items consecutively without a cleanup in between. Give your cutting board a good scrubbing before each new food task.

"Use a brush and plenty of detergent," advises food chemist Robert LaBudde, Ph.D., a consultant for the food industry. "Get it nice and foamy, which indicates that it's working. Then scrub every square inch of it." Follow with a bleach sanitizing solution, then rinse and air-dry or dry with a fresh towel.

Better yet, use two separate cutting boards as Dr. LaBudde does in his own kitchen, one for meat, chicken, and fish, the other for fruit, vegetables, and other items. You still need to keep the boards clean, but your cross-contamination risks are cut. It doesn't matter whether your board is wood or plastic. The only advantage of plastic is that it can be put into a dishwasher for a very thorough cleaning.

🍎 **Thoroughly clean fruits and vegetables.** Your best insurance against infectious organisms hiding in raw fruits and vegetables is a careful cleaning, says Dr. LaBudde. This helps remove pesticide residues, too. A wash in plain water and a scrub with a soft-bristled mushroom brush will do just fine, he says. Don't use soap, which adds residue of its own. The new vegetable washes are fine but not really necessary, he says. There's generally no

need, he says, to wash precut salads and other vegetables that come vacuum-packaged, as they're triple-washed right before they're packed.

5: cooking
Think Defensively

Nearly one-third of all cases of food poisoning at home are caused by inadequate cooking, says the USDA. Most illness-producing infectious microorganisms lurking in food can be stopped in their tracks with the right amount of heat. "You have to kill it in the skillet," says Dr. Snyder.

🍎 **Cook with enough heat.** Whatever cooking method you're using, from boiling to broiling, getting food up to an internal temperature of at least 165° (180° for chicken), the point at which microorganisms like *E. coli* 0157:H7 are killed, is crucial. That's the reason many recipes call for bringing food to a boil then taking it down to a simmer, which is still hotter than 165°.

A cooking thermometer is one of the best investments you can make when it comes to food safety, says Dr. Penner. Find one (it's different from an oven thermometer) at a hardware store or maybe even your supermarket. Put it into your food—a roast, a casserole, whatever—for a few seconds when you think the food is done. Don't check doneness by the color of a piece of meat, as was once advised, Dr. Penner says. Research has shown that color changes during cooking depend on

have a safe holiday

Food safety is important year-round, but during the holidays it becomes increasingly important because we're often preparing large, less easily managed meals and serving them to large numbers of people. These recommendations from the Illinois State University Extension and the USDA can help you have a healthier holiday.

● **Make room in your refrigerator.** An overpacked refrigerator isn't as efficient in keeping food cool, heightening the risk that pathogens will reproduce. Shop for just what you need.

● **Be extra-sanitary in the kitchen.** You may be in a hurry, but don't rush so much that you neglect to clean utensils, dishes, and cutting boards exposed to meat or poultry that could cross-contaminate other foods.

● **Prepare holiday turkey with caution.** Thaw turkey in its original wrapper in the refrigerator. Allow 24 hours per 5 pounds. (It could take up to five days to thaw a 24-pound turkey.) When cooking turkey, remember to remove the giblet package in the cavity prior to cooking. Also, stuff the turkey just before cooking or bacteria from the turkey can start multiplying in the stuffing. Roast turkey at a temperature of 325° or hotter. Never cook it at a lower temperature, and never cook it overnight. Check for doneness—180° or above—with a meat thermometer.

● **Serve in a timely manner.** You have no more than two to four hours to serve the meal then refrigerate or freeze the leftovers. After that, harmful bacteria can multiply to unsafe levels on perishable foods. On a buffet, use warming trays to keep hot foods hot and bowls of ice to nestle cold foods.

● **Refrigerate leftovers quickly.** Put leftovers in small containers so they cool quickly in the refrigerator. Freeze any leftovers that you won't use soon. And send your guests away with leftovers, too.

characteristics of meat such as its level of acidity rather than whether it is completely cooked or not.

🍎 **Make sure eggs are really done.** Proper egg cooking helps prevent *Salmonella* poisoning. Because it's hard to take the temperature of an egg, use these cooking guidelines from the USDA's Berry:

● Fried eggs should be cooked for two to three minutes on each side until the yolk begins to thicken; never cook them "sunny side up" on one side only.

● Cook scrambled eggs until they're firm throughout, not runny.

● Poach eggs over boiling water for a good five minutes.

● Soft-boiled eggs should be cooked in the shell in boiling water for seven minutes.

🍎 **Never, ever, eat raw eggs.** And never eat foods that contain them. This includes uncooked cookie dough, homemade ice cream, and homemade eggnog. Lightly cooked foods containing eggs, such as soft custards, meringues, and French toast can also be risky. You can avoid these problems by using pasteurized egg products, in which all the bacteria have been killed, instead of fresh eggs.

And if you're tempted by a restaurant item that you know might contain a raw egg (Caesar salad, for example), ask your server if it is prepared with raw eggs. If it is, don't order it. (And do say why.)

🍎 **Use your microwave with caution.** It's better not to microwave risky raw foods like meat, chicken, or fish because microwave ovens don't cook food evenly, explains Dr. Snyder. It's okay to heat the food to about 100° in a microwave, but then transfer the food to your stove to complete the cooking, he advises.

🍎 **Watch those nibbles.** To assure that you are not introducing pathogens to properly cooked food, do any taste-testing with a clean spoon.

6: serving
Use Extra Care

Having done everything that needs to be done to select and prepare safe food, now you are home free, right?

"That's a fallacy," says the USDA's Berry, "because the bacteria that can really cause a problem are always present in our environment. It's a given that they are going to make their way into prepared food."

For example, we all carry *Staphylococcus aureus* in our nose and throat and on our hands. Coughing or sneezing near prepared food or even simply handling it contaminates the food. This bacteria then proceeds to produce dangerous, invisible toxins as long as the food sits out at room temperature. And reheating the food doesn't kill the toxins.

In addition, if even a few pathogenic microorganisms like *Salmonella* survive the cooking process, as sometimes they do, they start growing when food cools below 130°. And they grow with a vengeance, because non-pathogenic bacteria, called "spoilage bacteria," were totally killed off in the cooking process. With the competition gone, illness-causing bacteria have the food all to themselves.

Hence, food sitting out for too long and leftovers can be even more dangerous than just-prepared foods. "Perfectly safe-looking food that stays out at warm temperatures for more than four hours can cause vomiting, diarrhea, and possibly paralysis," says Dr. Snyder. But you can take plenty of precautions to avert such problems.

🍎 **Keep hot foods hot.** Cooked foods of all sorts—meats, vegetables, casseroles, sauces, and more—should be left out on the table or kitchen counter absolutely no longer than four hours, says Dr. Penner. A two-hour time limit would be even safer, as many infectious microorganisms have a lag time of between two to four hours before they begin to multiply. Keeping food covered and using a hot plate help assure that food doesn't lose its heat quickly.

If you're preparing a variety of cooked foods and trying to get them to your dinner table warm all at the same time, hold some of them in your oven with the temperature set to 200° until you're ready for dinner, Dr. LaBudde suggests. This keeps them above bacteria-producing temperature but not so hot that they get overcooked.

Keeping your serving utensils in the hot food keeps them bacteria-free, too, says Dr. Snyder. (And be sure to use utensils rather than your hands so as not to introduce additional bacteria to the food.)

 Keep cold foods cold. Microorganisms start multiplying in cold foods once they get warm. Foods like cold cooked meats and lunch meat, milk, tuna salad, cold pasta, and cream-filled pastries are all at risk when their temperature rises above 50°.

Keep cold foods in the refrigerator or covered and on a bed of ice until serving and don't leave them out for more than two hours, advises Dr. Penner. This rule is particularly important during the summer.

 Refrigerate leftovers. Pathogenic microorganisms will multiply in food that is cooled too slowly, so get leftovers into your refrigerator promptly. Once the temperature gets down to about 40°, microorganisms quit multiplying and toxin-producing bacteria become inactive.

 Bring temperature down quickly. Divide leftover food into small quantities to help them cool more quickly, advises Dr. Penner. "Oftentimes people will make the mistake of putting a big pot of chili or stew in the refrigerator."

Instead, store leftovers in shallow containers no more than 2 inches tall or in zipper-type plastic bags. Cut foods like roasts into slices 3 inches thick or less. (Never mix fresh food into a container with old food, because any contaminants in the old food will spread to the new.) Then put the leftovers in the cooler back part of your refrigerator on a wire shelf or rack to expose the container bottoms to more cool air, which further cuts the cooling time.

 Use leftovers quickly. Label food containers with the name of the food and the date you put it in the refrigerator. Check them daily for spoilage and throw out anything that looks or smells suspicious. For food safety, leftovers should be used in less than 10 days, but the food will taste better if you use it within five days.

 Reheat at high heat. You may be tempted to pull leftovers out of the fridge and eat them straight from the container, but resist the urge. Infection-producing microorganisms that grew before you put it in the fridge are waiting for you. And bacteria like *Listeria monocytogenes*, which can kill you, continue to multiply even in the refrigerator. *Listeria* is killed only when food is heated.

Reheat leftovers to 165° to assure that pathogens are killed off. On the top of your stove, heat food to a boil or near-boil, then simmer, stirring to make sure it's heating evenly. In your oven, reheat at a temperature no lower than 325°. Use your thermometer to make sure the food has reached 165° before serving it. Microwaving leftovers is fine as long as you stir to reheat evenly and check the temperature at several points.

chapter 3

conditions
AND
diseases

{{ I look upon it, that he who does not mind his belly will hardly mind anything else. —Samuel Johnson }}

You're so relieved when your doctor reaches for her prescription pad. You've been putting off this office visit. Those troublesome symptoms—possibly the signal of something serious—have been nagging at you. But you've been dreading the thought of any kind of expensive, prolonged testing and treatment. So it's with a sigh of relief that you reach for the prescription. All you have to do is take... VEGGIES?

It's not all that unusual these days for doctors to dispense dietary advice along with, or even well before, they call for prescription medicines or surgery. Many is the person with heart disease, diabetes, high cholesterol, even headaches, who has sat across from a physician getting the standard less-fat, less-sugar, more-vegetables lecture. The message is now coming in loud and clear: Diet makes a major difference in your health. In fact, medical research is increasingly showing that simple dietary changes often can prevent disease, bring relief, and sometimes even cure specific diseases. Every year medical research reveals more about what to eat (and what not to eat) if you have a specific disease or condition. Here's a look at how changing your diet can help you heal.

aging

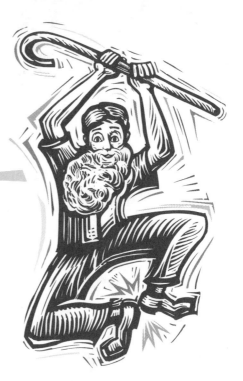

Concerned about aging? That makes you very current, modern, au courant. A concern for aging is a phenomenon of the 20th century. Up until this century, life expectancy hovered around 30 years, so pondering how to live a long life was literally wasted on the young. Today, people want and expect to live into their 70s or 80s. And those who balance good genes with good care can expect to live well past 100, possibly even to the maximum life span of 120 years.

People's health expectations have also undergone a significant change. More and more people not only want to live long, they want to live well during those extra years. There is every reason to believe that most of us can live long and be in good health—if we are willing to make changes in what we eat, how often and vigorously we move, and how we live our lives.

The more that people take charge of their lives and their health, the more likely the traditional view of the "elderly" person as feeble, frail, and ailing will dissolve into the distant past, much like the deadly threat of smallpox. That's because most of the diseases and dysfunction associated with aging—from heart disease, cancer, diabetes, and high blood pressure to cataracts, skin wrinkling, feebleness, and osteoporosis— are now recognized to have a significant lifestyle component. In short, it is not years alone that cause deterioration, but how you choose to live them.

What Does Aging Mean?

Starting somewhere between 20 and 30 years old, the body starts a gradual decline in many major systems, including the immune and muscular systems. The overall metabolic rate slows, the digestive tract becomes sluggish, and the endocrine (glandular) system slips, to name just a few of the aging processes. But people are generally not as concerned about this kind of aging as they are about illness and dependency as they get older.

"It is hard to separate out the issue of aging from the issues of disease," states Jeffrey Blumberg, Ph.D., professor of nutrition at the Jean Mayer USDA Human Nutrition Research Center on Aging at Tufts University in Boston. People experience an increased risk of diabetes as they age, for example. Blood pressure also rises, as do blood cholesterol levels and the risk for developing heart disease. Brittle bones (osteoporosis) are associated with advancing years. Reaction times also slow with age, and older people report they have more trouble remembering new names. This suggests an increased difficulty in processing new information for short-term memory.

In short, aging and age-related disease are closely linked, but entirely separate. More important, much of the aging process is within a person's control. Many of the above mentioned changes in body and mind are modifiable by making a few simple changes in diet and exercise. In other words, there's a whole lot you can do to hold off the aging process.

Nutritional Needs Increase with Age

Aging is a continuum, not a sudden event," says Robert Russell, M.D., professor of medicine and nutrition at Tufts University in Boston. "You don't wake up one morning to discover you're old. The same nutrition issues related to seniors—from heart disease to osteoporosis—have their beginnings in the middle years."

But you must get aggressive. Requirements for some nutrients are higher than previously thought and often higher than many people typically consume.

Vitamin D, a nutrient essential to the prevention of osteoporosis and possibly colon cancer, is a good example of how starting early can sidestep problems later on. The body can manufacture vitamin D when the skin is exposed to sunlight, but gradually loses this ability with age.

"A woman in her 20s can synthesize only 80 percent of the vitamin D that her body made when she was in third grade. By the time a woman is in her 70s, production has dropped to only 40 percent," says Dr. Russell. That means dietary sources of vitamin D become increasingly important as you age, and daily intake must remain at 400 international units (IU) or more, especially in the fifth decade and on. Yet, many adults don't drink four cups of milk every day. Milk is the only reliable dietary source of vitamin D—each cup supplies 100 IU of vitamin D.

Most women also need to be getting more calcium, which also comes from milk and other dairy products.

The B vitamins are another case in point. Three B vitamins—folic acid, vitamin B6, and vitamin B12—are essential for the prevention of heart disease. They keep levels of a compound called homocysteine low in the blood. If levels of this compound are allowed to rise, it contributes to heart-disease risk even in the absence of high blood cholesterol levels. Yet, up to 85 percent of women don't consume even recommended levels of vitamin B6. Up to 93 percent of women don't consume even one folic acid-rich vegetable on any one of four days (we should consume at least two dark green leafy vegetables daily). And people typically consume less vitamin B12 as they age even though their needs for this vitamin increase.

How do you make sure you're getting enough of these essential vitamins? Consume daily at least two dark green leafy vegetables, such as broccoli, spinach, romaine lettuce, or collard greens, for folic acid. Include several servings daily of foods containing vitamin B6 and B12, such as chicken, fish, extra-lean meat, or nonfat dairy products like milk and yogurt. Vitamin B12 status also should be monitored by a physician as a person ages, since deficiencies can go undetected, resulting in loss of mental function and memory.

Antioxidants: The Antiaging Vitamins

Aging is a multifactorial problem, but some aspects of aging and disease prevention are directly linked to nutrition, especially the antioxidants," says Dr. Blumberg. The link between the antioxidant nutrients and aging begins with free radicals, the classic villains of aging.

Free radicals are highly reactive oxygen fragments consumed in food, inhaled from air pollution, and generated in the body during normal metabolic processes. These free radicals attack and damage cells, their genetic code, and the protective coatings called membranes that surround every cell. Free radicals also impair energy production by damaging the cells' powerhouse centers (called the mitochondria). With thousands of free-radical attacks on each cell every day, over the course of decades the process results in fewer functioning cells and more damaged or abnormal cells. Because free radicals also attack the immune system, the body gradually loses its resistance to colds, infections, and disease. All of these processes have been identified as a normal part of biological aging.

Luckily, the body has an antioxidant system, comprised of vitamins, minerals, enzymes, and other compounds, that sweeps up and deactivates free radicals. The most potent of the dietary antioxidants are vitamin C, vitamin E, beta-carotene, selenium, and a group of health-enhancing compounds called phytochemicals found in fruits and vegetables, beans, garlic, and green tea. Stockpiling a strong antioxidant defense by consuming foods rich in the antioxidants helps slow or even halt free-radical damage to the tissues. And this helps prevent premature aging and age-related diseases, such as heart disease, cancer, arthritis, and cataracts.

The link is strong between antioxidants and aging. For example, nutrition intervention studies on more than 29,000 people between the ages of 40 and 69 years in Linxian, China, showed that taking a multiple vitamin and mineral supplement that contained the antioxidants, especially vitamin E, beta-carotene, and selenium, reduced the risk of premature death by 9 percent. It also reduced the risk for esophageal cancer by 17 percent and death from heart disease by almost 40 percent. A second study conducted by the same group found that antioxidant supplements also significantly lowered total mortality (by 13 percent), gastric cancer mortality (by 20 percent), and mortality from other cancers (by 19 percent).

In short, much disease is not a matter of age but a result of accumulating damage over time. If you stop the damage, you should stop, or at least slow, the aging clock. The sooner a person boosts antioxidant intake the better; however, it is never too late to strengthen the antioxidant system

make sure you get enough

Getting enough fruits and vegetables to help slow the aging process takes planning. Here are suggestions for increasing your intake of these nutrient-packed foods.

- Include at least two fruits or vegetables at every meal and two more for snacks.
- Include at least two servings daily of dark green vegetables, such as spinach, romaine lettuce, or chard, to ensure optimal intake of beta-carotene and folic acid.
- Include at least two items rich in vitamin C, such as citrus fruits or juice,

strawberries, or sweet peppers.
- Include at least five vegetables each week from the cabbage family, such as brussels sprouts, kohlrabi, asparagus, cabbage, broccoli, or cauliflower. These vegetables are chock-full of phytochemicals that lower your risk of developing cancer.

and help slow the damaging effects of free radicals.

How much of these substances do you need? The best place to obtain the entire orchestra of antioxidants is from fruits, vegetables, whole grains, and legumes. That's the very diet recommended throughout this book for preventing and helping to heal a wide variety of diseases. For the past 20 years, scientists worldwide consistently have found that people who eat lots of these plants have lower rates of cancer, heart disease, and disease in general. They also are more likely to maintain a desirable weight and live longer than people who shun these foods. While these foods are the diet's richest sources of vitamins, minerals, and fiber, more recent evidence shows there is more than just nutrients in plants. Research on animals has supported this theory and

has isolated certain phytochemicals that are particularly health-enhancing and disease-preventing.

Take cancer, for example, which is a multistep disease. At almost every step along the pathway leading to cancer, there are one or more phytochemicals, vitamins, minerals, and fibers in fruits and vegetables that slow or even reverse the process. People who eat the most fruits and vegetables are about half as likely to have cancer as people who eat the typical daily intake in the United States of two to three servings.

Although the recommended intake for fruits and vegetables is five servings a day, this is actually a minimum. Eight or more servings a day will provide a more optimal dose of the antioxidant phytochemicals, vitamins, and minerals. Whole grains are richer sources of many age-defying nutrients, like vitamin E, chromium, selenium, and zinc, than are refined grains.

should you supplement?

Even if you make perfect food choices every day, there still is reason to take a supplement.

Some antiaging nutrients are needed in amounts far greater than is realistically possible from diet alone. For example, the Alliance for Aging Research, a group of renowned scientists from major research institutions such as the University of California at Berkeley and Tufts University in Boston, recommends adults consume daily:

> 250 to 1,000 milligrams of vitamin C
>
> 100 to 400 international units of vitamin E
>
> 10 to 30 milligrams of beta-carotene

(People who smoke should consult with their physicians before supplementing with beta-carotene.)

Although you can meet the lower levels for vitamin C and beta-carotene by munching on six to eight fruits and vegetables every day, you must guzzle one cup of safflower oil or feast on 21 cups of spinach daily—not likely!—to consume even 124 international units of vitamin E.

Requirements for other nutrients, such as vitamin D and vitamin B12, escalate as we age, often to levels not likely to be achieved from food alone. Consequently, for people who cannot always eat perfectly or for those who want to ensure they receive an extra nutritional boost, there is reason to supplement—wisely and moderately.

So emphasize whole wheat breads, brown rice, and other whole grains and include at least six servings daily.

Legumes, especially soybeans, pack an extra nutritional punch because they are rich sources of two groups of phytochemicals called phytoestrogens and phytosterols that lower the risk of developing breast cancer and heart disease. (The phytoestrogens in soy products also might help curb hot flashes associated with menopause.) Preliminary evidence suggests that as little as 15 ounces of soymilk or 2 ounces of tofu daily is enough to reap the health benefits of these phytochemicals.

Another important dietary strategy is to avoid foods that generate free radicals, such as fried foods, processed foods made with oils, and fatty foods in general.

Lose the Fat

There is no other dietary guideline that has as great an impact on your health today and in the future as cutting back on fat—especially the saturated fats in meat and dairy products, and the hydrogenated fats in margarine and shortening. Diets that contain these fats are associated with increased risks for heart disease and possibly cancer. Several studies show that meat consumption in particular, with its high amount of saturated fat and cholesterol, also is correlated with heart disease in both men and women. In fact, disease risk increases as both the length of time and frequency of meat consumption increases. Consequently, people who adopt a vegetarian diet early in life have a lower risk of disease than do people who wait until after age 50 to switch from meat to beans.

In all fairness to meat, it might not be the harmful effects of a pot roast per se, but, conversely, the protective effects of other foods in the vegetarian diet that is the real issue. Studies on Seventh Day Adventists, a group with a high percentage of vegetarians and a low cancer rate, show that meat is not always a significant factor in the development of certain types of cancer. On the other hand, people who eat lots of fruits, legumes, and vegetables are at much lower risk for certain cancers, probably because they simply don't have as much room in their diets for fattier foods.

the three steps for

supplementing

Choosing the best supplement program is as easy as one, two, three.

1. Select a broad-range multiple vitamin and mineral supplement that provides approximately 100 to 300 percent of the Daily Value for all nutrients as listed on the label.

2. Supplement your multiple vitamin with extra calcium and magnesium. Size dictates that one-tablet-a-day multiples can never supply enough of these minerals. (The pill would be the size of a Ping-Pong ball!) Choose a calcium-magnesium supplement that provides approximately two parts calcium for every one part magnesium (for example, 500 milligrams calcium and 250 milligrams

magnesium). If your multiple vitamin (or your fortified cereal) does not contain vitamin D, make sure the calcium-magnesium tablet also comes with 400 international units of this vitamin.

3. If the multiple vitamin does not contain extra amounts of vitamin C, vitamin E, and the carotenoids, consider taking an antioxidant supplement containing just these nutrients.

Note: It's a good idea to ask your doctor about any supplements you're considering. Supplements in large amounts can interact with certain drugs. And some supplements are not appropriate for everyone.

Other fats also might escalate the aging process, at least as it applies to heart disease. For years we've been told to avoid butter and instead spread margarine on our toast, because butter is high in saturated fats, while margarine is made from heart-friendly vegetable oils. Or so we thought. More recent studies show that altered fats in margarine and shortening, called transfatty acids or TFAs, might be as bad as, if not worse, than butter. TFAs, in amounts typically consumed by Americans, alter metabolism and raise total blood cholesterol and LDL cholesterol (the "bad" cholesterol) in much the same way as saturated fats. Large amounts of TFAs also might lower HDL-cholesterol levels (the "good" cholesterol). Any or all of these changes produce the worst scenario for heart health.

In the Nurses' Health Study, conducted by Walter Willett, M.D., Dr. P.H., and colleagues at Harvard School of Public Health in Boston, the dietary intakes of 85,000 women were compared to disease rates. The researchers found that as intakes of TFA-containing foods, including margarine, cookies, biscuits, and cakes, increased, so did women's risk for heart disease. Women with the highest intakes had nearly twice the risk of women who ate few hydrogenated fats. More specifically, women who ate 4 or more teaspoons of margarine a day increased their risk of developing heart disease by 66 percent, compared to women who limited margarine to less than 1 teaspoon a month.

TFAs are in most foods that contain hydrogenated vegetable oils, from potato chips, cake frosting, and cookies to doughnuts, crackers, and prepackaged biscuit dough. It's easy to consume a TFA-rich diet if you include several convenience foods in the daily menu. "As far as we know, there is no safe dose for transfatty acids, but the lower the intake the better," concludes Willett.

trans—lating labels

Nutrition labels don't specify the amount of transfatty acids (TFAs) in the product, so you must do a bit of sleuthing to determine how much you're getting.

● Diet or whipped margarine contains less TFAs than tub varieties, and tub is better than stick margarine. (Look for brands that list water and/or liquid vegetable oil as the first ingredients.)

● Read labels and avoid foods that contain hydrogenated vegetable oils.

● Avoid foods fried in fast-food restaurants, from doughnuts to french fries. (Up to 40 percent of the fats in these foods can be TFAs).

● Make your own spread by whipping a stick of butter with a half cup of canola oil; store it in the refrigerator. This blend is lower in saturated fat than butter and is trans-free.

● Better yet, switch to olive oil and use it sparingly.

What is the bottom line when it comes to fat? Cut back on your total fat intake, whether it is from meat and fatty dairy products or highly processed convenience and fast foods. The general consensus is to keep total fat intake below 30 percent, but no lower than 15 percent, of your total daily calories. When you do use fat, make it olive oil, which is safe and might help reduce heart-disease risk.

Cut Calories, Extend Life

Calorie restriction is the only manipulation known in mammals to improve both life expectancy and life span," says George Roth, Ph.D., chief of Molecular Physiology and Genetics section of the National Institute on Aging in Baltimore, Maryland. All animals the researchers have studied, including mice, rats, hamsters, and monkeys, increase their life span from two- to four-fold when calorie intake is cut to 60 percent of what's called "ad libitum"—that's 60 percent of what the animals usually eat to feel satisfied and full. Cut the fat at the same time and the animals live even longer.

The benefits of semifasting for these animals far exceed just living longer. The hungry animals also are disease-free. Every age-related disease, from heart disease, diabetes, and cancer to memory loss and dwindling immunity, seems to vanish. Blood levels of the stress hormones and disease-causing free radicals also drop when calories are curtailed. Although poorly understood, restricting food might increase life span by decreasing free-radical reactions in the body, by altering hormone levels, or by lowering the metabolic rate (the rate of life). The secret is undernutrition, not malnutrition. This means that while calories are drastically reduced, the food the animals do eat still provides all the vitamins, minerals, fiber, and phytochemicals in optimal amounts for health.

It works for animals. Does it work for humans? Unfortunately, there is no direct evidence that serious calorie restriction will have the same effect on humans that it does on mice and monkeys. However, there is a wealth of indirect evidence. Obese people, for example, die at younger ages than do fit and lean (but not skinny) people.

On the other hand, drastic drops in weight have been linked to increased mortality, especially in middle-aged and older people. In short, if cutting calories works, it is only effective if done over the long haul.

A person's best bet is to achieve a lean and fit weight in the early years then maintain that weight throughout life. As Blumberg points out: "Both being too skinny or too fat increase a person's risk of dying early." So, strive for a healthy weight and avoid drastic changes in weight. Middle-aged and older people should boost their fitness level and attain a desirable weight by losing pounds gradually and permanently. (See "Overweight" on page 256 for strategies to accomplish this.)

Water, Water Everywhere

The body is mostly water. We start out life about 80 percent water and end our days with only slightly less fluid, or about 60 to 70 percent of our body weight. That major part of our bodies is in a constant ebb and flow. Even sedentary people lose about 2 to 3 quarts of water daily. Exercisers or people who live and work in hot climates lose even more. That means the average person must consume about a gallon of fluid every day to replace these losses.

Unfortunately, thirst is a poor indicator of fluid needs, especially as a person ages. Consequently, people at any age, but especially in the second 50 years, are susceptible to mild dehydration, which can undermine energy level and mental function, and increase stress on the body. To avoid dehydration, everyone should drink twice as much water as it takes to quench a thirst or at least eight glasses of water daily (or 1 cup of water for every 20 pounds of body weight).

Fruit juices and bottled water help supply some of that fluid, but not diuretic beverages such as coffee, tea, or alcohol, which only aggravate dehydration. Green tea is another way to add fluids. This beverage comes with the additional benefit of being chock-full of phytochemicals that help lower the risk of developing cancer. One way to ensure you reach the eight-glasses goal each day is to fill a pitcher with the day's allotment of water and keep it on your desk at work or the kitchen table at home. Your goal is reached when the pitcher is empty.

The Antiaging Diet

Preventing premature aging is a lifelong process that begins with a nutrient-packed diet and a daily exercise routine. The guidelines are simple and are based on the following principles:

Love those fruits and veggies. Include daily at least five, and preferably eight or more, servings of fresh fruits and vegetables to ensure optimal intake of vitamin C, beta-carotene, fiber, and the phytochemicals that aid in the prevention of disease.

Think green. Make sure at least two of your daily servings are dark green leafy vegetables to boost intake of folic acid, a B vitamin essential for the prevention of heart disease and possibly cancer.

Lower meat consumption. Replace meat with beans several times a week to maximize intake of the phytoestrogens that lower cancer risk (and possibly reduce hot flashes during menopause) and the phytosterols that lower heart disease and cancer risk. You'll also avoid the health risks associated with meat. The fiber in beans helps lower blood sugar and fats, thus reducing heart disease and diabetes risk.

Drink your milk. Include at least three low-fat, calcium-rich foods (preferably milk, to ensure optimal vitamin D intake) in the daily diet to build and maintain strong bones.

Use whole grains. Emphasize whole over refined grains to increase intake of chromium and other trace minerals essential for immune function and blood sugar regulation.

the antiaging diet

What does an anti-aging diet look like? Here's an example of how to apply the anti-aging dietary guidelines.

Breakfast:
1 whole wheat pita, cut in half, warmed, and filled with:
Eggbeaters (½ cup) scrambled with: ½ cup chopped frozen spinach
1 ounce low-fat cheese
1 clove garlic, minced (optional)
salt and pepper to taste
Topped with 2 Tbsp. salsa
Green tea with lemon

Midmorning Snack:
1 slice banana bread topped with:
1 Tbsp. fat-free cream cheese
1 medium nectarine
1 glass water

Lunch:
Tuna salad:
2 cups romaine lettuce
¼ cup thinly sliced carrots
¼ cup canned kidney beans, drained
1 6-ounce can water-packed tuna, drained
2 Tbsp. low-calorie Italian dressing
1 medium apple
8 ounces sparkling water with lime or green tea

Afternoon Snack:
Carrot-raisin salad with:
1 cup grated carrots
1 Tbsp. raisins

2 Tbsp. fat-free mayonnaise
½ tsp. lemon juice
salt and pepper to taste
3 fat-free whole wheat crackers
1 cup nonfat milk blended in a blender with 1 tsp. vanilla extract, ¼ tsp. nutmeg, 1 packet sugar substitute, and 1 ice cube

Dinner:
1½ cups bean and vegetable soup (add 2 minced garlic cloves)
1 piece (2½×2½×1½ inches) cornbread (made with oil and nonfat milk)
Tossed salad:
1 cup leaf lettuce, chopped
¼ cup canned mandarin orange slices, drained, or fresh raspberries
4 mushrooms, thinly sliced
2 Tbsp. red onion, thinly sliced
2 Tbsp. fat-free raspberry vinaigrette salad dressing

Evening Snack:
1 cup fresh strawberries
¼ cup fat-free chocolate syrup
1 cup nonfat milk, whipped in a blender with cinnamon, sugar substitute, and 1 ice cube.
Sparkling water

Total: 1,913 calories; 23% protein; 20% fat (44 grams); 57% carbohydrate

Shun excess calories. Limit useless calories from fat, sugar, and alcohol. Consuming more calories than needed to maintain a desirable weight only fuels the aging process.

Review your supplements. Consider taking a moderate-dose multiple vitamin and mineral supplement, as well as a calcium and magnesium supplement and extra antioxidants. (See "Should You Supplement?" on page 62.)

Go for garlic. Include garlic several times each week to provide other health-enhancing phytochemicals. "Garlic appears to have a beneficial effect in stimulating immune function and lowering blood cholesterol levels even when consumed in moderate amounts of one to two cloves a day," says Dr. Blumberg.

Drink lots of water. Drink at least eight glasses a day.

Move that body. Exercise daily for at least 30 minutes. More is even better. Build strength and flexibility with weight lifting and stretches, while boosting endurance and cardiovascular (heart and blood vessel) function with aerobic activities, such as walking, bicycling, and swimming. People can slow the aging process—even reverse it to an extent—with exercise. A weekly routine that includes some weight-bearing exercise, such as walking, jogging, or swimming, with some strength-training exercise, such as weight lifting, maintains strong bones, reduces heart-disease and cancer risks, boosts the immune system, helps maintain a desirable weight, reduces the risk of dependency or frailty later in life, and is essential to grasping the vitality to enjoy those extra years. In fact, unfit people at any age can cut in half their risk of dying prematurely by adding exercise to their daily routine. Biologically speaking, active people are two decades younger than their sedentary counterparts.

healing diet

PROBLEM FOODS	GOOD FOODS
Fried and fatty foods	Dark green, leafy vegetables
	Garlic
	Green tea
	Nonfat or low-fat dairy products
	Soy products
	Variety of fruits and vegetables
	Whole grains

BEST ADVICE: Achieve a desirable weight and keep it there permanently. Drink plenty of water. Exercise every day.

anemia

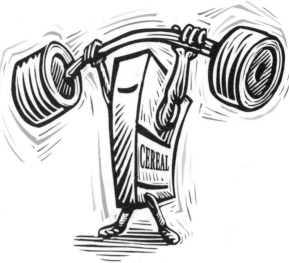

Laura can't remember when she wasn't tired. She finds herself out of breath just climbing the flight of stairs to her apartment and often has trouble concentrating at work. She also battled one cold after another last winter. Laura blames her lethargy on getting older and being too busy, but she might be suffering from a common nutrient deficiency— anemia. That means she really would benefit far more from an iron-rich snack at midday rather than her usual cup of coffee.

Anemia Basics

Anemia is a blood condition. In someone with anemia the number or size of red blood cells is below normal. Or else the amount of an iron-rich protein called hemoglobin within those cells falls below normal. (Hemoglobin gives blood its red color.) What does this have to do with being out of breath or feeling lethargic?

Your red blood cells carry oxygen from your lungs to all the tissues of your body. Your red blood cells also transport the waste product carbon dioxide from your tissues back to your lungs to be exhaled. A drop in red blood cells means the heart, muscles, brain, and other tissues in the body are literally starved for oxygen.

All the symptoms of anemia mirror this tissue suffocation, including lethargy, general weakness, shortness of breath after minor physical effort, and poor concentration.

Dizziness, fainting spells, apathy, irritability, or poor regulation of body temperature are other possible symptoms. The complexion may be pale and, like Laura, a person with anemia might be prone to colds or infections.

During pregnancy, anemia increases the risk for spontaneous abortions, low-birth-weight babies, and premature births. Anemia during the first few months or years of life can compromise intellectual development.

In advanced cases, people with anemia crave nonfood items, such as chalk, ice, or dirt (a condition called pica). Other possible symptoms are thin and flat fingernails, a smooth and waxy tongue, and stomach disorders.

Ironing Out Anemia

Doctors know that anemia can develop for a variety of reasons, including excessive or chronic bleeding (such as a bleeding ulcer) or repeated blood donations. More often than

iron deficiency versus anemia

When you consider the population as a whole, iron deficiency is an even greater problem than anemia. Somewhere between 7 and 12 percent of women and children are anemic. But as many as 25 percent of the general public and up to 80 percent of exercising women are iron deficient.

What's the distinction between anemia and iron deficiency? Anemia is the final stage on the continuum of iron deficiency. Long before a person develops anemia, iron stores have drained, which results in similar symptoms of tiredness, reduced resistance to colds, and poor concentration. A person can be iron deficient for months, years, even decades without knowing it. That's because routine blood tests for iron status, such as the hemoglobin and hematocrit tests, reflect only a person's risk for anemia.

If you suspect that you are either anemic or iron deficient, you should see your doctor. Your doctor will have your blood tested with any of several tests that detect the amount of iron in your blood. What do those lab values mean and how do you know if you are normal, borderline, or deficient? Here's a quick glance at the different tests and what values for iron mean.

Test	What the Numbers Mean
Serum Ferritin:	Normal values: 40 to 160 micrograms/liter Iron depletion: 20 micrograms/liter Iron-deficiency anemia: fewer than 12 micrograms/liter Iron overload: more than 400 micrograms/liter
Transferrin Saturation:	Normal value: 20% to 50% Iron depletion: 30% Iron-deficiency anemia: less than 10%
Total Iron Binding Capacity (TIBC):	Normal values: 300 to 360 micrograms/deciliter Iron depletion: 360 micrograms/deciliter Iron-deficiency anemia: 410 micrograms/deciliter
Hemoglobin:	Normal values: 12 to 16 grams/deciliter Iron-deficiency anemia: fewer than 12 grams/deciliter
Hematocrit:	Normal value: 37% to 47% Iron-deficiency anemia: less than 37%

not, however, the cause is dietary. Many people simply don't consume enough iron-rich foods. Over the course of months or even years, this poor iron intake gradually leads to anemia.

Those people most prone to iron-deficiency anemia include infants, children, women during the childbearing years, and the elderly.

Iron needs are high for infants and children because of their rapid growth rates, but finicky eating habits and small tummies often collide with high iron needs, resulting in deficiency.

Women's daily iron requirements are high to make up for monthly blood loss from menstruation.

Yet women often consume insufficient food, especially iron-rich foods, to make up for these losses.

And the elderly often lose the taste for meat and other iron-rich foods, placing them at ever increasing risk for deficiency unless alternative iron sources are found.

In addition, as we age, our stomachs get less and less acidic. That means that iron and other blood-building nutrients like vitamin B12 are not as well absorbed as they were in earlier years.

On the other hand, men consume considerably more food in general than do children and women and have much lower iron needs. So men are at low risk for developing anemia.

When men do develop anemia, it is often an indication of internal bleeding from another condition, such as stomach ulcers.

Women just past the age of menopause, because they no longer menstruate, also are at low risk of iron deficiency as long as they consume otherwise nutritious diets.

Who Needs More Iron?

Iron deficiency is the most common cause of anemia and is the most common nutrient deficiency in the United States. Premenopausal women are at particular risk, especially those who:
● exercise.
● have been pregnant within the past two years.
● consume fewer than 2,500 calories daily.

And let's face it. It's not at all unusual for women to consume fewer than 2,500 calories a day. In fact, women average only 1,600 calories a day. A well-balanced diet supplies 6 milligrams of iron for every 1,000 calories, according to Fergus Clydesdale, Ph.D., professor and head of the Department of Food Science at the University of Massachusetts in Amherst. Based on this ratio, women should be consuming at least 2,500 calories daily to meet their daily requirement of 15 milligrams. (And iron requirements are even higher for women with heavy menstrual losses or who use intrauterine devices for birth control.) It's no wonder women average 8 to 10 milligrams of iron daily. Most women are shortchanging themselves when it comes to iron intake.

Women of childbearing age who exercise regularly are at even higher risk for iron-deficiency anemia. The body has elevated oxygen needs during exercise. At the same time, exercise causes increased iron loss through urine and sweat. All this simply means that people who exercise need more

how much iron do YOU need?

The average iron intake is 6 milligrams for every 1,000 calories eaten. Research shows that some groups, such as menstruating women, especially women using an IUD as a birth control device, require twice the recommended amounts of iron to reach optimal iron stores. It is very difficult for a pregnant woman or a woman who is nursing to consume enough food to meet her daily iron requirements. That's why physicians usually recommend a supplement that contains 30 to 60 milligrams of elemental iron.

The Daily Value for iron that is used on food and supplement labels is 18 milligrams, and that's more than enough to meet almost everyone's needs. The Recommended Dietary Allowances (RDA) for iron are:

	Age	Iron (milligrams)
Infants/Children		
	birth to 6 months	6
	6 months to 10 years	10
Young Adults and Adults		
Males	11 to 18 years	12
	19+ years	10
Females	11 to 50 years	15
	51+ years	10
Pregnant		30
Nursing		15

iron. Consequently, iron-deficient exercisers experience reduced muscle strength, tire easily, and recover slowly after exercise.

"Exercise is where low tissue stores of iron will show up," says registered dietitian Jan Johnson-Shane, Ph.D., R.D., professor of nutrition at Illinois State University in Normal. "Low iron intake can result in compromised blood levels of iron." Insufficient iron might inhibit the ability to increase exercise capacity, she adds.

The kinds of food choices one makes also make a difference when it comes to having enough iron stores in the blood. In an effort to reduce fat intake and improve health, most Americans have cut back on meat. Consequently, many people consume up to 95 percent of their total day's iron from plants (i.e., fruits, vegetables, cooked dried beans and peas, and grains). What needs to be taken into consideration here is that the body absorbs iron from meat (with 20 to 30 percent absorption) much better than it can absorb iron from plant sources (only 2 to 7 percent absorption).

Dr. Johnson-Shane has studied the beneficial effect of red meat on iron status. "It's important to look at the total fat intake, with red meat being only one source of fat in the diet," she says. "If the serving is small, say 3 ounces, and extra-lean cuts are used as a side dish, rather than the main course, then red meat is an excellent source of iron while still falling within the guidelines of a low-fat diet."

It's important to understand that you can be iron deficient long before you actually develop anemia. And ideally, you can prevent anemia by dealing with the problem early on. (See "Iron Deficiency Versus Anemia" on page 70.)

Getting Enough Iron

For people at high risk for iron deficiency or anemia, the first line of defense is to increase the intake of iron-rich foods. Here's how:

 Know your best sources for iron. You should include three or more of the following in the daily diet: extra-lean red meat, legumes, dark green leafy vegetables, organ meats, and fish. Also, consider including iron-fortified foods in the diet.

 Look for iron-fortified foods. "The incidence of anemia has decreased in recent years, more than likely as a result of iron fortification of foods," says Dr. Clydesdale. "It's not only safe, but probably necessary, for women to select fortified food products. How else can women get enough iron?" All ready-to-eat cereals are fortified with iron, as are products made with enriched grains—white bread, noodles, rice, and pasta.

 Consider a supplement. Although this book recommends getting your nutrients from foods, this is one case where a supplement may be in order. If your daily calorie intake regularly falls below 2,500 and you are an adolescent girl or a premenopausal woman, you might consider taking a moderate-dose multiple vitamin and mineral that contains 10 to 18 milligrams of iron. Ask your pediatrician about iron supplements for your children.

Warning: Do **not** take high doses of iron unless your doctor tells you to. Taking more iron than you need won't provide additional health benefits and could be harmful.

Boosting Iron Absorption

There's more to getting enough iron than just eating iron-rich foods. Iron status, in fact, may balance between iron-inhibitors and iron-enhancers in the diet. Here's the way to help tip the scale in your favor:

 Balance meats and grains. Consume small amounts of extra-lean (9 percent fat or less) meat with large amounts of iron-rich grains, vegetables, and beans. The iron in meat helps increase absorption of iron in plants (for example, chili with beans).

 Reach for the C. Always eat a vitamin-C-rich food with iron-rich foods, since vitamin C increases iron absorption (for example, orange juice with a turkey sandwich).

 Use those iron pots. Cook acidic foods, such as spaghetti sauce, in cast-iron cookware. The iron leeches from the pot into the food and boosts the iron content of the meal several-fold.

the woman's iron-rich diet

Children, women, and seniors need to include several iron-rich foods in the daily diet. Even then, if an adult consumes fewer than 2,000 calories or a child eats fewer than 1,500 calories, it might be difficult to get enough iron from food alone. Here's a sample day's menu that meets a woman's iron needs:

Food	Amount	Iron (milligrams)
Breakfast:		
Oatmeal, cooked	1 cup	1.59
Nonfat milk	1 cup	0.10
Whole wheat toast	2 slices	2.10
Jam, all fruit	1 tsp.	0.07
Orange juice	6 ounces	0.34
Midmorning Snack:		
Raisins, seedless	½ cup	1.71
Almonds	1 Tbsp.	0.32
Lunch:		
Black bean soup	1 cup	2.15
Whole wheat bread	2 slices	2.10
Cheese, low-fat	2 ounces	0.14
Strawberries	1 cup	0.57
Carrot salad	1 cup	0.37
Afternoon Snack:		
Yogurt, nonfat	1 cup	0.20
Apricots	2	0.38
Dinner:		
Oyster stew	2 cups	2.1
Whole wheat roll	1	0.84
Spinach salad	1 cup	1.52
Broccoli, cooked	⅔ cup	0.51
Late-Night Snack:		
Three-bean salad	½ cup	1.61

Total:
Calories: 2,050
Iron: 18.7 milligrams
Vitamin C: 272 milligrams

% calories from protein: 18
% calories from carbohydrates: 61
% calories from fat: 21

🍎 **Time your supplements.** Take iron supplements on an empty stomach and avoid taking calcium or zinc at the same time you take iron, since these minerals reduce iron absorption.

🍎 **Watch those beverages.** Drink tea and coffee between meals, not afterward. The tannins in these beverages reduce iron absorption up to 70 percent.

🍎 **Help those whole grains.** Whole grain tortilla; biscuits; muffins; and pita bread, crackers, and other unleavened whole grains contain a substance called phytate that inhibits iron absorption. This is only a problem when these products are the main source of grain in the diet, and it can be counteracted by including vitamin-C-rich foods with the meal (for example, bean burrito made with whole wheat tortilla and vitamin-C-rich cilantro and tomatoes).

Other Nutrients and Anemia

Iron might hold center stage when it comes to anemia, but it isn't a solo act. Several other nutrients are important in the manufacture and maintenance of red blood cells, including folic acid and vitamin B12. Inadequate intake of either of these B vitamins results in large, misshapen cells and a type of anemia called macrocytic anemia. An inability to absorb vitamin B12, which is especially common in the elderly, results in a type of anemia called pernicious anemia.

Here's a look at the individual nutrients and what you need to do to make sure you're getting enough of each.

Folic Acid

Folic acid is of particular concern. Dark green leafy vegetables are the best dietary source of this B vitamin. However, many people opt for french fries instead of spinach, so their diets fall far short of optimal for folic acid.

🍎 **Go for the green.** Everyone needs at least one serving (two is even better) daily of a green, leafy vegetable, such as spinach, chard, collard or beet greens, broccoli, or kale. Orange juice and cooked dried beans and peas also are good sources of folic acid.

Vitamin B12

Vitamin B12 is found only in foods of animal origin, such as extra-lean meat, chicken, fish, milk, or dairy products. So strict vegetarians could be lacking in this vitamin unless they choose vitamin-B12-fortified foods.

🍎 **Watch intake as you age.** Vitamin B12 requirements increase with age to compensate for reduced absorption, so make sure you consume at least two to three servings of vitamin-B12-rich foods after age 65 or take a moderate-dose multiple vitamin and mineral that contains at least 3 micrograms of this vitamin. In some cases, a physician might recommend vitamin B12 shots or a nasal spray for those people who do not absorb the vitamin.

Copper, Vitamin C, and Vitamin B6

Copper, vitamin C, and vitamin B6 also are needed for the formation of red blood cells. Long-term poor intakes of these nutrients result in anemia.

🍎 **Keep things in balance.** Make sure you consume lots of copper-rich foods, such as whole grain cereals, legumes, and dark green leafy vegetables, and accompany each meal with a vitamin-C-rich fruit or vegetable. These include broccoli, cantaloupe, strawberries, oranges, grapefruit, sweet peppers, and pineapple. Vitamin B6 is best obtained from protein-rich foods, such as chicken, fish, and milk, and is found in bananas, legumes, nuts, and avocados.

All in all, anemia is an easily preventable disorder. So, don't take feeling poorly lying down. Have your blood values tested and improve your dietary habits, and you'll be amazed at your newfound vim and vigor!

healing diet

PROBLEM FOODS	GOOD FOODS
Whole grain tortillas, biscuits, muffins, pita bread, and crackers	Dark green, leafy vegetables
	Foods high in vitamin C
	Fish
	Iron-fortified foods
	Lean red meat
	Legumes

BEST ADVICE: If you suspect anemia or iron deficiency, see your doctor for a blood test. Take steps to get more iron into your daily diet.

arthritis

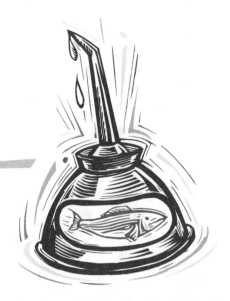

If you have arthritis, you've probably heard that certain foods will help relieve arthritis pain. Or that others will aggravate it.

Perhaps you've heard that you should avoid all vegetables in the nightshade family (potatoes, sweet peppers, tomatoes, eggplant). Or that you should drink a mixture of apple-cider vinegar and honey once a day. There are a lot of dietary recommendations out there aimed at people who are desperate to find some relief from the pain and inflammation of this condition. Do any of them really work?

Although there's no medical evidence to support any of these particular claims, in some cases a diet change can help with arthritis, says David Pisetsky, M.D., Ph.D., professor of medicine at Duke University Medical Center in Durham, North Carolina.

Here's the lowdown on the connection between arthritis and foods.

A Word on Don'ts

Before we talk about foods that might help relieve arthritis symptoms, let's focus on what you shouldn't eat. The one thing that's clear is that if you're overweight, shedding a few pounds can be of great benefit in preventing and relieving arthritis symptoms.

"If you lose weight, you can reduce the chance of developing osteoarthritis of hip or knee," says David Hellmann, M.D., professor

of medicine at Johns Hopkins University in Baltimore, Maryland. This is partly because extra weight puts additional stress on these joints with every step you take.

In an extensive study based at the Boston University Arthritis Center, women who lost around 11 pounds cut their chances of developing arthritis by one half, and later research indicated that a 10-pound gain significantly increased the odds of getting osteoarthritis.

Other studies have linked obesity to osteoarthritis in the hands. This suggests stress on the joints is not the only possible explanation for connection between excess weight and arthritis. It appears that extra body fat can affect cartilage in ways not yet understood.

Watch those extra pounds. It's clear that maintaining your ideal weight is best, says Dr. Hellmann. If you're overweight, nutritionists suggest you lose weight slowly, no more than 1 or 2 pounds a week. Eat lots of fruits, vegetables, and whole grains, recommends Beth Carlton, R.D., a registered dietitian in Sacramento, California. Limit fatty meats, rich sauces, sodas, butter, cookies, and pastries. Drink eight glasses of water a day, and if you snack, choose foods such as plain popcorn,

what type of arthritis
do you have?

Arthritis is a catchall term that simply means inflamed, stiff, and painful joints. There are many causes for this condition and many different forms that it can take. The most common types are osteoarthritis and rheumatoid arthritis, which are quite different.

Most people with arthritis have osteoarthritis, commonly known as the "wear-and-tear" disease. Our joints are designed with a spongy material called cartilage to cushion our bones.

As we get older, the cartilage can get chipped or worn away through normal wear and tear—or it can be damaged in an accident. Most of us have some signs of this kind of arthritis in our knees by the time we are 40. In severe cases, the pain can even keep you from moving your joints.

Joints also have a lining called the synovial membrane that pumps out a lubricating fluid that keeps the joint moving smoothly. In rheumatoid arthritis, this membrane swells and thickens painfully. Rheumatoid arthritis is an autoimmune disease. This means that for some reason, the immune system that normally protects you instead "attacks" your body. In the case of rheumatoid arthritis, the immune system is attacking the synovial membrane. Without treatment, problems can spread to cartilage and bones and, in severe cases, affect other parts of the body as well.

Other forms of arthritis or related ailments include gout, Lyme arthritis, fibromyalgia, polymyalgia rheumatica, and lupus.

carrot sticks, or fruit. (See "Overweight" on page 256 for a detailed look at how to lose excess weight.)

The Vitamin Picture

Along with paring down those pounds, there are a few nutrients you need to pay special attention to, among them vitamin D and all the vitamins known as antioxidants.

Because vitamin D is essential for forming bones, lack of it may affect bone and the cartilage that covers it. What happens in the bone itself seems to influence the progression of the disease, explains Timothy McAlindon, M.D., assistant professor at Boston University Medical Center and vitamin D researcher.

Several studies, in fact, have suggested that vitamin D can slow osteoarthritis. One study linked low intake of vitamin D with the progression of osteoarthritis in the knee. Researchers X-rayed the knees of 556 men and women then X-rayed them again eight to nine years later. They found that the people who took in the least vitamin D (3 to 170 international units) were three times more likely to have their osteoarthritis worsen. The ones getting the recommended daily allowance of 400 international units or more had the fewest problems.

Another study by Nancy Lane, M.D., at the University of California at San Francisco, suggests that vitamin D helps protect against the progression of hip osteoarthritis.

How much vitamin D is enough? Dr. McAlindon's study found that benefits started at 400 international units daily.

● **Catch some rays.** You can manufacture your own vitamin D by getting 10 to 15 minutes of sun exposure a day.

● **Digest some D.** You can also get vitamin D from tuna, salmon, and fortified milk.

The Need for Vitamin C

Another study led by Dr. McAlindon found that people getting lots of vitamin C were one third as likely to have their knee osteoarthritis worsen. Dr. McAlindon concluded, "High intake of antioxidant micronutrients, especially vitamin C, may reduce the risk of cartilage loss and disease progression in people with osteoarthritis." (Antioxidants are substances that neutralize free radicals—molecules that cause damage to the body's cells. Vitamin E is also an antioxidant.)

"Antioxidants might help because they mop up free radicals, and free radicals could theoretically do damage to cartilage components," says Dr. McAlindon. "Vitamin C has many properties, and it clearly could be beneficial when trying to repair cartilage."

● **Get more vitamin C.** The study suggested that at least 100 milligrams daily

of vitamin C—about the amount in a couple of oranges—could help reduce risks.

Dr. McAlindon noted that the most impressive results occurred when people got their vitamin C through food: "I advise people to eat more fresh fruits and vegetables." Antioxidants abound in fresh fruits and vegetables such as sweet peppers, carrots, and sweet potatoes.

Nutrients for Rheumatoid Arthritis

If you have rheumatoid arthritis, you may want to take particular care in your food choices. This and other inflammatory diseases are often treated by steroids, which unfortunately interfere with calcium absorption. So people taking moderate to high doses of steroids have more risk of osteoporosis, a thinning of the bones that can lead to debilitating breaks.

The good news, however, is that extra calcium plus vitamin D can help slow or even reverse bone loss in people receiving corticosteroids for rheumatoid arthritis, according to a study at the Medical College of Virginia in Richmond. In the two years of the study, people on corticosteroids who were getting 1,000 milligrams of calcium and 500 international units of vitamin D daily had slight gains in bone density. Those without the calcium and vitamin D lost as much as 2 percent of bone density.

● **Drink your milk.** Current daily recommendations are that people ages 19 to 49 should get 1,000 milligrams of calcium a day. That amount increases to 1,200 milligrams for those 50 and older. You can get roughly 1,000 milligrams of calcium from 2 cups of milk and 8 ounces of yogurt.

🍎 **Know where to find your calcium.** "Dairy foods are the best sources of calcium, of course," says Susan I. Barr, Ph.D., R.D.N., a professor of nutrition at the University of British Columbia in Vancouver. "The best nondairy sources include fortified products such as calcium-fortified orange juice and calcium-fortified soy drinks," she says. Also good are canned fish (but you have to eat the bones!) and dark leafy greens.

🍎 **Get the big picture.** Some research also has suggested that people with rheumatoid arthritis are low in a number of crucial vitamins and minerals. When 48 people with rheumatoid arthritis were studied for five days, it turned out that only about half of them ate enough folic acid and only around one-fourth had enough calcium and vitamin E. Only one in 10 had enough zinc, and six of 100 had enough selenium.

The researchers advised that people with rheumatoid arthritis increase their dietary intake of these nutrients, and doctors agree that good nutrition is crucial in this disease.

Here are some sources of these nutrients:

Folic acid: Fortified cereals, fresh spinach, wheat germ

Vitamin E: Wheat germ, whole grains, eggs

Zinc: Lean beef, poultry, milk, whole grains

Selenium: Fish, shellfish, whole grains

The Benefits of Fatty Acids

We're used to thinking of anything with the word "fatty" as bad. But fatty acids are in fact important nutrients. Some are called EFAs, for essential fatty acids.

A number of medical studies suggest that fatty acids, especially the omega-3 variety found in cold-water fish, can help ease the inflammation of rheumatoid arthritis.

"In rheumatoid arthritis, high-fish diets have made a very slight difference in some patients," says Dr. Hellmann. "Omega-3 fatty oils have been shown in several studies to make a very modest improvement."

One study done in Denmark, for example, tested 51 people with active rheumatoid arthritis and found that they had significant improvement of morning stiffness and joint tenderness after just 12 weeks of taking supplementary fatty acids.

And a year-long New Zealand study of 90 people with active rheumatoid arthritis found improvement with a daily dose of the fatty acid found in cold-water fish. By the third month, people had as much as a 25 percent improvement in symptoms, and nearly half of them were able to reduce the dose of their medications.

Dr. Hellmann, however, stresses that in his clinical experience improvement from fish oil appears to be slight. "No patient in 20 years of my practice has noted an improvement while eating lots of fish or while taking fish oil supplements," he says. And in real life it would be unpalatable or

food links to bouts of gout

If you've ever had a gout attack, you won't forget it. This stabbing pain comes on suddenly, often at night, and most often in the big toe. There's no doubt that gout is linked to diet, although it's not the only cause.

These painful attacks are brought on by an excess of a substance called uric acid that collects as crystals in joints in the feet. Some people simply produce too much uric acid, and others may have too much because of kidney problems. A similar condition, called pseudogout, affects large joints such as the wrists and knees.

To help avoid gout:
● Avoid foods high in purines, such as sardines, anchovies, sweetbreads, brains, kidney, and liver.
● If you're overweight, shed some pounds. Being overweight can increase your risk of gout.
● Avoid alcohol, which is not only high in purines but also keeps you from getting rid of them through your urine.

difficult to reach the levels that were taken in some of these studies.

● **Get friendly with fish.** The Arthritis Foundation suggests that a reasonable compromise is eating at least two meals of fish a week. The ideal is to eat even more than that. Salmon, sardines, herring, mackerel, cod, and haddock are high in the important fatty acids.

Trying Out a Vegetarian Diet

Are you ready to give up steaks forever? Probably not. But how would you feel about putting meat behind you if you found that it lessened the pain of rheumatoid arthritis? A few studies have suggested that a vegetarian diet may help do just that. In one study done in Finland, 43 people with rheumatoid arthritis who followed an uncooked vegan diet—eating only foods of plant origin—showed some signs of improvement.

Another, more extensive study found significant improvement in people with rheumatoid arthritis who followed a carefully controlled vegan diet for a year, then went on a vegetarian diet that included dairy products. The people on this diet experienced fewer tender joints, and less pain and morning stiffness. A follow-up a year later found that the benefits were still present regardless of the diet the people were then eating.

The problem in applying these and similar studies to life in the real world is that the studies called for strict diets that required careful monitoring. And researchers made sure that the people following these diets got adequate nutrients. A well-designed vegetarian diet can be healthy for anyone, however, and the Arthritis Foundation suggests that it just might help with your arthritis.

If you'd like to try a vegetarian diet but are uncertain about how to make sure that you're getting proper nutrition, ask your doctor to recommend a registered dietitian to help you make the switch.

healing diet

PROBLEM FOODS	GOOD FOODS
Alcohol	Fish
Foods containing fat or salt	Milk and other dairy products
	Whole grains, fruits, and vegetables

BEST ADVICE: Achieve and maintain an ideal weight for your body.

asthma

Ask someone who has asthma to describe the feeling of an attack, and you'll probably hear that it's like trying to breathe through a straw. People with asthma have to work that much harder to catch their breath.

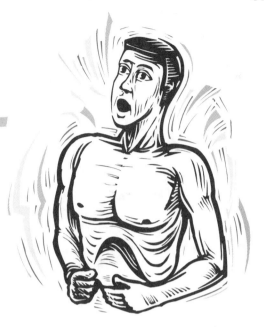

What Is Asthma?

Asthma occurs when the bronchial passages in the lungs constrict, or narrow, making it harder for air to flow in and out of the lungs. The lungs of people with asthma are too sensitive, reacting to such triggers as cold weather, pet dander, smoke, dust, exercise, stress…or something they ate.

Triggers change from person to person. Everyone experiences the disease in his or her own way. So anyone who has asthma has to pay close attention to when and where the symptoms flare up. The number one symptom of asthma is repeated coughing. Other symptoms include wheezing, shortness of breath, and tightness in the chest.

The number of people with asthma in the United States has increased by almost 40 percent from 1990 to 1994, according to the Centers for Disease Control and Prevention. Almost 15 million Americans now have this disease. Women are more likely than men to develop asthma and more likely to die of the disease.

Another segment of the population that has been hit with the disease is children. Asthma has become the most chronic disease of childhood, and it's the number one cause of school absenteeism, accounting for more than 20 percent of missed school days. Researchers suspect the reason for the increase in childhood asthma is indoor pollution—a collection of cigarette smoke, pet dander, chemicals, and dust. People spend more time indoors than they did 25 years ago.

Asthma researchers have only recently addressed the underlying cause of asthma—inflammation of the airways. According to guidelines released in 1997 by the National Heart, Lung, and Blood Institute, the most effective way to minimize the severity of asthma and prevent acute attacks is by using a daily anti-inflammatory steroidal medication, such as corticosteroid. Unlike short-acting inhalers, which are used at the onset of symptoms, the inhaled steroids are taken on a regular schedule to control inflammation. Short-acting bronchodilators, also known as "rescue" medication, are still the best for rapid relief of asthma attacks when they occur.

Diet and Asthma

If you have asthma, there are two things about what you eat that should concern you. One is the role of a well-balanced diet in maintainng a healthy immune system. (For a detailed look at how to eat to keep your immune system performing at its best, see page 203.) And the other is your personal food trigger(s). Certain foods are more likely to bring on an asthma attack, while others might help temporarily control an attack.

"Six to eight percent of people with asthma have attacks that are brought on by food allergies," says Marc S. McMorris, M.D., an allergist at the University of Michigan Health Systems in Ann Arbor. "These asthmatics always suffer from eczema as well. Food allergies are more common in children with asthma."

Some food is just more apt to cause an allergic reaction. The most common foods that can bring on an asthma attack are milk, eggs, nuts, peanut butter, shellfish, soy, and wheat. "The recommendation these days is for persistent asthma attacks you look at food as the cause," says Dr. McMorris. "We then test the patient's reaction to the most common allergic foods." He recommends not doing your own food testing: "The safest approach is to go to the doctor."

If your doctor recommends that you avoid any of these foods to keep asthma attacks at bay, you'll have to be really vigilant. What you're eating is not always obvious. All fresh pasta and some pasta fillings are made with eggs, for example. Many dishes in Greek and Chinese restaurants are prepared with eggs, and egg whites are often used to create a shine on baked goods. The answer is to become food savvy. Read food labels carefully and ask the right questions when dining at a restaurant or a friend's home.

Here are some other dietary strategies for preventing asthma to consider:

Take a careful look at citrus. What could possibly be wrong with a morning glass of orange juice? For some people with asthma, citrus fruits—such as oranges, grapefruits, tangerines, limes, lemons, and clementines—can trigger an attack. If you suspect that citrus might be troublesome, mention your concern to your doctor.

Watch those additives. It's impossible not to find a food in your pantry that hasn't been spiked with additives, preservatives, or other nonfood ingredients. Since people with asthma are never quite sure which of these additives might bring on an attack, the safest bet is to eat as few processed foods as possible and buy foods with the fewest ingredients listed on the label. But even fresh produce can cause a reaction because of pesticides and insecticides. If you suspect that you're pesticide-sensitive, try organic fruits and vegetables that are pesticide-free and see if that helps.

Suspect sulfites. Used to preserve food and wine, sulfites are a common trigger of asthma. If you want to know if a food contains sulfites, look for bisulfite, potassium

the heartburn connection

If you have asthma, chances are pretty good that you also have bouts of heartburn—also known as reflux. A condition that causes stomach acid to migrate into the esophagus, reflux occurs in about half of all people who have asthma.

"Asthma changes the dynamics of the chest," says Marc S. McMorris, M.D., an allergist at the University of Michigan Health Systems. "It flattens out the diaphragm so the stomach acid doesn't have to go all the way up the esophagus to cause reflux."

Reflux during sleep can contribute to nocturnal asthma. The best way to prevent reflux is by avoiding heartburn-causing foods such as spices, tomatoes, and caffeine. It also helps to abstain from all food and drink within three hours of bedtime.

Elevating the head of your bed 6 to 8 inches also helps. (Use blocks under the bed's legs, not a pillow.) Using one of the several reflux medications available over the counter or by prescription also provides relief.

metabisulfite, sodium bisulfite, sodium sulfite, or sulfur diozide on the label.

Foods with sulfite include processed potatoes, shellfish, dried fruit, some tomato sauces, cider, vinegar, pickles, salad dressings, processed soups, beer, and wine.

Consider yeast. This staple of bread and coffee cake won't bring on a full-blown asthma attack, but it can certainly cause chest congestion.

Pay attention to how you feel after ingesting any products containing yeast. Yeast is also found in certain tomato sauces and beer. If you're extremely sensitive to yeast, you may be able to detect its presence by smell.

Don't rely on just coffee. You may have heard that a strong cup of coffee can get you through an emergency situation. Coffee and tea open up bronchial passages because theophylline, a close relative of caffeine, is a standard bronchodilating medication.

Don't let yourself count on it. Elise Solsin, a nutritionist at Mt. Sinai Hospital in New York City, has asthma. When she was caught away from home without an inhaler, she drank a cup of coffee instead.

"It worked for me," says Solsin. "It got me through the next couple of minutes. But this doesn't mean I would recommend it to my patients. In fact, I tell them not to use coffee or tea to control asthma."

Ask your doctor about caffeine, even as an emergency substitute, before using it. Chances are he or she won't endorse its use.

healing diet

PROBLEM FOODS	GOOD FOODS
Alcohol	Whole grains
Citrus fruit	Fruits
Eggs	Vegetables
Food additives	
Milk	
Nuts	
Peanut butter	
Shellfish	
Soy	
Yeast	
Wheat	

BEST ADVICE: If you have asthma, you should be under a doctor's care. If you suspect that food may be triggering asthma attacks, discuss it with your doctor.

cancer

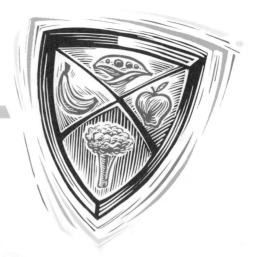

The best way to prevent cancer in your lifetime: Go to the grocery store. Buy some bananas, broccoli, and a cart full of other fruits and vegetables. Eat as many as you can today. Then do the same thing tomorrow. Repeat every day for the rest of your (very healthy) life.

Sound too simple to be true? Consider this: Scientists now estimate that unbalanced diets are the leading culprit behind at least one-third and maybe up to two-thirds of all cancer. In fact, the quarter of Americans who eat the fewest fruits and vegetables have double the cancer rate for most types of cancer of the 25 percent of folks who eat the most. If you don't smoke—smoking is the leading cause of about one-third of cancers—eating more of the right foods (and fewer of the wrong ones) is the best protection money can buy.

"Changing their diet is one of the most significant ways people who don't smoke can reduce their risk for cancer," maintains registered dietitian Abby Bloch, Ph.D., coordinator of clinical research at the GI Nutrition Service at Memorial Sloan-Kettering Cancer Center in New York City. "There are hundreds upon hundreds of compounds that work together in plant foods like grains, fruits, and vegetables that provide a protective milieu inside our bodies so our cells can stay healthy and function normally. First and foremost, we need to eat more of those foods."

10,000 Hits a Day: How Food Helps

To better understand how food fends off cancer, it helps to understand the kinds of assaults your body faces each day and how it defends itself.

Cancer-triggering enemy number one is a group of molecular marauders known as free radicals. Every bit as dangerous as their name implies, free radicals are oxygen molecules that have lost an electron and become unstable. So, they run rampant in your body, attacking your healthy cells in hopes of stealing electrons and stabilizing themselves. Unstopped, free radicals trigger a chain reaction that eventually damages your cell's DNA and paves the way for tumors or cancer. Scientists estimate that our bodies take about 10,000 free radical attacks every day.

Though you can avoid some free radicals by steering clear of cigarette smoke, prolonged sun exposure, and pollution, which accelerate free radical production, you can't avoid these molecular pirates entirely. We create them with every breath we take. The trick is to neutralize them before they do their dirty work. And the best way to do that is with antioxidants.

what's a serving?

For optimal cancer protection, many doctors recommend eight servings of fruits and vegetables every day. Though that sounds like a lot, it's really not when you consider how small a serving is. One serving for fruits and vegetables equals:

1 medium fruit
½ cup of cut fruit
¾ cup of 100 percent fruit juice
½ cup raw or cooked vegetables
1 cup raw leafy vegetables
½ cup of cooked beans or peas

Sit down to a lunch of bean chili, a side salad with vegetable toppings, and a piece of fruit, and you've already eaten four servings in just one meal.

Antioxidants are nature's knights in shining armor. They're compounds found in food, such as vitamins C and E, and carotenoids like beta-carotene and lycopene that literally step between free radicals and your healthy cells. These compounds offer their own electrons to convert free radicals back to stable oxygen molecules before they can do any damage.

This antioxidant protection is just one way food protects us from cancer, says Thomas J. Slaga, Ph.D., chair of the Center for Cancer Causation and Prevention at the AMC Cancer Research Center in Denver. The other is by helping your body cleanse itself of carcinogens, or those thousands of cancer-causing compounds you come in contact with every day. "The whole plant kingdom is blessed with chemicals that enhance your body's ability to produce the enzymes you need to detoxify cancer-causing agents," says Dr. Slaga. "It's just your job to eat these fruits, grains, and vegetables."

Unfortunately, though the National Cancer Institute has been advising people to eat at least five servings of fruits and vegetables a day, most of us fall short, says Dr. Bloch. "It's astounding. Fruits and vegetables are the best foods you can include in your diet. Yet, only 10 percent of the population eats five a day. From a cancer protecting perspective, we'd actually like to see people eating eight servings a day," she says. "It's really not that hard. You just have to think ahead and make some minor changes to how you eat."

Food for Protection

If the bad news is that people aren't eating enough of the foods that fight cancer, the good news is that scientists are finding protective powers in more foods every day, so you have dozens to choose from as you start including them.

Aim to eat a variety of the foods mentioned in this chapter, including them in your diet as often as you can, advises Charles Myers, M.D., director of the cancer center at the University of Virginia Medical

Center in Charlottesville. "When it comes to having an impact on cancer reduction, these foods are more powerful than chemotherapy. That's how important they are."

🍎 **Have fruit on hand.** One of the most overlooked cancer-fighting food groups is fruit, says Dr. Bloch. "Fruits are typically very rich in antioxidant vitamin C, and right now only about a third of Americans get the 200 milligrams of vitamin C they need for optimal health," she says. "Plus, if you don't eat fruit, you're missing out on some terribly important antioxidants, like terpenes in cherries, quercetin in red grapes, and limonene from citrus fruits."

Many of these fruit compounds not only prevent tumors, but they also have actually shrunk existing tumors in laboratory studies. They're so effective that when researchers in the Netherlands compared the rate of cancer deaths among more than 2,000 men over a 14-year period, they found that across the board, the men who ate the most fruit had the lowest risk of dying from cancer. "If you have a glass of orange juice in the morning, and then a banana later in the day, you're already at two servings," says Dr. Bloch.

🍎 **Eat a very vegetable dinner.** "I recommend that people have at least one vegetarian dinner a week," says Dr. Bloch. "It starts them thinking in the right direction—vegetables first." Vegetables fight cancer in all the ways you can fight cancer, quenching free radicals, eliminating toxins, and helping your body produce the enzymes it needs to neutralize dangerous carcinogens, says Dr. Myers. Since they all have unique protective properties, try to include as many different-colored vegetables in your diet as possible;

that way you'll be eating a variety of protective compounds, he says.

Red vegetables like tomatoes, for instance, contain lycopene. Researchers at Harvard found that when men ate two to four servings of lycopene-rich foods a week, they were 34 percent less likely to develop prostate cancer. Dark green vegetables, like spinach, contain lutein, and orange vegetables like carrots are rich in beta-carotene, which appears to fight against breast and other types of cancer.

These vegetables not only work well separately, they may work even better when they combine forces. In one study at State University of New York at Buffalo, researchers compared the diets of about 300 middle-aged women with breast cancer against the diets of the same number of women without cancer. The cancer-free women ate significantly more vegetables and had much higher blood levels of protective compounds like vitamin C, beta-carotene, zeaxanthin, and lutein.

🍎 **Include the crucifers.** When it comes to cancer-fighting vegetables, crucifers may be king. Vegetables like broccoli, brussels sprouts, and cabbage contain two separate compounds—indole-3-carbinol (I3C, for short) and sulforaphane—that help sweep up cancer-causing substances before they have a chance to do any harm. "These compounds are very strongly protective," says Dr. Bloch. Plus, these vegetables contain other antioxidants like vitamin C and beta-carotene, she notes. "The crucifers are a powerhouse of a food group."

Researchers in the Netherlands have found that in the overwhelming majority of cases, the more cruciferous vegetables folks eat, the lower their risk for cancer, especially lung, stomach, and colorectal cancer.

🍎 **Substitute with soy.** You've probably heard how the drug tamoxifen protects against breast cancer. Soy may offer similar benefits without the side effects. Soy foods like soybeans and tofu contain an estrogen-like plant chemical (phytoestrogen) called genistein that seems to act enough like estrogen to allow it to stick to estrogen receptors on breast cancer cells. But it's not enough like estrogen to actually get inside the cell. So, it just sits there, blocking the way, preventing real estrogen from getting inside the cell and promoting tumor growth. Researchers believe soy foods could be the reason that Asian women, who eat soy-rich diets, have significantly lower rates of breast cancer than American or European women.

The easiest way to work soy into the typical American diet is to substitute soy foods for dairy foods and meats. You can buy soy milk, soy burgers, even soy hot dogs. "The best part is if you switch from a red-meat based diet to a soy-based diet, you're swapping cancer-causing foods with cancer-preventing foods," says Dr. Myers.

🍎 **Go big on beans.** Beans are not only filled with fiber, which studies show protects against colorectal cancer, but they also contain compounds like lignans, isoflavones, saponins, and protease inhibitors, which seem to keep normal cells from turning cancerous and prevent cancer cells from growing, says Dr. Bloch.

"People shy away from beans because of their gas-producing reputation," she adds.

"But if you start eating beans, you start producing the enzymes you need to digest them, so that won't happen.

"In the meantime, you can buy flavorless products like Beano so you can eat them without worrying. (Beano is a product, available in your local drugstore, that can help you digest beans without producing gas.) Beans are so easy to add to your diet. Eat them in soups. Or use beans instead of meat in tacos."

🍎 **Go for garlic.** Garlic and onions are well respected for their benefits against heart disease but often overlooked when it comes to their cancer-fighting prowess. The same compounds that make you cry when you start slicing onions are the ones that may stop cancer-causing chemicals in their tracks, say scientists. There are substances in garlic that rival chemicals used in chemotherapy, like diallyl trisulfide, which flat-out kills human lung cancer cells.

"Like beans, it's incredibly easy to add onions and garlic into your diet. Add them to pasta, put them in soups, or use them on sandwiches," says Dr. Bloch.

🍎 **Favor flavonoids.** There's definitely something to that timeless apple-a-day theory. Apples are likely so good for you because they contain colorful compounds called flavonoids. Also found in foods like onions, berries, broccoli, green beans, and sweet peppers, as well as tea and red wine, these tiny color crystals pack a stunning antioxidant punch. In a 24-year study of nearly 10,000 men and women, Finnish researchers found that those who ate the most flavonoids in their diet were 20 percent less likely to develop cancer than those who ate the least.

Even more remarkable: The biggest flavonoid eaters also had a 46 percent lower risk for lung cancer. And regular apple eaters had the lowest lung cancer risk of the bunch—68 percent lower than people who ate apples infrequently.

🍎 **Crunch on carotenoids.** There are more than 500 of these bright orange contenders against cancer. Carotenoids, like beta-carotene, lycopene, and lutein, are found in bright red, yellow, and orange fruits and vegetables like carrots, cantaloupe, pumpkin, watermelon, sweet peppers, and tomatoes, as well as in dark leafy green vegetables like spinach and broccoli—you just can't see the orange color in these foods because the green pigment chlorophyll covers it up. Carotenoids help block cancer on two levels. One, they're some of the most potent antioxidants on the block. Two, some of them stop cells from proliferating—an important step in cancer development.

"Lycopene, which is found in tomatoes, is probably the most active," says Myers. Harvard researchers found that men who ate numerous servings of lycopene-rich foods, including tomato sauce, were less likely to develop prostate cancer.

Guava, pink grapefruit, and watermelon are also good sources.

🍎 **Take time for tea.** "Some folks thought the green tea theory sounded flaky when it first came out," says Dr. Myers. "But the scientific literature is overwhelming. Researchers have identified the active ingredient. It's a phenolic compound that actually triggers death in a large range of human cancer cells." Population studies have shown that green tea drinkers lower their risk for certain cancers, particularly those of the colon, rectum, and pancreas.

Though black tea contains some phenols, green tea is the best choice for cancer prevention, adds Dr. Myers. "These phenolic compounds are sensitive to oxidation, and black tea is heavily oxidized during processing. The greener the better.

Adding lemon juice also helps prevent the protective compounds from oxidizing." You can get a whopping 300 to 400 milligrams of phenols in just one cup of brewed green tea.

🍎 **Fill up on fiber.** It's all about what's known as "gut-transit time." The more fiber you eat, the bulkier your stool, and the less time it takes for waste products to be evacuated from your system. Not exactly table talk, to be sure, but it is cancer-prevention talk. Fiber is the indigestible part of plant foods that moves through your system, sweeping up toxins and adding weight to your stool. When you eat lots of fiber, you remove more carcinogens, cholesterol, and other toxic elements from your body more quickly. This dramatically lowers your risk for cancer, especially colorectal cancer.

Foods chock-full of fiber include all-bran cereals and beans, which contain between 5 and 10 grams a serving. You also get lots of fiber from fruits, vegetables, and whole grains like barley. "Optimally, we try to get people to eat 35 grams of fiber a day. But very few people eat anywhere near that.

Most Americans eat about 10 grams," says Bloch. "Because it can be a little hard on your digestive system if you're not used to it, I tell people to build fiber in their diet slowly. Start by working up over a couple of weeks to 20 grams. Then aim for 35."

🍎 **Make room for milk.** Researchers have found that women living in sunny, Southern climates like Atlanta or San Antonio are 30 to 40 percent less likely to get breast cancer than their Northern counterparts. Researchers suspect that the benefit may be from all the vitamin D the Southerners are soaking up every day. Vitamin D appears to hinder the growth of breast cancer cells in laboratory studies.

What does this have to do with diet? Well, sunshine isn't the only vitamin D source. Milk is, too, and a good one at that. Scientists followed close to 5,000 women for about 16 years, and they found that those who got 200 or more international units of vitamin D in their diets had a 30 percent lower risk of breast cancer than women who get less than 50 international units. Milk, fatty fish, and fortified breakfast cereals are some of the best sources.

🍎 **Get some glucarate.** Finally, stocking up on fruits and vegetables, especially apples, grapefruits, and bean sprouts, can boost the amount of a relatively unknown but mighty compound called glucarate in your diet, says Slaga. "Glucarate enhances the whole detoxification system that takes dangerous cancer-causing agents and neutralizes them," he says. "It's just another benefit of eating a plant-based diet. People should aim to get five servings of fruits and vegetables at the very least, preferably more."

How Food Hinders

A discussion on food and cancer wouldn't be complete if it didn't include the foods that don't protect against, but promote cancer. Though they're few, they tend to be the ones people gravitate toward, says Dr. Bloch. "Americans make the mistake of putting meat, processed foods, and fatty snacks before vegetables, fruits, and grains in their daily diet. So, they're not only getting fewer of the foods that help, but they're getting more of the foods that harm."

Certain foods, like saturated fat, facilitate the cancer process by actually encouraging cancer cells to grow and proliferate, explains Dr. Myers. "Obviously, this is a situation you want to avoid." That said, here are some foods to consider trimming from your diet.

🍎 **Cut the fat.** This is the biggie. "Fat, especially fat from red meat, whole-fat dairy foods, eggs, and creamy salad dressings, is converted to a substance called arachnidonic acid in the body," explains Dr. Myers. "And it's arachnidonic acid that stimulates the growth of most cancers in test-tube studies." High-fat diets also increase the production of hormones like estrogen and testosterone, which can increase the risk of breast and prostate cancer. "Even skin cancer is more common among people eating high-fat diets," adds Dr. Myers.

You should limit your intake of all kinds of fat to about 20 to 25 percent of total calories. And try to choose monounsaturated

weighty issues

One of the side benefits of eating a high-fiber, plant-based, cancer-protective diet is that you'll likely eat fewer calories and lose weight, too—both important factors for keeping cancer at bay.

"There is no question that eating too many calories and being 20 percent heavier than your ideal body weight—which a third of the population now is—increases your risk for cancer," says Abby Bloch, R.D., Ph.D., coordinator of clinical research at the GI Nutrition Service at Memorial Sloan-Kettering Cancer Center in New York City.

Low-fat, high-fiber foods fill you up without all the excess calories, she says. "Add exercise and you'll increase your cancer protection even more."

---

fats from vegetable sources like olive oil and omega-3 fatty acids from such fish as salmon, whenever possible, says Dr. Bloch. "These fats may actually have a protective effect in small doses. But if you're making them 45 percent of your diet, they'll do more harm than good."

Hold the pickles. A pickle now and then on the side of a sandwich is fine. But eating pickled food all the time can put your stomach at risk, says Dr. Slaga. "In Asian countries, where many of their daily staples are pickled, a process that produces harmful chemicals, there is a much higher incidence of stomach cancer than we have here," he says. "Our rates have dropped dramatically since the 1900s when we began to have better ways of preserving and storing food, like refrigeration."

Be careful at the barbecue. You may like the taste of charcoal-broiled food. But too much time at the backyard barbecue can expose you to the same cancer-causing chemicals as smoking cigarettes, warns Dr. Myers. "Grilling food causes certain compounds in meats to change into heterocyclic amines, which can cause cancer," he says. "A six- to eight-ounce charred steak could contain the same level of some of these dangerous chemicals as a couple of packs of cigarettes."

One way to protect yourself and still enjoy your barbecued chicken is to marinate the meat in olive oil and lemon juice first, says Dr. Myers. "The vitamin C in the juice prevents the formation of these dangerous compounds." Other studies have shown that marinades of cider vinegar and mustard also do the trick.

Use meat for flavor. All the meat we Americans eat is a major contributor to our cancer rates, says Dr. Bloch, not just because it contains saturated fats and other cancer-causing compounds, but because it squeezes out all the protective foods from our diet. "The best advice I can give people when it comes to meat is to reverse their thinking. Instead of picking a meat to put in the center of the meal and complementing it with vegetables, pick a vegetable or two and use meat to flavor them," she says. "It's like chicken and broccoli in a Chinese restaurant. The broccoli is the feature; the chicken the accent."

healing diet

PROBLEM FOODS	GOOD FOODS
High-fat foods (especially red meat, full-fat dairy, and creamy salad dressings)	Beans and legumes
Charcoal-barbecued food	Fruits
	Low-fat dairy products
	Soy
	Tea, especially green tea
	Vegetables

BEST ADVICE: Eat a high-fiber, plant-based diet, rich in fruits, vegetables, and grains. Swap meat for soy foods like tofu on a regular basis. Drink plenty of green tea.

celiac disease

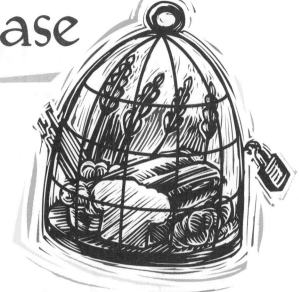

When Yogi Berra made his now famous remark that "it's not over until it's over," he could have been referring to the process of digestion instead of baseball. "Food can be chewed, swallowed, and broken down by the stomach, but if its nutrients don't get absorbed into the bloodstream by the small intestine, it might as well not have been eaten at all," says Ivor D. Hill, M.D., chief of the Division of Pediatric Gastroenterology and Nutrition at the Bowman Gray School of Medicine in Winston-Salem, North Carolina.

And this, unfortunately, is precisely what happens to people with celiac disease, also known as sprue. Although rare (affecting only about one in 5,000 Americans), the condition causes the fingerlike projections (villi) on the interior surface of the small intestine to shorten and collapse to the point of losing their absorptive abilities. "The result is that a person with a serious case of the disease can virtually be starving to death despite eating a very healthful diet," Dr. Hill says.

Short of that, people who have this condition can experience a wide variety of symptoms capable of making their lives uncomfortable, to say the least: muscular weakness, chronic diarrhea, excessive gas and abdominal bloating, stomach cramps, achy bones, uncontrollable weight loss, mental confusion, ringing in the ears, headaches, and even a blotchy and itchy skin condition known as dermatitis herpetiformis. Left untreated, the disease can lead to even more conditions, including anemia, cirrhosis of the liver, diabetes, brittle bones, and increased risks of intestinal cancer.

Gluten and Genetics

What causes celiac disease? And who's at risk? The cause of the disorder was unknown until 1950 when a Dutch physician observed that children suffering from celiac disease in Holland improved dramatically when wheat was removed from their diets in response to the grain shortages experienced during World War II. The offending agent soon was identified—a water-insoluble protein in wheat known as gluten—and suddenly people worldwide with celiac had the "cure" they were looking for. Simply by avoiding gluten, most people with celiac can be symptom-free within just four to six weeks.

"Sprue is an excellent example of the power of knowledge," says Michael Oppenheim, M.D., author of *The Complete*

forbidden foods

As you'll see, this list makes it clear that the key to avoiding gluten in processed foods is to inspect labels very—repeat, very—carefully. If in doubt, call a food's manufacturer. Celiac disease definitely is a condition where safe is infinitely better than sorry.

- All breads, cereals, pastas, or baked goods made from or containing wheat, rye, barley, or oats.
- Canned or processed fruits prepared with wheat, rye, barley, or oat products (check labels). All fresh, frozen, or canned fruits not containing these additives are allowed.
- Canned, frozen, or processed vegetables prepared with any form of wheat, rye, barley, or oats (check labels). All fresh, frozen, or canned vegetables not containing these additives are allowed.
- Canned or dry mixed soups containing grain-based thickeners or seasonings (check labels). Soups made fresh without any grain-based ingredients are permitted.
- Ice creams, puddings, sherbets, or icings containing emulsifiers, starches, stabilizers, thickeners, vegetable gums, or malt extracts derived from grains.
- Beverages: Postum, instant tea, coffee, or powdered fruit juice mixes containing grain derivatives; also beer and other alcoholic beverages made from grain, such as whiskeys and "pop" wines fortified with grain alcohol.
- Seasonings: some curry powders, chili seasonings, chutneys, gravy extracts, meat sauces, catsups, mustards, flavored vinegars, soy sauces, and peanut butters containing grain-based derivatives.
- Salad dressings containing grain-based ingredients.

Book of Better Digestion. "It can be a terrible disease if not treated properly, but otherwise just a mild annoyance."

Exactly why certain people find themselves "annoyed" by sprue remains in question. Some research has suggested that a virus or bacterium may spark the condition, which appears—as with allergies and rheumatoid arthritis—to be an autoimmune disease. In other words, the body reacts to gluten by signaling the immune system to attack the cells lining the small intestine's walls. Certain surgeries (gallbladder removal, for example) also have been suspected of triggering the condition, as have various diseases of the intestinal tract and even some antibiotic medications.

What research has been able to pin down is a strong genetic component to the disease: It's been found to occur in as many as one in 300 people of Northern European descent, yet is rare to nonexistent among Asians, Blacks, Jews, and people of

Mediterranean descent. It also tends to run in families, with odds of one in 10 that it will occur in siblings and children of people who have celiac. The disease can develop at any period during life, but does so most often during infancy (which can stunt growth) and again during middle age. Women, for unknown reasons, have been found to have celiac disease twice as frequently as men.

"We suspect, however, that the number of cases that get diagnosed may in fact be just the tip of the iceberg of a much larger problem," Dr. Hill says. "This probably is true in the United States, especially, where symptoms of nutritional deficiency caused by malabsorption tend not to be so obvious given our excessive caloric intakes."

Abstinence Is the Best Medicine

If celiac disease is suspected, a number of diagnostic procedures may be performed to confirm it, including blood tests, stool examinations, X-rays, or even a tissue biopsy of the lining of the small intestine itself.

If the condition is found, you can say farewell not just to your morning toast, but to a veritable cornucopia of other gluten-containing foods as well. "A celiac sufferer really needs to become a gluten sleuth," Dr. Hill says. "Gluten in one form or another is present in so many different foods now that only by being very careful to read labels and sometimes even checking with food manufacturers can one be totally certain of avoiding trouble."

The most obvious gluten villains are foods such as breads, cereals, and baked goods that are made from wheat directly,

but foods made from other gluten-bearing grains (barley, rye, and oats) also must be avoided. After these most obvious offenders, however, things can get a bit tricky because gluten "quite literally can hide in everything from soup to nuts," Dr. Hill says. It can be in cheese, ice cream, luncheon meats, canned soups, condiments, salad dressings, some instant coffees, and even grain-based liquors and beer. Even some wines, if they've been fortified with grain alcohol, need to be nixed.

Ways to Escape for Good

A lot of patients are left wondering, 'Gosh, well then what can I eat?'," says Dr. Hill. "But the diets we come up with for them invariably turn out to be quite acceptable."

They're especially acceptable considering the results: "People who follow their gluten-free diets strictly can be free of symptoms within just a few weeks," says Dr. Hill. "Better yet, any damage done to the small intestine usually also gets reversed if the diet is continued."

Check out these gluten-dodging strategies with that bit of good news in mind.

🍃 **Become a gluten sleuth.** People with celiac "must learn to avoid gluten with the same fervor they would rat poison," says University of Iowa gastroenterologist Joseph Murray, M.D. This means avoiding not just gluten's most obvious sources such as cereals, baked goods, pastas, and breads, but also reading the ingredients labels of all processed foods and sometimes even

for more
information

There are a number of good organizations that can help you with issues ranging from the best gluten-free recipes to the latest updates on the gluten contents of hundreds of processed foods:

The Celiac Sprue Association, P.O. Box 31700, Omaha, NE 68131-0070

The American Celiac Society-Dietary Support Coalition, 58 Musano Court, West Orange, NJ. 07052

The Celiac Disease Foundation, 13251 Ventura Blvd., Studio City, CA 91604

The Gluten Intolerance Group of North America, P.O. Box 23053, Seattle, WA 98102-0353

checking with a food's manufacturer. "The ingredients used in processed foods can change, so it's important to remain as informed as possible," Dr. Murray says.

🍎 **Learn gluten's many faces.** Don't expect the word "gluten" always to pop out in boldly cautionary letters, Dr. Murray warns. Seemingly innocent ingredients such as malt, maltodextrin, hydrolyzed vegetable protein, modified food starch, diglycerides, and caramel coloring can in fact be gluten hot beds.

🍎 **Know the price of cheating, even "just a little."** It can be tempting to stray, especially since adverse reactions usually are not experienced right away. Discomfort might not be experienced at all if the amount of gluten eaten has been small, but this does *not* mean that damage is not being done. "Whether symptoms occur or not, the small intestine of most celiac patients suffers damage with any amount of gluten that's

ingested at all," Dr. Murray says. This is why adherence to a gluten-free diet must be so strict, he says. "Even the smallest relapse can deprive the small intestine of the gluten-free environment it needs to heal."

🍎 **Eat as healthfully as possible.** "Because food choices do become limited, it's important for people with celiac to make the foods they *can* eat as nutritious as possible," Dr. Hill says. This means plenty of fruits and vegetables, potatoes, rice, lean meats, and fish.

🍎 **Play it safe with a good multiple vitamin.** "Even when a person is following a strict gluten-free diet and his or her condition is in remission, nutrients still may not be getting fully absorbed, so fortifying the diet with a good vitamin supplement can be a good idea," Dr. Hill says. This goes for iron especially, he says, which can help prevent the anemia commonly associated with celiac disease.

🍎 **Don't smoke.** Studies show that people with celiac are at an increased risk for developing cancer of the small intestine, so smoking—a proven carcinogen—should be banned right along with gluten to help reduce this risk, Dr. Hill says.

🍎 **Get yourself a good cookbook.** People with celiac disease can allow themselves to feel deprived, or they can feel *challenged* in a positive way, Dr. Hill says, and it's the latter of these responses, of course, that's preferable. "A lot of people have shown incredible imagination in keeping their palates pleased, and some very good cookbooks have come of this resourcefulness," he says. (Some titles to consider: *The Gluten-Free Gourmet* by Betty Hagman and *Special Diet Solutions—Cooking Without Wheat, Gluten, Dairy, or Refined Sugar* by Carol Fenster, Ph.D.)

Tips for Fine-Tuning

Aside from exercising the precautions above, there are additional steps you can take to be doubly protected from gluten's harmful effects:

🍎 **Don't automatically assume all rice and soy beverages are safe.** Some use a production process that incorporates enzymes extracted from barley.

🍎 **Beware of unhealthy advice from health-food stores.** Wanting to make sales,

some will push products (spelt and kamut, for example) that are thought to be safe but are not.

🍎 **Be vigilant against bread crumbs.** They can find their way into or onto sticks of butter, cutting boards, countertops, toasters, and jars of mayonnaise and jam.

🍎 **Be especially careful when eating out.** In addition to requesting a gluten-free meal from the start, try to avoid fried or grilled foods that may have shared space with a gluten-containing food in the deep-fryer or on the grill.

🍎 **Curb your confidence in corn.** Corn itself is permissible, as is corn meal if it's pure, but some commercially packaged brands are blended with wheat. Read the label carefully to be sure or call the manufacturer to be more certain yet.

🍎 **Leave no cap unturned.** Check for gluten in medicines, toothpastes, mouthwashes, and even in the adhesive on envelopes and stamps.

healing diet

PROBLEM FOODS	GOOD FOODS
There are a tremendous number of foods to avoid in order to promote healing. See "Forbidden Foods" on page 96.	Fruits
	Vegetables
	Lean Meats
	Fish
	Potatoes
	Rice

BEST ADVICE: Be a gluten sleuth; find out all the places that gluten can lurk. Get yourself a good gluten-free cookbook (or two or three). If you smoke, quit. And do take a multivitamin supplement.

colds

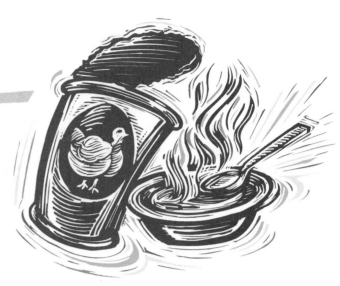

Is it feed a cold, starve a fever? Or is it the other way around?

If you're like most of us, you probably never can remember which way that phrase goes. That's OK because the truth is a sick body shouldn't be starved. Even when you're sick and the absolute last thing you want to do is eat, your body needs food for energy. Many people are tempted to eat very little or not eat at all when they're stricken by a cold. Big mistake!

Generally, a bland diet is best when you're not feeling at your best. But did you know that when you are sick with a cold, certain foods actually can help you feel better? Not only that, eating right can go a long way towards keeping you from catching colds in the first place.

Cold Facts

But before we talk about the foods that are best for dealing with a cold when you have one, let's look at some of the facts about colds. There are about 200 known forms of the rhinovirus, the microbe that accounts for about 40 percent of cold viruses. The average adult catches four to six colds per year. At a recovery rate of five to 10 days per cold, that could add up to almost two months of sick time. It's no wonder we spend so much time talking about and trying to figure out how to avoid the sneezes and coughs of the common cold.

If you are one of those lucky people who never gets sick, it means that your immune system's three modes of defense against germs—the skin, the mucous membranes that line the respiratory and digestive tracts, and the white blood cells—are working effectively.

Even the healthiest immune systems can be vulnerable to cold viruses, and that's because these viruses are very tough creatures, and they spread easily. Here's how: Someone at your office sneezes or coughs into his hand then touches a doorknob with that hand. You touch that doorknob then put your hand to your eye or nose. Guess what? You've caught your coworker's cold.

Another factor that contributes to the number of colds you catch is the time of year. Common wisdom among doctors is that people catch more colds in the winter because we spend so much time indoors and are exposed to the coughs and sneezes of others. Parents and schoolteachers of young children are also more at risk because children are particularly susceptible to viral infections.

to C or not to C

Talk to five doctors and you're likely to hear five theories on the effectiveness of this vitamin.

Most doctors will allow that vitamin C can sometimes lessen the symptoms and shorten the duration of a cold, but there's no scientific proof that even hefty doses can prevent a cold.

"A huge number of people take the vitamin for colds, but in carefully monitored studies, I haven't found it effective," says Steven R. Mostow, M.D., chairman of the department of medicine at Rose Medical Center in Denver. "Now Linus Pauling would tell me that I need to test larger doses of the vitamin, but in large doses, like 1,000 milligrams every four to six hours, you get another problem: stomach upset."

One study of British men who were vitamin-C-deficient does support Linus Pauling's contention that larger doses of the vitamin are what it takes. When the men increased their C intakes to at least 1,000 milligrams a day, the number of colds they caught reduced by 30 percent. These men were deficient to begin with, however.

But vitamin C levels decrease when people are stressed, and stress does put people at risk for catching a cold.

So what does this all mean for you? It certainly can't hurt to supplement your diet with 60 to 200 milligrams of vitamin C a day during cold seasons. If you're taking the vitamin for the first time, start out with a lesser dose to see how it reacts on your stomach.

You also can be more vigilant about the kinds of fruits and vegetables you eat by choosing those that are high in vitamin C. Some good choices include oranges and orange juice, grapefruits, mangoes, papaya, asparagus, and kale.

The good news in all this is that your immunity increases each year. You catch fewer colds as you age. "The clear advantage to getting older as far as colds go is that you catch fewer colds," says Steven R. Mostow, M.D., chairman of the department of medicine at Rose Medical Center in Denver. "You become immune to each of the 200 viruses as you wade your way through them."

Seeking Relief

There are two very effective ways to avoid catching a cold. First, if you smoke, quit immediately. Smoking increases inflammation of the upper respiratory tract and lessens the effectiveness of the body's natural defenses. Second, wash your hands often, especially after shaking hands with someone who has a cold or after sneezing or blowing your nose.

A study reported in the *New England Journal of Medicine* found a link between psychological stress and the likelihood of developing a cold. The equation is simple: The more stress you're under, the more colds you develop.

There is no cure for the common cold, but there are remedies that can shorten the illness and relieve some of the symptoms. Most of us reach for over-the-counter relief, probably because these medications make us feel better rather quickly. Antihistamines and decongestants attack congestion, while aspirin, acetaminophen, and ibuprofen relieve aches.

Foods that Clobber the Cold

Researchers also know that certain foods can help prevent colds and provide some relief from symptoms. Here's an evaluation of the foods that are believed to work best when you're fighting a cold or trying to avoid getting sick.

Strive for five. There is no better way to bolster your immune system than by incorporating at least five servings of fruits and vegetables into your daily diet. A strong immune system could stave off a cold from striking you in the first place. And it certainly will give you more ability to fight the colds you do catch.

Forget crash dieting. Losing more than 1 pound a week by dieting can suppress the function of one type of immune cell, according to a study of obese women done at Appalachian State University in Boone, North Carolina. The cells that were affected, T-cells, are white blood cells that target and kill microbe-infected cells.

Researchers noted that the suppression was only temporary, but still caution against losing more than a pound a week on a diet.

Pick papaya. A 3.5-ounce serving of this sweet, melonlike fruit provides 100 percent of the recommended daily allowance for vitamin C and 10 percent of your daily folate needs. Despite their exotic image, papayas are easy to find in most supermarkets year-round.

Go exotic. By habit most of us turn to orange juice when we come down with a cold, but the lesser-known passion fruit and guava can be just as good for you.

Passion fruit helps soothe a sore throat. And, ounce for ounce, guavas, which are similar to melons, have triple the vitamin C of oranges.

Get straight As. Vitamin A has been shown to improve the disease-fighting ability of skin and mucous membranes, and is necessary for production and activity of several types of white cells. The best food sources are green and yellow vegetables, including carrots (raw are better than cooked), spinach, and winter squash.

Spice up your life. Consume something with a little zing, especially foods made with chili peppers, hot mustard, or horseradish, to help clear congestion.

Hot spices help drain the upper respiratory passages.

Get plenty of fluids. Has your doctor ever told you to drink a lot when you're sick with a cold? The reason is the liquid keeps mucous membranes moist, enabling them to trap cold viruses and dispose of them before they can infect more of your cells. The most recommended fluid is water, but diluted fruit juices, seltzer, decaffeinated coffee, and tea work, too. Aim for eight glasses a day. Drinking enough fluids is especially important in the winter when indoor and outdoor air are much drier.

🍎 **Forget about alcohol.** The one fluid you definitely want to avoid when sick with a cold is alcohol. Several studies indicate that alcohol seems to impair the immune system's ability to wipe out cells infected with the cold virus. It's best to save that beer or glass of wine for days when you're feeling well.

🍎 **Think zinc.** No cold remedy has gotten more attention in the past few years than the mineral zinc. One study, done in 1997, found that zinc lozenges taken within 24 hours of a cold's onset can resolve symptoms within four days. According to study coauthor Michael Macknin, M.D., of the Cleveland Clinic Foundation, zinc blocks the cold virus's ability to adhere to the lining of the respiratory tract.

"The results of the study were very dramatic," says Dr. Macknin. "But they don't prove that zinc works. The findings need to be confirmed." To achieve the desired effect from the zinc, you need to take one 13.3-milligram lozenge every two hours while you're awake.

The problem is that taking too much zinc can backfire by lowering the body's copper levels, which decreases your ability to fight infection. Also, in 20 percent of the study's patients, the lozenges caused mild

calling all grandmas

There isn't a grandmother around who doesn't recommend chicken soup for a cold. Well, guess what? You should listen already.

A study performed by Steven R. Mostow, M.D., chairman of the department of medicine at Rose Medical Center in Denver, compared the effectiveness of homemade chicken soup to acetaminophen for relieving cold symptoms. Amazingly enough, the soup shortened the course of the cold and alleviated symptoms far more effectively than did the acetaminophen.

The theory is chicken soup soothes sore throats and clears congestion. (By the way, canned chicken soup didn't work as well.)

queasiness when taken on an empty stomach. And many nutrition experts are not convinced that zinc helps at all. So instead of the lozenges, you could try increasing the amount of zinc-rich foods in your diet. Steak, pork, crab, wheat germ, brown rice, and oatmeal are high in zinc.

🍎 **Try a little warm salt water.** Gargling with an 8-ounce glass of warm water and a few teaspoons of salt makes a sore throat feel better and drains clogged sinuses. You need to gargle at least three times a day.

🍎 **Have a nice cup of tea.** Tea contains theophylline, a natural substance that opens up congested air spaces and helps drain upper-respiratory passages. The warmth of the tea also soothes a sore throat. A little honey can help stimulate mucus production and reduce the throat tickle that accompanies many colds.

Herbs to the Rescue

There isn't all that much you can do for a cold, beyond riding it out. However, there are a few herbs that might prove helpful.

Echinacea. This herb has its share of believers and doubters. Those who swear by it believe that echinacea contains substances capable of strengthening the immune system and thus may help the body ward off an infection by a cold or flu virus. The herb is sold in tincture, pill, and tea form. Although its effectiveness is up for debate, most doctors agree that if taking it makes you feel better, then you should take it.

Goldenseal. This plant contains an antibiotic substance, berberine, that, like echinacea, is said to stimulate the immune system. Many health-food stores sell echinacea drops that also contain goldenseal.

Eucalyptus. Available in health-food stores, this herb is a favorite remedy of nutritionists for loosening tight coughs. They brew its leaves into a strong tea. The leaves also can be used in a steam vaporizer to relieve coughs. Eucalyptus is found in cough drops and cough suppressants.

Garlic. As unpleasant as it might sound, garlic is most effective for a cold when eaten raw, since cooking alters some of the herb's active ingredients. Garlic contains selenium, a natural immune system booster. It acts as an expectorant when consumed in a tea or used with warm water for gargling. Try throwing a handful of minced garlic on top of a serving of pasta. (You might find yourself enjoying it.)

Ginger. Ginger tea is recommended for getting rid of chills, relieving sinus and chest congestion, and countering nausea. You can get the same benefits by grating fresh ginger into the foods you prepare.

Licorice. A common component of Japanese herbal remedies, licorice extract is believed to boost immunity. It also can be used as an expectorant for upper-respiratory congestion.

Peppermint. Peppermint tea taken at the first sign of a cold can alleviate symptoms of viral infection, including cough and fever.

healing diet

PROBLEM FOODS	GOOD FOODS
Alcohol	Fruits
	Vegetables
	Oranges
	Papaya

BEST ADVICE: Have some chicken soup and get plenty of rest.

constipation

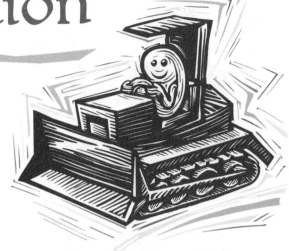

Constipation happens to just about everyone from time to time. Only rarely is it serious and only rarely does it require complicated treatment. Still, for many people, constipation occurs...well, with regularity.

It might be helpful here to start with a basic definition. Nowhere is it written in stone that people must have a bowel movement every day, explains Steven Peikin, M.D. , professor of gastroenterology at the Robert Wood Johnson Medical School at Camden, in New Jersey. In fact, he says, studies show wide differences in how often people move their bowels—from several times a day to only once or twice a week. So consider yourself normal, whatever your schedule, he says, provided you experience no discomfort.

It's only when you cease having bowel movements as often as is normal for you that you become constipated. And a prolonged bout can definitely cramp your style. Along with hardened, difficult-to-pass stools, you may experience bloating, abdominal pain, and lack of energy.

For anyone with an occasional complaint, there's a simple and usually fast cure: more fiber. Just a bowl of bran cereal or a plateful of fruit can often clear up constipation in a matter of hours. Should that fail, fiber-rich bulk laxatives, such as Metamucil, that are available over the counter will usually do the trick.

Causes of Constipation

Before getting into exactly how fiber works its magic and how to increase the fiber content of your diet, it helps to know just what causes constipation in the first place.

Lots of things, it turns out. Constipation can accompany premenstrual syndrome. It can result from taking over-the-counter medications, such as aluminum-based antacids or even iron and calcium supplements. Other major culprits include prescription drugs, such as high blood pressure medications and antidepressants.

One 1995 study found a surprising reason why infants may develop constipation: Some are allergic to cow's-milk protein. Putting infants on a diet free of cow's-milk protein worked the cure with 21 of the 27 babies in the study.

In the elderly, lack of exercise often results in constipation. Seniors, like many people who have trouble moving their bowels, often turn to over-the-counter laxatives for relief, maybe a bit too often, explains Peikin.

Habitual laxative use can lead to a condition called "cathartic colon" or "lazy bowel," he explains. That is, the muscles in the colon actually grow dependent on laxatives to produce a bowel movement.

Look at your busy schedule as another possible cause. Constipation affects people who travel frequently, as well as people constantly on the go at work and home.

Still other people experience frequent bouts of constipation followed by periods of diarrhea. And this can be a sign of irritable bowel syndrome (IBS), a chronic, though not serious condition.

Fat Slows You Down

If you want to know the most common cause of constipation, look no further than your diet, says Dr. Peikin. For starters, people simply eat too much fat. Ideally, your diet should contain no more than 30 percent of calories from fat.

To be fair, human beings naturally crave fatty foods. In fact, evolution has designed the small intestine to absolutely adore foods that are high in fat, and for good reason. Fatty foods are loaded with energy, something our cave-dwelling ancestors could always make use of. So when fat-loaded meals reach the small intestine, the fat—think of it as high-powered fuel—gets soaked up like grease through a sponge.

How does this cause constipation? Once all the fat has been absorbed by the small intestine, very little food matter remains. And what little is left passes to the large intestine. The large intestine does two important jobs: One, it absorb some of the water contained in the food it receives; two, it passes any indigestible food on as waste. When the large intestine receives very little food to begin with—as happens when you eat high-fat meals—it doesn't sense that it's full. So it doesn't void this small amount of food matter as waste. Who rushes to empty a half-full trash container?

The result is that the undigested food simply sits there, while its water content is systematically siphoned off. This in turn causes the stools to harden, and it makes them difficult to pass. Voilà, constipation.

When you diet, basically the same thing happens. The large intestine receives less food, and the little that does arrive simply sits there. Also, if you're dehydrated from exercise or whatever reason, the large intestine will seek to replace the moisture your body needs by working especially hard to siphon water from the food it receives.

Fabulous Fiber

Although a diet that's high in fats and low on fluids can cause constipation, eating lots of fiber and drinking plenty of fluids will do just the opposite.

But what exactly is fiber? Scientifically speaking, fiber consists of complex

recommended number of
daily fiber servings

The recommended number of fiber servings we should eat each day depends on our age, sex, and level of activity.

	Age	Grains	Vegetables	Fruits
Children	1-3	6	3	2
	4-6	7	3.3	2.3
	7-10	7.8	3.7	2.7
Females	11-50	9	4	3
	51+	7.4	3.5	2.3
Males	11-14	9.9	4.5	3.5
	15-18	11	5	4
	19-50	11	5	4
	51+	9.1	4.2	3.2

Serving Sizes

Grains: 1 serving = 1 slice bread; 1 ounce ready-to-eat cereal; ½ cup cooked cereal, rice, or pasta

Vegetables: 1 serving = 1 cup raw leafy vegetables; ½ cup other vegetables, cooked or chopped raw; ¾ cup vegetable juice

Fruits: 1 serving = 1 medium apple, banana, orange; ½ cup chopped, cooked, or canned fruit

Source: U.S. Department of Agriculture

carbohydrate molecules. Think of them as long, bulky strands of beads. They're found only in plant foods, namely in whole grains, fruits, vegetables, beans, nuts, and seeds.

Why fiber works so well is simple. Unlike fats, which get quickly sopped up in the small intestine, the complex bulky carbohydrate molecules in fiber can't be absorbed at all. Our digestive system lacks the enzymes to break them down. As far as your small intestine is concerned, these fibrous foods are utterly worthless. So the small intestine quickly passes them on to the large intestine. The large intestine can't do much with the fiber either. And the fiber's very bulk—remember those long, bulky carbohydrate molecules—causes the large intestine to feel full quickly and pass the fiber on through the colon. Moreover,

fiber foods

Fiber content varies widely from food to food. Just two plums have a whopping 3.2 grams of fiber, for example, but 15 grapes have less than half a gram. When planning meals, pick generously from these foods.

Food	Serving Size	Total Fiber in Grams
Breads		
French	1 slice	0.9
Oat bran muffin	1	1
Pumpernickel	1 slice	2.7
Tortilla (flour and corn)	1	0.7
White, enriched	1 slice	0.6
Whole wheat	1 slice	1.5
Pasta and rice		
Egg noodles	¼ cup	0.4
Spaghetti, cooked	½ cup	0.9
White rice, cooked	½ cup	0.1
Wild rice, cooked	½ cup	0.4
Cereals		
All bran	⅓ cup	8.6
Oat bran, dry	⅓ cup	4
Wheat germ, plain	3 tablespoons	3.9
Fruit		
Apple, raw, with skin	1	2.8
Grapefruit, raw	½ medium	1.4
Grapes, raw	15 medium	0.4
Pear, raw, with skin	1 medium	2.9

fiber itself hoards water—up to 15 times its own weight, as a matter of fact. This water adds still more mass to fibrous waste, which makes it pass through the digestive system all the more quickly.

Note: Because fiber retains so much water, it's important to drink plenty of fluids when you're on a high-fiber diet. Doctors recommend eight to 10 glasses per day, which can include water, milk, juice, soup, or whatever.

Sticking to a high-fiber diet and drinking plenty of fluids will cause your digestive system to function at an optimal level. That is, foods will take a good 18 to 24 hours on average to pass completely through your system.

The U.S. Dietetic Association recommends eating 20 to 30 grams of fiber

Food	Sering Size	Total Fiber in Grams
Fruit (*continued*)		
Plums, raw, with skin	2 medium	3.2
Prunes, dried	3	17
Raspberries, raw	1 cup	3.3
Nuts		
Almonds, roasted	1 whole	0.6
Peanuts, roasted	10	0.6
Pecans	2 whole	0.5
Walnuts	2 whole	0.3
Vegetables		
Beans, green, frozen	½ cup	1.6
Broccoli, cooked	½ cup	2.5
Brussels sprouts, cooked	½ cup	3.8
Okra, cooked	½ cup	4.1
Potato, white, baked	1 medium	3.8
Squash, winter, cooked, sliced	½ cup	3.6
Tomatoes, raw	1 medium	1
Turnips, cooked	½ cup	4.8
Beans and peas		
Beans, kidney, cooked	½ cup	6.9
Beans, lima, cooked	½ cup	4.3
Lentils, cooked	½ cup	5.2
Peas, black-eyed, cooked	½ cup	3.1
Peas, split, cooked	½ cup	3.1

Source: Iowa State University Extension Service

per day. Most experts concur with this amount, and some cancer researchers urge you to eat up to 35 grams per day. Unfortunately, only one in five Americans actually eats that amount, according to estimates by the USDA.

And yet, the USDA advises, to receive that amount of fiber each day, all you'd need to eat would be two to four servings of fruit, three to five vegetable servings, and six to 11 helpings of grains. You can easily meet your daily fiber quota by the following:

- Add a banana to your bran cereal.
- Snack on an apple.
- Eat a salad for lunch with a whole grain roll.
- Enjoy a normal dinner with a side dish of vegetables and fruit for dessert.

Notice the different kinds of fiber in this simplified meal plan. Doctors once

too much, too fast

Got constipation? Eat more fiber.
Sounds easy. When some people learn this key to regularity, they use it a little too well.

Devouring big platefuls of beans, fruits, and vegetables, when you're not used to these foods, can overwhelm the bacteria in the large intestine and result in painful intestinal gas, especially if you're constipated.

It's better to introduce fiber a little at a time, advises Steven Peikin, M.D. , professor of gastroenterology at the Robert Wood Johnson Medical School at Camden, in New Jersey. "If you're eating 10 grams a day now, you can increase that amount to 20 or 30 grams without much problem," he says. Gradually increase your fiber intake to give your system a chance to become accustomed to it.

advised their patients with chronic constipation to dive into bran as the single and best source of fiber. But now they recommend eating a diet heavy on different kinds of fiber.

"No one knows whether one specific type of fiber is more beneficial than another since fiber-rich foods tend to contain various types," says registered dietitian Joyce Saltsman, Ph.D., a nutritionist with the U.S. Food and Drug Administration's Office of Food Labeling. In fact, fiber comes in two basic varieties: water soluble and water insoluble. As you probably guessed, water soluble fibers mix up just fine with water; water insoluble fibers don't. Most plant foods contain some of both kinds.

Insoluble fibers work the hardest at relieving constipation by adding bulk to the stool. Some common foods rich in insoluble fiber include wheat and corn bran, dried beans, carrots, potatoes, broccoli, and leeks, even popcorn.

Foods containing soluble fiber include oat and rice bran, citrus fruits, apples, pears, strawberries, cauliflower, and corn, as well as the seeds and skins of many fruits and vegetables. When these fibers reach the large intestine, they are acted upon by bacteria in a process known as fermentation. Though fermentation does cause intestinal gas, researchers believe the process also helps create well-formed and easily passed stools.

Fortify with Fiber

It's all well and good to say eat more fiber, but how exactly can you make that a daily habit? Here are some suggestions:

Become a high-fiber shopper. Make a habit of checking food labels for fiber content. When the product advertises that it's a "good" source of fiber, it means you will receive 2.5 to 4.9 grams of fiber for each serving.

Foods that claim to be "rich" or "high" in fiber are required to have at least 5 grams per serving. The cereal aisle in your supermarket contains the best selection of foods high in fiber.

🍎 **Fruitify your mornings.** Start the day off with fruits like oranges, grapefruit, and melon. Add still more fiber with a bagel or whole wheat toast.

🍎 **Pack snacks that pay you back.** Apples, oranges, and pears make for great snacks. Be sure to eat the skins, too. An apple with skin, for example, contains 2.8 grams of fiber. A peeled apple contains 2.4. Other fiber-rich snacks include nuts, sunflower seeds, crackers made with whole grains, and uncooked vegetables.

🍎 **Supercharge your sandwiches.** Make the switch to whole grain breads. Just one slice of pumpernickel bread contains 2.7 fiber grams. Boost the fiber still more by piling on veggies like tomatoes, cucumbers, and bean sprouts.

🍎 **Boost your salads.** Already rich in fiber, garnish salads with nuts, beans, and sprouts.

🍎 **Fiberize baked goods.** Spoon 2 to 3 tablespoons of unprocessed wheat bran into casseroles and homemade breads. This adds up to 4 grams of extra fiber per serving.

🍎 **Maximize main meals.** Feast on potatoes, skins and all. Or serve whole grain

regularity
the natural way

If a bowl of fruit or extra-large helping of vegetables doesn't help relieve constipation in the short term, try some of the foods that are natural laxatives.

● **Try prunes.** Prunes make up many people's second line of defense. Besides containing fiber, prunes possess a natural laxative called isatin. Isatin can also be found in dried fruits such as apricots and figs.

● **Have a cup of coffee.** Caffeine stimulates the muscles in the intestines. But if you don't like caffeine, try adding the juice from half a fresh lemon to a cup of hot water.

● **Change temperature.** Try drinking a cup of coffee or some other hot drink, then drink something cold immediately afterward. The extreme temperature change sometimes stimulates the colon.

wheat pasta. One cup cooked pasta contains 3 to 8 grams of fiber.

Heap on servings of vegetables, nuts, beans, and lentils. One cup of leafy vegetables has roughly the same amount of fiber as ½ cup of other kinds of vegetables (either cooked or raw) or ¾ cup of most any vegetable juice.

🍎 **Get double benefits from desserts.** Serve fruit by itself or use it to top off yogurt and ice cream dishes.

healing diet

PROBLEM FOODS

Fatty foods
Meat
Processed foods

GOOD FOODS

Beans
Fruits
Vegetables
Whole grains

BEST ADVICE: Eat a high-fiber, plant-based diet, rich in fruits, vegetables, and grains. Drink plenty of water and other fluids.

dental caries

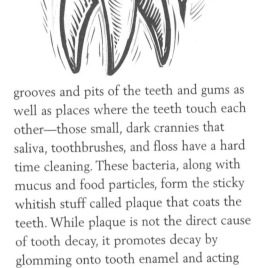

You call them cavities. Your dentist calls them dental caries. Whatever you call those little (and sometimes not so little) holes that penetrate your tooth's enamel, they are unwanted, unpleasant, and often painful.

Tooth decay is actually a disease. In fact, until the last 20 years or so, it was the most common disease in the United States. Almost all kids had at least a few cavities. Today more than half of all 12-year-old children are cavity-free. But plenty of kids—and a fair share of adults—still get cavities.

The fact is, a lot of cavities simply do not have to happen. They can easily be prevented. How?

You've undoubtedly heard that sugary treats are the main culprit in causing tooth decay. In fact, you probably had it drilled (pardon the pun) into you as a child: Candy Equals Tooth Decay. Although sugar does play a role in causing tooth decay, it's not the whole story. To get the full picture, it helps to understand what causes tooth decay in the first place.

The Bacteria Acid Factory

Tooth decay requires three ingredients: germs, food, and unprotected teeth, according to Thomas McGuire, D.D.S., leading authority on dental wellness and author of *Tooth Fitness*. The mouth, like most of the body, swarms with bacteria. These germs especially like to colonize the grooves and pits of the teeth and gums as well as places where the teeth touch each other—those small, dark crannies that saliva, toothbrushes, and floss have a hard time cleaning. These bacteria, along with mucus and food particles, form the sticky whitish stuff called plaque that coats the teeth. While plaque is not the direct cause of tooth decay, it promotes decay by glomming onto tooth enamel and acting like an acid factory, explains Dr. McGuire.

The germs in plaque can digest only the tiny molecules of simple sugars, such as sucrose (table sugar). So, does that mean you have to worry only about sugar? No way. The larger molecules of fats and proteins and starches are way too big for the bacteria in your mouth to eat. But they have help. Amylase, an enzyme in your saliva, for example, breaks down starches into other simple sugars, like maltose, glucose, and fructose. And these molecules *are* small enough for the bacteria to eat. As these bacteria digest sugar, they ferment it, giving off powerful acids strong enough to dissolve the minerals in tooth enamel—the hardest substance in your body.

What all this means in practical terms is that candy isn't the only culprit. Healthy foods like bread, pasta, and rice can cause tooth decay, too. And so (oh, my gosh) can fruits and vegetables.

The acid bath that bacteria create while eating part of your meal is still not the end of the story, however.

The third requirement for creating cavities is unprotected teeth. Teeth go unprotected for a number of reasons:
● genetics (you can inherit weak enamel)
● inadequate fluoride
● nooks and crannies created either by nature or by dental work, such as fillings, crowns, and bridges
● poor oral hygiene habits
● an inadequate supply of saliva, caused by illness or certain medications.

"Today we know that dental caries is a site-specific disease," according to Stephen Moss, D.D.S., division head of Growth and Developmental Sciences at New York University College of Dentistry and chairman and professor of the Department of Pediatric Dentistry. "There is no one specific cause." Cavities occur because of some disruption in the tooth's environment that allows the tooth to be bathed in acid hour after hour and day after day, he says.

When a cavity develops, you know that either the enamel lacks enough fluoride protection or that saliva simply can't get access to the site.

Saliva is your best natural ally in preventing tooth decay, says Dr. Moss. He calls saliva a liquid form of enamel. It acts on the teeth like the bloodstream acts on cells. Saliva brings nutrition, carries away waste, and continuously repairs the enamel with its load of calcium and fluoride. The fluoride your dentist applies, or that you get from your toothpaste, simply helps your saliva work better.

Preventing Cavities

The best ways to prevent cavities are by now etched in your consciousness:

● Brush twice a day, morning and night.
● Floss at least once a day.
● Visit the dentist regularly for checkups and professional cleanings.

But what about diet? Diet is key in preventing caries, too. *Directly or indirectly, all tooth decay is related to diet.*

Researchers have even tried to classify foods according to how much potential they have for causing tooth decay.

Problem Foods

Every dentist tells us to cut down on sweets and between-meal snacks. And it stands to reason that sticky foods, like raisins or caramels, would linger longer in your mouth, fermenting and promoting decay. But research tends to complicate the traditional advice.

One study done at the Forsyth Dental Center in Boston, for instance, found that starchy foods (especially cooked starches) may cause even more trouble for teeth than sugary foods. Researchers found that potato chips and saltines promoted worse decay-causing conditions than sugary foods like cookies, caramels, and chocolate bars. Foods that combine starches and sugar, like doughnuts, were also worse for teeth than sugars alone.

Protective Foods

Other foods seem to exert a protective effect on teeth. Studies have shown that aged cheeses, like cheddar and Swiss, Edam, Gouda, provolone, and Gruyère, eaten along with sugary foods can counteract the cavity-causing effects of those foods. The chewiness and taste of these cheeses stimulate saliva flow, and the calcium and phosphates they contain form a protective barrier against plaque that helps slow mineral loss from your tooth enamel.

European studies have found that licorice—the real thing, not most licorice-flavored candy sold in the United States, which is flavored with anise—has antiseptic properties in the mouth. Licorice root, which is available in most stores that sell herbs, makes a pleasant-tasting tea.

Japanese researchers have found that polyphenols (powerful antioxidants) in oolong tea inhibited tooth decay in rats. Green tea has also been found to reduce cavities. It contains polyphenols as well, and its tannins have an antiseptic effect in the mouth. Green tea also contains fluoride.

A number of studies show that chocolate may also help combat cavities. Not only does cocoa contain bacteria-inhibiting tannins, but it is also alkaline—a chemical property that helps neutralize mouth acids.

Several studies have found that peanuts seem to neutralize acids in the mouth. Researchers note that fats in peanuts,

chocolate, and other foods coat the teeth, protecting them from acid, and may also kill germs in the mouth. (It certainly sounds like one of the better candy choices—for your teeth, if not your waistline—might be chocolate-covered peanuts.)

Dentists say that crude fiber, found mainly in raw fruits and vegetables, helps clear acid-forming carbohydrates out of the mouth quickly.

Despite these generalizations, attempts to classify foods as good or bad for your teeth have failed. As Dr. Moss puts it, it's not so much what you eat as much as how often you eat during the day that promotes tooth decay. Your teeth can't read labels, says Moss. They don't know the difference between milk, cereal, and cookies. Bacteria need only small amounts of sugar to reach maximum acid production. It's a myth that more sugar makes more cavities.

So there is really no such thing as a good food or a bad food when it comes to your teeth. Take all such lists, including the one on page 116, with a grain of salt.

A food's cavity-causing potential is determined more by how often you eat it and how long it sticks around in your mouth than by how much sugar it contains. For example, most soft drinks contain a lot of acid-forming sugar, but they don't stick to teeth as much as hard candy does. Sipping a soda throughout the day, however, is more damaging to your teeth than drinking it with lunch. Sipping it through a straw will do less harm than swigging it from a can.

Foods for a Healthy Smile

So what dietary tactics should you and your family adopt to protect your teeth? Here's what Drs. McGuire and Moss and many other dentists recommend.

🍎 **Feed your children a balanced diet high in vitamins and minerals.** Calcium, phosphorus, and fluorides build strong teeth in children up to age 16 or so, whose teeth are still forming. See that they get plenty of calcium-rich foods, such as milk, yogurt, and cheese. Vitamins A and C, found in rich supply in fresh fruits and vegetables, promote healthy gums and keep your immunity to bacteria strong.

🍎 **Enjoy high-fiber foods.** The fiber in foods gently helps scrape your teeth clean as you chew.

🍎 **Protect your teeth from sugar.** Studies have found that more than 95 percent of children's snacks contain carbohydrates or sugars that can create an acid bath for the teeth, according to Dr. Moss. If you or your children must eat starches or sweets between meals, brush or rinse those teeth vigorously with warm water soon afterward. A warm rinse will help dilute the acids in your mouth and rinse away food debris.

🍎 **Chew sugarless gum when you can't brush.** Chewing stimulates saliva flow, and the xylitol sweetener in sugarless gum may inhibit bacterial growth in your mouth.

🍎 **Look out for hidden sugars.** Many cough syrups and lozenges, breath mints, and antacids contain sugar. Treat them like candy and brush or rinse out your mouth after using them.

🍎 **Use a straw.** To minimize contact with acids and sugars in sodas and juice, sip them through a straw.

🍎 **Don't put a baby to bed with a bottle of juice or milk.** The worst cavities that dentists see in babies and very young children come from regularly going to bed with a bottle in the mouth. This creates a daily acid bath that destroys the teeth. If the baby must have a bottle at bedtime, make sure it's water.

healing diet

PROBLEM FOODS	GOOD FOODS
Sugary snacks	Cheese
Sodas	Dairy products
Starchy foods	Fruits and vegetables containing vitamins A and C
	Green tea

BEST ADVICE: Follow each meal with a good brushing. If you are in a place where you simply can't brush, rinse your mouth with warm water. Use a straw to drink sodas and juices.

depression

Do you dig a container of chocolate ice cream out of the freezer whenever you're feeling depressed? Or reach for an oversize bag of chips? If so, you're not alone.

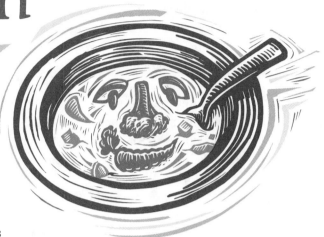

There is simply no denying that food and mood are connected. Medical researchers have even found a connection between diet and serious depression (diet is not the whole story).

Talk to anyone who has suffered from serious depression and you'll hear them recount black moods often accompanied by inexplicable bouts of sadness, insomnia, crying, and lethargy.

Depression makes you irritable. It messes with your sex drive. It can affect your concentration. It can bring on feelings of guilt, worthlessness, and alienation. And it often disturbs your eating patterns.

Approximately 17.6 million adults in the United States experience depression each year. Depression is one of the top 10 most likely reasons for someone to consult a family physician, and it costs our economy more than ulcers, diabetes, arthritis, or high blood pressure.

In most people depression is mild. They can still function but do so at a lower capacity and at a slower pace.

"Treatment for depression is relatively quick and painless," says Richard O'Connor, Ph.D., a psychotherapist in Lakeville, Connecticut, and author of *Undoing Depression: What Therapy Doesn't Teach You and Medication Can't Give You.* "The newer medications are very effective. Psychotherapy is just as effective. The two together are effective with 90 percent of patients."

According to Dr. O'Connor, who has battled depression himself, many people are reluctant to seek help for depression. "In a way, the reluctance to seek help is a symptom of the disease," he says. "Everybody I know who's depressed still struggles with the feeling that he ought to be able to snap out of it himself. Depression is an illness. It happens to the best people, and it can be overcome with help."

Food and Mood

Reasons for becoming depressed vary from individual to individual. In some people, depression is inherited. In others, depression begins after a devastating or catastrophic event occurs. No matter how depression begins, there are certain factors that can influence it even more—including diet.

Food is one thing that can affect anyone's mood. "Poor dietary habits are common in depressed people," says Stephanie Dixon, R.D., a nutrition consultant in San Francisco. "Certain dietary habits are definitely associated with mood changes. People turn to pasta or desserts when they're depressed. And because these foods have a deep effect on brain chemicals, they affect your mood. If someone is depressed, it's wise to see if their diet has something to do with it."

Think for a minute about what you eat each day. A few cups of coffee can make you jumpy and short-tempered. A chocolate bar provides an energy high for a while, but once the effect wears off, you feel more tired and sluggish than before you ingested the sugar. A bowl of pasta calms you at first, then makes you feel drowsy.

A glass or two of wine makes you feel relaxed and less uptight, but later you feel tired and cranky. A lunch eaten at a fast-food restaurant tastes great going down, but hours later you suffer from an energy low.

All this happens because the brain's neurotransmitters, which regulate behavior, are controlled by what you eat. The neurotransmitters are dopamine, serotonin, and norepinephrine. When your brain produces serotonin, tension is lowered. When the brain produces dopamine or norepinephrine, you feel alert and are able to think and act quickly.

The foods directly linked to these neurotransmitters are carbohydrates and proteins. Eating carbohydrates alone seems to have a calming effect, while proteins increase alertness. But carbohydrates and proteins aren't the only foods that influence depression.

Feel-Better Foods

Here's a look at how you can use certain eating behaviors and foods to help deal with depression.

 Eat a well-balanced diet. "People with depression don't know how to take good care of themselves," says Dr. O'Connor. "We don't know how to eat right. We have to practice eating healthy food in moderation at regular times."

The best way to maintain a healthy diet is by eating at least three different kinds of foods at each meal. During the day, try to have at least five servings of whole grains and cereals, two to four of fruits, three to five of vegetables, two to three of dairy and two to three of meat. Sound difficult?

It really isn't once you put your mind to it. Say your typical breakfast consists of a low-fat muffin and a cup of coffee. Add a piece of fruit or a glass of orange juice and a carton of low-fat yogurt or a glass of milk to your meal and you now have a breakfast that consists of a grain (could be more than one serving, depending on the size of the muffin), a fruit, and a dairy product.

 Stick to small meals. To regulate mood swings, Dixon suggests eating four to six small meals during the day instead of three large meals. Eating small meals keeps your blood sugar levels on an even keel. "A big meal of 1,000 calories or more affects mental alertness," she says. "You feel great right after the meal and then you become sluggish 30 minutes later."

Eating small meals throughout the day also prevents the peak-and-valley feeling.

When you only eat three meals a day, you run out of energy between each feeding. You're probably familiar with the 3 p.m. lull. Your body needs fuel and doesn't want to wait until dinner to get it.

👋 **Make sure you're eating enough.** If you expend an enormous amount of energy in the morning, don't skimp on breakfast. You've got to have a good breakfast, otherwise you're asking for mood swings and fatigue in the afternoon.

Here's a suggested day of meals from Dixon: Start with a breakfast of cereal with milk and a piece of fruit. Eat a mid-morning snack of a bagel with a piece of fruit. Make lunch a serving of linguine with clam sauce and a salad. Eat a mid-afternoon snack of pretzels with carrot and celery sticks. End the day with a dinner of grilled chicken, a baked potato, steamed broccoli, a piece of fruit, and some milk.

👋 **Balance your carbohydrates.** Consuming a pure carbohydrate, such as a bagel or a bowl of pasta, triggers an increase in the neurotransmitter called serotonin. And this will affect your mood. Carbohydrates have a calming effect. In fact, too many can leave you feeling sleepy and energy-starved. A better balance is achieved when you combine carbohydrates with some protein, which promotes alertness. Eat a turkey sandwich on a bagel, for instance.

depression
and weight gain

Do psychological disturbances cause some people to become fat? The answer varies greatly depending on whom you ask.

"It might be more of a situation of what came first, the chicken or the egg," says Richard O'Connor, Ph.D., a psychotherapist in Lakeville, Connecticut, and author of *Undoing Depression: What Therapy Doesn't Teach You and Medication Can't Give You.* "I know that depressed people don't eat as well as nondepressed people. We eat comfort foods, lose self-discipline, and overeat."

"When I see someone not eating well, I look to see if depression has some bearing," adds Stephanie Dixon, R.D., a nutrition consultant in San Francisco. Correcting bad eating habits isn't the remedy, but if you're depressed you usually don't care about dieting."

Depression also could very well be a consequence of being fat in a society that worships slimness. Having others reject you because you're overweight definitely causes unhappiness, which in turn may make it harder to lose the weight.

Or add some shrimp or grilled chicken to your pasta.

You also can tailor your diet to how you're feeling. If you're particularly anxious, you may want to consume more carbohydrates than protein. If you're feeling lethargic, eat a meal that's higher in protein than carbohydrates.

herbal relief

It's being heralded as the herb of the moment, but people have been ingesting St. John's wort—a yellow-flowered plant—for some 2,000 years. The herb has been popular in Europe for about 15 years as a natural remedy for depression. It's now just as popular in the United States thanks to a 1997 review in the *British Medical Journal*. The review chronicled 23 studies involving 1,757 patients in which St. John's wort (*Hypericum perforatum* as scientists call it) worked three times better than a placebo. The herb also produces fewer side effects than synthetic antidepressants.

How does it work? St. John's wort appears to affect the brain in the same way Prozac does—by prolonging the activity of the mood-enhancing brain chemical serotonin. "Of my patients who are using St. John's wort, most are reporting mild improvement," says Dr. O'Connor. "From what I understand, there's reason to believe that it may be of some help for mild cases of depression. However, people who are severely depressed or are taking a prescription antidepressant should be discouraged from stopping their current medication and taking St. John's wort without consulting their doctor first."

🍎 **Say no to fat.** When you're feeling depressed, comfort foods are what you crave. Food high in saturated fat—fast-food hamburgers and fries, a pint of premium ice cream—may taste great going down, but you'll end up feeling more depressed in the long run. Fatty foods slow the body down. You feel tired and sluggish. That's because fats inhibit the synthesis of neurotransmitters by the brain by causing the blood cells to clump together. The result is poor circulation, particularly to the brain.

🍎 **Watch that sugar.** The body's reaction to sugar is quick and simple. Eat a slice of cake or a handful of cookies and initially you feel great. Your dark mood is suddenly gone and you're full of energy. But this high you're

feeling is quickly accompanied by fatigue and a return of your depression.

Dixon doesn't counsel her nutrition clients away from desserts entirely, but she does warn them of the perils. "I tell them to enjoy dessert if they feel like it, but to remember how it will bring them up and then right down again," she explains. "It may seem to relieve their depression at first, but the aftermath can leave them feeling worse than they originally did."

Another problem with sugar foods is the calories and the accompanying weight gain. "Sugar keeps you satiated for a while, but later you feel bad about yourself," says Dr.

O'Connor. "You're angry at yourself for pigging out again. Plus the added weight contributes to depression."

🍎 **Get enough iron.** Low reserves of iron can make you sluggish and lacking in concentration. Iron is also important for regular functioning of the nervous system. To boost your iron intake, Dixon suggests eating lean cuts of beef, lamb, and pork, and the dark meat of chicken or turkey three to four times per week.

Look for bread and cereal with the words "iron-enriched" or "iron-fortified" on the label. It's best to eat these foods with a source of vitamin C (orange juice with your cereal, tomato on your turkey sandwich) to enhance iron absorption. Also, refrain from drinking coffee or tea with all your meals since these beverages interfere with iron absorption. In addition to lean meat, the best food sources for iron are prunes, apricots, spinach, green peas, and broccoli.

🍎 **Use caution with caffeine.** Caffeine can make depression worse. Heavy coffee drinking brings on symptoms that mimic an anxiety attack, including headache, jitteriness, upset stomach, and difficulty sleeping. Studies indicate that psychiatric patients who drink a lot of caffeine-containing beverages tend to be more depressed than other patients.

"Too much caffeine can contribute to the feeling of being out of control," says Dr. O'Connor. "You're put on a cycle of going up but then coming down."

If you're depressed, it's best to limit or entirely stop your caffeine intake. Don't stop your caffeine intake cold turkey because you're likely to suffer a withdrawal headache. The best way to wean yourself off caffeine is gradually. Reduce the number of cups of coffee, tea, or soda by one or two a day until you're totally off caffeine.

Replace your caffeinated beverages with the following: decaffeinated coffee or tea, herbal teas, hot water with a lemon wedge, broth, or warm cider.

Better yet, instead of a coffee break, try an exercise break. A quick walk outside—or around the office—is better than another cup of coffee or tea. In addition, exercise, even moderate amounts, raises self-esteem and gives you an energy boost.

🍎 **Say no to alcohol.** You had a terrible day, and there's no one around to talk to. You're feeling down and helpless. So you pour yourself a glass of wine.

After the second glass, you start feeling a bit better. You begin to forget your problems. So you pour yourself another glass, then another. Soon that good feeling vanishes, and you're just tired and cranky. The sadness returns, too.

"Alcohol is a no-no if you're depressed," says Dr. O'Connor. "It's a depressant. Alcohol's first effect on the system is to depress your inhibitions, but after 30 minutes it depresses the rest of you. Your judgment becomes depressed, and you begin to do things you aren't proud of. And that just eats away at your self-esteem and makes you more unhappy."

Alcohol is also dehydrating. That effects the body by making you tired. If you do drink an occasional beer or glass of wine, drink plenty of water also. Match each glass of alcohol that you drink with the same amount of water.

healing diet

PROBLEM FOODS

Alcohol
Coffee and tea
Fatty foods
Sugary foods

GOOD FOODS

Foods containing iron, such as
    lean red meat
Vegetables

BEST ADVICE: Everyone experiences the blues from time to time. But if you get into a depression that just won't quit, see your doctor for treatment.

diabetes

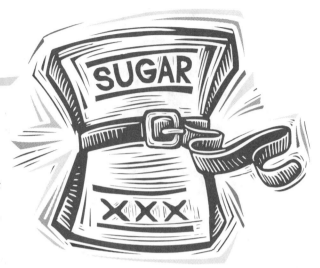

The disease didn't stop Cézanne from creating his colorful French masterpieces. Nor did it hamper the inventive mind of Thomas Edison. And it wasn't about to interfere with the lilting voice of jazz great Ella Fitzgerald. What health challenge did all these famous people have in common? Diabetes—and they all lived full, prolific lives in spite of it.

Diabetes is a disease in which the body does not produce or properly use insulin, a hormone that is needed to convert sugar, starches, and other food into energy.

Without enough insulin, your body cannot move blood sugar into the cells. Sugar then builds up in the bloodstream, causing your blood glucose level (or "sugar") to rise too high.

Many people with diabetes live happy, healthy lives. However, if glucose levels are not properly managed, serious complications can arise, such as heart attacks, strokes, blindness, kidney disease, nerve disease, and sexual dysfunction.

The cause of diabetes is a mystery, although both genetics and environmental factors, such as obesity and lack of exercise, appear to play roles.

Types of Diabetes

There are two main types of diabetes: Type 1 (once called juvenile-onset or insulin-dependent) diabetes, is an autoimmune disease in which the body does not produce any insulin. This kind of diabetes most often occurs in children and young adults. People with type 1 diabetes must take insulin injections every day. About 10 percent of people with diabetes have type 1.

Type 2, or non-insulin-dependent, is a metabolic disorder resulting from the body's inability to make enough, and/or properly use, insulin.

About 90 percent of people with diabetes have type 2, making it the most common form of the disease. About 15 million Americans have this type, but only two-thirds even know it.

The number of Americans with diabetes has risen almost 50 percent since 1983 and has tripled since 1958, according to a survey by the National Institute of Diabetes and Digestive and Kidney Diseases. Researchers point to increased rates of obesity and of lack of exercise, both of which can raise the risk of type 2 diabetes.

Are You at Risk?

If caught early enough in the initial stages, type 2 diabetes can be treated with a healthy diet and regular physical activity.

Here's a quick test to help you determine if you are at risk for diabetes:

Type 1:
● Do any of your sisters or brothers have type 1?
● Do either of your parents have this type?

Type 2:
● Are you older than 45?
● Do you have a family history of diabetes?
● Are you overweight?
● Do you lead a sedentary lifestyle?
● Do you have low HDL cholesterol?
● Do you have high triglycerides?
● Do you belong to the following racial and ethnic groups—African Americans, Hispanic Americans, Asian and Pacific Islanders, or Native Americans?
● Did you have diabetes while you were pregnant?
● Did you have a baby weighing 9 pounds or more at birth?

If you said yes to any of these questions, discuss your risk of diabetes with your physician. The American Diabetes Association (ADA) suggests everyone older than 45 be tested every three years with a simple fasting blood glucose test.

The Team Approach

If you have diabetes, you are not alone in your health care. There is a whole host of health professionals who can help you pave the path to vibrant health and wellness. No matter which type of diabetes you have, you should be under the medical supervision of a diabetes management team. The members of this team are based on your specific needs.

Everyone who has this disease should see a diabetes specialist, such as an endocrinologist, at least once every six months. You should also periodically see a nurse educator and a registered dietitian.

If you feel the need for it, your team could also include an exercise physiologist, social worker, psychologist, or other mental health professional to help you cope with the stresses and challenges of living with a chronic condition. Some people also find consulting a member of the clergy helpful.

Everyone with diabetes should visit an ophthalmologist for an annual eye exam to make sure any eye problems associated with diabetes are caught early and treated before they become serious.

Take Charge with Proper Nutrition

A major key to treating diabetes is following a meal plan specific to your individual profile—your glucose metabolism, tastes, lifestyle, and other medical conditions. The goal of this plan is to keep blood-sugar levels as close to normal as possible.

"Nutrition plays an integral role in the health and well-being of people with diabetes," says registered dietitian Joan Hill, director of Educational Services and Programs at the Joslin Diabetes Center in Boston. "The food choices you make are

symptoms **of diabetes**

Since millions of people may have diabetes and not know it, it pays to familiarize yourself with the following warning signs. In most cases, there are no symptoms at all. People can live for months, even years, without knowing they have the disease. Contact your physician if any of these symptoms occur:

- Frequent urination
- Unusual thirst
- Frequent infections
- Extreme hunger
- Blurred vision
- Unusual weight loss

- Cuts/bruises that are slow to heal
- Extreme fatigue
- Tingling/numbness in the hands or feet
- Irritability
- Recurring skin, gum, or bladder infections

extremely important for blood glucose management, as well as reducing the risk factors for complications from diabetes."

Basically, what's healthy for you is what's healthy for anyone who wants to eat well. Focus on eating less fat and fewer sugary foods, and adding a variety of fresh fruits, vegetables, whole grains, lean meats, poultry, and fish.

Your individual food plan should give you enough calories to stay at a healthy weight for you. This is a weight you can achieve and stay with, and one that you and your diabetes management team agree on.

Here are some tips to help you make smart food choices, so you can maintain control of your diabetes.

Know your numbers. "You need to be directly involved in your diabetes care," urges Hill.

"Negotiate with your health care team so they know which foods you like and which foods you don't particularly care for."

Foods that have the greatest impact on blood sugar levels are those that are richest in carbohydrates.

The percentage of carbs recommended in the diet varies, depending on whether a person wishes to lose weight and how often that individual exercises. Ask your health care professional what percentage of your total daily calories should come from carbohydrates. (One gram of carbohydrate provides 4 calories.)

Get the right amount of protein. For most people with diabetes, the ADA recommends getting up to 20 percent of the daily calories from protein (poultry, fish, dairy, and vegetables). If you have kidney disease, talk to your doctor about lowering your protein intake. (One gram of protein provides 4 calories.)

Watch those fats. A healthy intake of fat is 30 percent or less of the daily calories.

diabetes & pregnancy

If you are a woman with diabetes and wish to start a family, your future has never looked brighter.

However, it is important to check with your doctor for specific guidance at this time. "Maintaining excellent blood glucose control is critical to forming a healthy fetus, especially in the first 12 weeks of pregnancy," says registered dietitian Joan Hill, director of Educational Services and Programs at the Joslin Diabetes Center in Boston. "Try to have good control at least three months prior to pregnancy."

While you are pregnant, you need a diabetes treatment plan that helps keep your meals, exercise, and insulin in balance. This plan will change as your pregnancy progresses.

You will also need to test your blood glucose often and keep a record of your test results. With your blood glucose in the near-normal range and good medical care, your chances of a trouble-free pregnancy and a healthy baby are nearly as good as they are for a woman without diabetes.

Gestational Diabetes

About 5 percent of pregnant women develop gestational diabetes, a condition that will disappear when the pregnancy is over. The American Diabetes Association recommends that all pregnant women should be screened for gestational diabetes (also called hyperglycemia) between the 24th and 28th weeks of pregnancy. By then, the placenta has begun to make the hormones that lead to insulin resistance.

Women who have had gestational diabetes are at increased risk for later developing type 2 diabetes.

Less than 10 percent should come from saturated fats (animal products). Up to 10 percent should come from polyunsaturated fats, which are found in plant products, fish, and other seafood. Keep in mind that each gram of fat provides 9 calories, which is more than double as many calories as a gram of carbohydrate or protein.

Keep cholesterol down. Daily cholesterol intake should be 300 milligrams or less. Cholesterol is found in animal products such as dairy products, egg yolks, and meats.

Get your weight where it belongs. Most people with type 2 diabetes are overweight. Lose the excess weight, and you may be able to reduce your medication or stop taking it all together.

The best way to lose weight is to eat fewer calories and increase your activity level. Minor changes can help. For example, cutting out 250 calories per day and walking briskly for 20 minutes three to five times a week may be all you need to do to control weight and blood glucose levels.

"Losing just 10 to 20 pounds improves blood glucose and blood fats in people with diabetes," says registered dietitian Nadine Pazder, spokesperson for the ADA and certified diabetes educator. "Some people look at the 40 to 50 pounds they need to lose and get discouraged," says Pazder. "They feel it's hopeless, so they don't even try. They need to set small, realistic goals, such as losing 5 to 7 pounds. Once they do that, they can keep going until they've reached their healthy weight."

Make small changes. "Fat is calorically dense, so even cutting small amounts of fat from the diet can help," says Hill. "One of my patients always used cream in his coffee, and he drank about eight cups a day. So I asked him to switch from cream to whole milk. He actually lost weight just from making that minor substitution."

Play cards. With steak, that is. On average, Americans eat too much fat. To reduce our risk of heart disease, the nation's top killer, we need to eat less saturated fat and cholesterol. "People with diabetes are at a greater risk of cardiovascular disease and stroke, so they have even more reason to watch their fat intake," says Hill. "A quick and easy way to cut down on fat is to reduce the size of meat on your plate. The next time you're eating, choose a cut that is the size of a deck of playing cards."

Broaden your horizons. "I advise my patients to substitute a large steak with a smaller piece of meat cut into strips and tossed into a stir-fry with plenty of vegetables," explains Hill. "It's also a good idea to start thinking this way when you're eating out."

Fish for health. Triglycerides are a type of blood fat associated with an increased risk of heart attacks and hardening of the arteries. In a small Canadian study of people with type 2 diabetes, participants lowered their triglyceride level when they took omega-3 fatty-acid supplements. However, according to the ADA, fish oil supplements can raise blood glucose and are not recommended because they are not standardized, and some don't even contain omega-3 fatty acids.

"To keep the benefits of omega-3 fatty acids," advises Hill, "incorporate more cold-water fish in your diet, such as salmon, tuna, bass, mackerel, sardines, herring, bluefish, and halibut."

Fill your plate with veggies. "Vegetables are a great source of an array of nutrients, without adding many extra calories," says Hill. "Cover half your plate with a wide variety of vegetables, one-quarter with complex carbohydrates, and the remaining quarter with meat."

Examples of complex carbohydrates include grains (barley, buckwheat, millet, oats, quinoa, rice, rye, and triticale), pasta, bread, potatoes, and beans.

Have a bowl of beans. Several studies have shown that a high-fiber diet reduces the body's demand for insulin. "Fiber is very important for people with diabetes," says Hill. "Fiber fills you up, so you'll eat less, and is not broken down to blood glucose." High-fiber foods also help lower cholesterol.

Good sources of fiber include beans, peas, apples, barley, carrots, prunes, figs, and oat bran.

kids with diabetes

If your child has type 1 diabetes, you know what a challenge it can be to keep him or her on a strict diet. Here are some menu planning tips from the Juvenile Diabetes Foundation International:

Breakfast. It's okay to serve your child presweetened cereals. Just be sure to watch the overall amount of carbohydrates for the day. For example, 1 ounce (¾ cup) of S'Mores Grahams has 24 grams of carbohydrates. One ounce (¾ cup) of Cap'n Crunch Peanut Butter Crunch has 21.6 grams of carbs. And 1 ounce (1 cup) of Rice Krispies has 24.8 grams of carbs. So while you might eat more Rice Krispies by volume, you'd actually get fewer carbohydrates by eating the Peanut Butter Crunch.

Lunch. Is your child getting bored with the same old peanut butter sandwich for lunch? Here are some other good protein sources to provide a little more variety: Cheese, hard-cooked eggs, cottage cheese, sugar-free yogurt, ham, turkey, and a kid-favorite—nachos.

Dinner. Between after-school extracurricular activities, special occasions, and holidays, it's tough to feed kids dinner at the exact same time every day. The dinner meal is important because it affects the time you give insulin so it will stay in the child's system throughout the night. If you know your child is not going to be able to eat dinner at the regular time, change what you provide for lunch and the timing, to keep blood sugar on an even keel. For a 3 p.m. Thanksgiving dinner, for example, encourage your child to have a snack at lunch. Give the evening insulin at the usual dinner time and the evening snack at the usual evening time.

🍎 **Reach for cereal.** The Nurses' Health Study is an ongoing research project that has followed more than 120,000 women since 1976. According to one report from the study, women who ate more fiber, especially fiber from breakfast cereal, had a lower risk of type 2 diabetes. Breakfast cereals come in a wide variety of tastes and shapes, and they are a quick and easy way to sneak fiber into your diet any time of the day or night.

Check the labels the next time you're shopping. Choose cereals that contain at least 5 grams of fiber per ½-cup serving.

Time it right. "An excellent way to help prevent the spikes and lows in glucose levels is to eat at the same time every day," says Hill. "Aim for at least three meals a day. You can also reduce the size of each meal and work in snacks."

For example, for breakfast you might have a small bagel with low-fat cream cheese, half a grapefruit, and coffee, then at mid morning have a slice of whole wheat toast with low-fat cheese. "Just be careful not to exceed your calorie budget for the day," she adds.

Know your A-C-Es. In a study done in England, doctors examined blood samples from 28 people with type 1 diabetes and 24 people with type 2 diabetes. Researchers concluded that people with diabetes have impaired protection from antioxidants. These include vitamins A, C, and E. This impairment may increase their chances of developing complications from diabetes.

Good food sources of vitamin A include carrots, pumpkin, and sweet potatoes. Vitamin C can be found in cherries, orange juice, and red bell peppers. Vitamin E can be found in vegetable oils and wheat germ.

Consider chromium. This mineral helps your body metabolize carbohydrates and fats. If you don't have enough chromium, your body has a difficult time regulating blood sugar.

"In preliminary research, chromium supplements look promising, but more studies are needed," says Hill. Discuss taking chromium supplements with your doctor.

The RDA for chromium is 50 to 200 micrograms. Good food sources of chromium include whole grains, fortified cereals, spinach, and carrots.

healing diet

PROBLEM FOODS	GOOD FOODS
Fatty foods	Breakfast cereal
Sugary foods	Fish
	Fruits
	Lean meats
	Vegetables
	Whole grains

BEST ADVICE: Enlist the help of a health professional to create a dietary program custom tailored to meet your individual needs.

diverticulitis

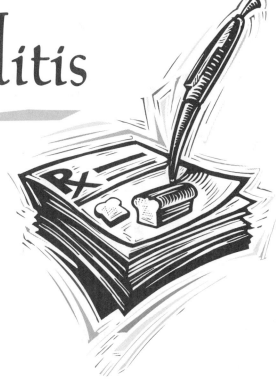

How about this for irony? The very foods that cause diverticulitis are the foods doctors prescribe as a short-term cure.

Before delving into the details about the strong connection between diet and this common condition, you need the answer to one important question: Exactly what is diverticulitis? It occurs when tiny sacs (diverticula) develop in the large intestine. Since these sacs are painless, most people are unaware they have them. And yet they're very common in people ages 50 and older. By some estimates nearly half of Americans older than 60 have diverticula, enough that this condition has its own name—diverticulosis.

It could well be the most common disease that no one knows they have. However, with 15 to 20 percent of diverticulosis cases, the diverticula become infected. That's when you develop diverticulitis. And, if you have it, you definitely know that something is wrong.

Symptoms of diverticulitis include persistent and often severe abdominal pain, fever, rectal bleeding, nausea, and cramping. Some say an attack of diverticulitis feels similar to appendicitis, except with diverticulitis, the pain occurs on the left side or the lower abdominal region, instead of the right side where the appendix is located. Since these symptoms can also point to more serious conditions such as a tumor, it's vital that you see a doctor if you experience lengthy and acute abdominal pain. (Don't try to diagnose this one yourself.)

Feasting on Fat

If you visit your doctor with these symptoms, you will very likely get a blood test to see if infection is present. The doctor will also examine your abdomen for tenderness. And with imaging technologies such as ultrasound your doctor can actually see the diverticular sacs. Once your doctor is sure you have diverticulitis, you'll probably get a prescription for antibiotics to fight the infection and, hopefully, a few days' rest at home. A brief hospital stay is possible.

Now here's where diet enters the picture. While you're recovering, you may be told to avoid foods entirely for a short period or else stick to a liquid diet. Later, your doctor may prescribe a diet that's high in fats. So expect to subsist on creamy soups, mild spaghetti, and the like until the infection heals. At the same time you'll be asked to avoid fruits, grains, vegetables, and other high-fiber foods. Sounds like just the opposite of what all the health-food articles have been saying for years, doesn't it?

Here's the reason: High-fiber foods can't be absorbed by the small intestine. And so they pass rapidly to the large intestine, where they're finally discharged as waste. Because these fibrous foods are so bulky, they stretch and strain the large intestine in the process. Not a good thing when the large intestine is infected.

A low-fiber diet does just the opposite. Fats and proteins become quickly absorbed in the small intestine. This time only a little food matter remains. And as with fibrous foods, this material also moves on to the large intestine. But since the remainders of a high-fat diet don't take up as much space, this food matter tends to linger a lot longer in the large intestine before being passed on as waste. Because the food simply sits there, the large intestine gets the rest it needs to heal properly.

Fiber Fallacies and Facts

Low-fiber foods have proved such an important part of treating people with diverticulitis that doctors once believed a low-fiber diet might actually prevent future attacks. Remember the old-fashioned name for fiber—roughage? Well, researchers once thought that fiber was too rough for people with diverticulitis. They theorized that coarse, fibrous grains, vegetables, and the like could actually abrade the lower intestinal walls and create conditions that lead to infection. For that reason, people with diverticulitis were once warned to forever afterward steer clear of popcorn, tomatoes, and grapes. It was thought the kernels and seeds might scratch the intestinal wall.

All that has changed. Now researchers know that just the opposite is true. When the antibiotics finally kill off a diverticulitis infection, doctors now gradually switch their patients back to high-fiber foods. With the lower intestine now nicely healed, the last thing your doctor wants is for low-fiber food matter to linger there.

And here's why: Doctors now realize that foods that do linger in the large intestine tend to get trapped by the diverticula. That can ultimately lead to infection and another potentially painful bout of diverticulitis. The bulky fibers come to your rescue and clear out other food matter that otherwise might linger in the large intestine.

Little wonder researchers at the USDA and elsewhere recommend that you get 20 to 35 grams per day of fiber—about twice what most Americans eat. If that sounds like you'll be downing bowl after bowl of wheat germ, never fear. It's fairly easy to get this much fiber if you eat the right kinds of foods, namely lots of fruits, vegetables, and whole grains.

Here's an example of a simple one-day menu, adapted from *Gastrointestinal Health*, by Steven Peikin, M.D., that more than fills the fiber quota:

Breakfast:
½ melon
2 oatmeal raisin muffins
2 teaspoons margarine
1 cup 1% low-fat milk

Lunch:
Turkey soup
1 slice corn bread
1 peanut butter bar
1 cup 1% low-fat milk

Dinner:
Fettuccini with clam sauce
1 whole grain roll
1 teaspoon margarine or butter
Spinach salad
1 peach

Calories: 2,011
Fat grams: 52
Fiber grams: 24

There are a number of other easy ways to fortify your diet with fiber, says Dr. Peikin. Here are a few:

Forget the white stuff. Switch to whole grain breads and rolls. And serve whole wheat pasta.

Go for nuts. Add nuts and beans to soups, salads, and casseroles.

Love that fruit. Reach for fruit when you want a snack. Eat fruit for dessert often and top off other desserts with fruit.

Don't get dehydrated. As you raise the fiber content of your diet, drink lots of fluids. Fiber absorbs up to 15 times its weight in water, and that's water that would otherwise go straight to your system.

So drink at least 8 cups per day to make up the difference.

(See "Constipation," which begins on page 105, for additional tips on adding fiber and keeping things flowing smoothly.)

Be there for the long haul. Barring surgery, any diverticula that you have will be with you for life.

That's why anyone with diverticulitis should commit to a high-fiber diet for the rest of their lives, says Dr. Peikin.

In fact, this is just the kind of food humans were designed to eat, he says. Studies as far back as 1983 show that Japanese people who came to America experienced more diverticulitis as their diet shifted away from traditional fibers found in rice and vegetables and toward a Western diet made up more of meats and full-fat dairy products. Similar studies looked at the high-fiber diet of rural African populations where diverticulitis is very rare. By comparison, disease levels have climbed among urban Africans who eat more meats and fatty processed foods.

As Dr. Peikin explains it: Human beings simply haven't evolved yet to handle the high-fat diet that's part of modern society. Maybe in 100 generations our digestive systems will have adapted enough so that they thrive on fast-food burgers and double cheese pizzas. But until then, it's better to stick with the fiber.

healing diet

PROBLEM FOODS	GOOD FOODS
During and immediately after an attack:	**During and immediately after an attack:**
Beans	Fasting, followed by a liquid
Fruits	diet, then a diet high in creamy
Nuts	soups and dairy products
Vegetables	
Whole grains	**Long-term:**
	High-fiber foods
Long-term:	
Full-fat dairy products	
Excessive amounts of meat and	
processed foods	

BEST ADVICE: If you believe you have diverticulitis, see a doctor for diagnosis before embarking on any dietary change.

134

fatigue

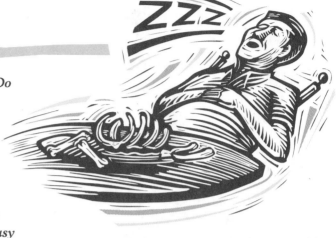

Has your energy level taken a hike? Do you need a cup of coffee in the morning to kick-start your day and another cup midmorning to help keep you going? Do you have trouble concentrating after lunch or often skip activities in the evening because you're too worn out? Do you blame your lack of oomph on your busy schedule? Do you assume you were born this way, or, worse yet, that you're just getting old? Think again.

Fatigue is a symptom of many emotional, mental, and physical disorders, and its causes vary from poor nutrition, inadequate sleep, and stress to overwork, infection, and disease. This is probably why it is one of the most common health complaints. However, the answer to waning energy could be as simple as what and when you eat.

Eat Breakfast

People who skip breakfast struggle more with weight problems and low energy later in the day than do people who take time to eat, according to C. Wayne Callaway, M.D., associate clinical professor of medicine at George Washington University in Washington, D.C. "You can't measure a person's perceived energy level, but you can measure metabolic rate, which is lower in breakfast skippers compared to

people who take time to eat a morning meal," says Dr. Callaway.

Why is breakfast the best antidote for exhaustion? This is the only time during the day that eight, and perhaps 10 or more, hours have gone by between meals. "By sunrise, the body is essentially fasting and that first meal of the day literally breaks the fast," says Gretchen Hill, Ph.D., associate professor at Michigan State University in East Lansing. During the hours since dinner, and even while sleeping, the body still needs fuel to keep the heart beating, nerves transmitting messages, eyes blinking, and cells dividing and growing—in other words, all the millions of metabolic processes that combine to keep you alive need fuel.

Much of that fuel comes from readily available stores of glucose in the blood, liver, and muscles. More than half of your glucose reserves are drained by morning and need a kick-start that only comes from eating a carbohydrate-rich meal. Allow even four hours to pass between meals and blood sugar levels drop, resulting in fatigue, poor concentration, irritability, and lethargy. Double the time to eight or even 12 hours,

what is
chronic fatigue syndrome?

Chronic Fatigue Syndrome (CFS) is intense, disabling fatigue that severely restricts daily activities for weeks, months, or even years. CFS affects about 1 percent of Americans, two-thirds of which are young, middle-class women. Other symptoms of CFS include persistent flulike aches, mild fever, sore throat, swollen lymph nodes, muscle weakness, muscle fatigue (especially after exercise), headaches, joint pain, depression, sleep disturbances, and inability to concentrate.

A diagnosis of CFS is usually made when an individual has multiple symptoms persisting for up to six months; however, the cause of this disorder remains unknown.

Researchers have several theories regarding CFS. Some suspect the cause to be a viral infection and note that a serious infection of some type is often present before CFS develops. Other researchers report disturbances in blood pressure or the immune system, such as suppression of immune system cells. Still other researchers note that people with CFS have some symptoms in common with psychiatric disorders and that some people with CFS benefit from antidepressant drugs.

There are no foolproof dietary solutions to this condition. The theory that avoiding all funguslike foods (such as mushrooms and yeasted breads) curbs symptoms has not been supported by research. A person with CFS should follow the dietary guidelines for preventing and treating general fatigue and consult a physician for other therapies.

and you can imagine the energy-draining effects of failing to stop and refuel.

You might feel fine, full of energy, and raring to go for the first few hours after you wake up even if you skip breakfast. That burst of energy comes from a mind and body revved from a good night's sleep. This initial energy glow wears off, however, as the morning's demands stress a body already running on fumes. "While breakfast increases the metabolic rate by 25 percent, which is one of the reasons why people report they feel better after eating in the morning, skipping breakfast slows the metabolic rate and leaves a person feeling tired, sluggish, even cold," says Dr. Callaway. By afternoon, even if you eat a relatively good lunch in an effort to boost lagging energy levels, you never will regain the day-long energy you would have had if you'd taken five minutes to eat breakfast.

🍎 **Do eat breakfast.** If you are a seasoned breakfast avoider, Dr. Callaway recommends

what's your excuse?

Whatever the excuse for not eating breakfast, it isn't worth the cost to your health, energy level, and waistline. Here are the top three reasons why people skip the most important meal of the day, as well as the reasons why those excuses aren't good enough:

Excuse Number 1: "I don't have time to eat in the morning."

It takes only five minutes to prepare a healthful breakfast. If you are pressed for time, prepare your breakfast the night before, then be a "dashboard diner" and take your breakfast with you in the morning.

Excuse Number 2: "I'm not hungry in the morning."

You should be hungry in the morning, since it has been eight or more hours since the last meal. If you're not hungry, it's probably a result of ignoring hunger pangs, so they eventually went away. Or, it could be a sign of overeating the night before, so that you've set up a vicious cycle of skipping breakfast then overeating the rest of the day. Start eating a light breakfast, even if you are not hungry, and stop to refuel frequently during the day.

Within three weeks you will reset your appetite clock to wake up hungry and ready for breakfast.

Excuse Number 3: "I'm hungry all day if I eat breakfast."

Increased hunger is not caused by breakfast. Rather, take a look at the foods you choose. Sugary foods eaten alone, whether they are sugar-coated cereals and doughnuts or fruit, don't stick with you and leave you hungry within an hour or so after breakfast.

Instead, combine complex carbohydrates with protein foods, such as whole wheat toast topped with a slice of cheese, along with fruit to curb hunger and stay satisfied longer.

Hunger attacks soon after breakfast also could be a sign you didn't eat enough the day before. Irregular eating habits cause fluctuations in blood sugar and brain chemistry, which put a damper on your energy level and trigger hunger. In both cases, a nutritious breakfast followed by several small meals and snacks throughout the day is the best way to maintain steady blood sugar and energy levels.

that you start eating breakfast, even if you aren't hungry.

🍎 **Give it time.** "It takes two to three weeks to reset the appetite clock," says Dr. Callaway. After that, you should notice a

boost in energy and less problems with overeating later in the day.

🍎 **Don't be so sweet.** Avoid high-sugar breakfasts, such as doughnuts and coffee, that provide an initial energy boost but leave you drowsy within a few hours. Instead, choose meals with a mix of protein and starch that will maintain blood sugar (and energy) levels throughout the morning. Examples include egg substitutes and toast, whole grain cereal and milk, or an English muffin with low-fat cheese and orange juice.

🍎 **Use your imagination.** Don't feel that your first meal of the day has to look like a typical American breakfast. Try nontraditional foods, such as leftover pizza, toast and soup, or a sandwich.

Eat to Sleep

Ninety-five percent of adults experience some form of insomnia during their lives, and missing a good night's sleep leaves you less than energized the next day. Insomnia is a complex issue with numerous causes, but sometimes the answer to your sleep problems might start at the dining table, not in the bedroom. (See "Insomnia," which begins on page 209, for a more detailed look at the intricate connection between diet and poor sleep.)

🍎 **Watch that caffeine.** A cup of coffee or tea or even a glass of cola or a chocolate doughnut is a quick pick-me-up that might do you in. "People snack on chocolate or drink coffee during the afternoon and then wonder why they can't sleep at night," says Robert Sack, Ph.D., professor of psychiatry and director of Adult Sleep Disorder Medicine at the Oregon Health Sciences University in Portland. "Even small amounts of caffeine can affect sleep architecture, especially in people sensitive to the effects of caffeine."

If you are a coffee drinker troubled by sleep problems, try eliminating caffeine. If you feel and sleep better after two weeks of being caffeine-free, then avoid caffeine permanently. You can try adding back one or two cups after the two-week trial, but cut back if insomnia reappears.

🍎 **Go easy on alcohol.** A nightcap may make you sleepy at first, but you'll sleep less soundly and wake up more tired as a result. Alcohol and other depressants suppress a phase of sleeping called REM (rapid eye movement) where most of your dreaming occurs. Less REM is associated with more night awakenings and restless sleep. One glass of wine with dinner probably won't hurt. However, avoid drinking any alcohol within two hours of bedtime and never mix alcohol with sleeping pills.

🍎 **Eat a light evening meal.** What and how much you eat for dinner could be at the root of your insomnia. Big dinners make you temporarily drowsy, but they also prolong digestive action, which keeps you awake. Instead, eat a light evening meal that includes a small serving of protein-rich chicken, extra-lean meat, or fish to help curb middle-of-the-night snack attacks.

🍎 **Think twice about spice.** Spicy or gas-forming foods also might contribute to sleep problems. Dishes seasoned with garlic, chilies, cayenne, or other hot spices can cause nagging heartburn or indigestion, and the flavor-enhancer MSG (monosodium glutamate) causes vivid dreaming and restless sleep in some people. Gas-forming foods or eating too fast can cause abdominal discomfort, which in turn interferes with sound sleep. Try avoiding spicy foods at dinner time. Limit your intake of gas-forming

stamina-building
meals and snacks

The basic principles of eating for energy are not complicated, but they can take some getting used to. Here are some good, quick answers to that all-important question: What should I eat for my next meal?

Good-Start Breakfasts:
- A toasted frozen whole wheat waffle topped with fat-free sour cream and fresh blueberries
- A flour tortilla filled with cottage cheese and fresh fruit, warmed in the microwave
- A low-fat whole wheat bran muffin with applesauce and yogurt
- An English muffin topped with 1 ounce fat-free cheese and broiled until bubbly, served with a glass of orange juice
- A bowl of Nutri-Grain, Shredded Wheat, or Grape-Nuts with low-fat milk and fresh fruit

Energy-Boosting Lunches:
- Two tortillas filled with shredded carrots, zucchini, fat-free refried beans, and salsa, served with low-fat milk and fruit
- A cup of vegetable soup and a grilled-cheese sandwich on whole wheat bread, served with sliced tomatoes and orange juice
- A tuna sandwich on rye bread with sliced cucumbers, served with fresh fruit and low-fat milk

Snacks:
- Fresh strawberries, blueberries, or blackberries
- Light microwave popcorn, natural
- Fresh kiwi dunked in yogurt flavored with shredded orange peel, poppyseed, and cinnamon, or fresh kiwi mixed with low-fat kiwi-strawberry yogurt
- Fresh fruit and nonfat milk smoothies
- Dried apricots and almonds mixed with low-fat granola
- One-half honeydew melon filled with nonfat yogurt
- One-half papaya filled with cottage cheese
- Carrots dunked in peanut butter
- Crisp vegetables dunked in curried nonfat yogurt dip

foods to the morning hours and thoroughly chew food to avoid gulping air.

🍎 **Use food to soothe the savage breast.** The evening snack might be the best alternative to sleeping pills. An all-carbohydrate snack, such as crackers and fruit or toast and jam, triggers the release of serotonin, which aids sleep.

"According to our studies," comments Gary Zammit, Ph.D., director of the Sleep Disorders Institute at St. Luke's Hospital in New York City, "a light carbohydrate-rich snack an hour or so before bedtime might help some people sleep longer and more soundly." A glass of warm milk, a protein-rich beverage, probably doesn't affect serotonin levels. But the warm liquid does soothe and relax and provides a feeling of satiety. Any of these effects might also help facilitate sleep.

Quick-Fix Quackery

Ever notice how people in commercials for candy or soft drinks are so perky? The implied message is that a quick (and sweet) pick-me-up will get you going, but in reality these foods and beverages are likely to produce a short-term high followed by a long-term crash.

A sugary snack can send some people on a blood sugar roller coaster that leads to fatigue. Researchers at Kansas State University in Manhattan measured mood in 120 women who drank 12 ounces of water or beverages sweetened with either artificial sweetener or sugar. After 30 minutes, the women who drank the sugar-sweetened beverage were the drowsiest.

Larry Christensen, Ph.D., chairman of the Department of Psychology at the University of South Alabama in Mobile, has studied the effects of coffee and sugar on mood. (A sugary snack combined with coffee is a typical coffee break pick-me-up.) Dr. Christensen reports that many people experiencing depression note improvements in energy levels when they eliminate either sugar or caffeine from their diets.

"Fatigue and feeling down in the dumps are primary characteristics of a sugar-sensitive person," says Dr. Christensen. "People usually react to either caffeine or sugar. Seldom are people sensitive to both."

Some people are so sensitive to sugar or caffeine that even two cookies or one cup of coffee affects their energy level.

Why do sweets bring you down? For one thing, unlike starch, which slowly releases carbohydrate units, called glucose, into the blood, sugar dumps rapidly into the bloodstream causing a dramatic rise in blood sugar. To counteract this rise, the pancreas quickly releases the hormone insulin, which hustles excess sugar from the blood into the cells. Consequently, blood sugar drops, often to levels lower than before the snack. Sugar also triggers the release of the brain chemical serotonin that can make you feel relaxed or drowsy within an hour or two after the snack. Finally, women who snack on sweets are likely to consume inadequate amounts of energizing nutrients, such as vitamin C, the B vitamins, magnesium, potassium, and zinc.

🍎 **Snack defensively.** Rather than fuel fatigue with these quick fixes, snack defensively.

Choose nutrient-packed, time-released carbohydrates, such as whole grain crackers or breadsticks, low-fat granola, or a soft microwave pretzel for between-meal snacks.

Ironing Out Fatigue

If your energy level is in perpetual low gear, your problem could be a lack of iron, especially if you are a teenager, a woman during the childbearing years, pregnant, or breast-feeding. Children can also be low in iron. Although only 8 percent of women are anemic, as many as 80

the 10 energizers

Do you work with, or against, your energy level? "Yes" answers are energy boosters; "no" answers are energy drainers.

1. Do you eat at least five small meals and snacks throughout the day, including breakfast? (Eating every four hours provides a steady supply of fuel to sustain a high energy level.)

2. Do you consume at least 2,000 calories each day of fresh fruits and vegetables, whole grains, low-fat milk products, and other nutrient-packed foods? (Too few calories means too little fuel and nutrients, which can leave you low on energy.)

3. Do you avoid overeating in the evening?

4. Do you limit caffeinated beverages to three 5-ounce servings or less each day?

5. Do you limit sugar intake and eat only small amounts of sugary foods with a meal?

6. Do you drink at least six glasses of water each day? (Chronic low fluid intake can result in mild dehydration and fatigue.)

7. Do you avoid quick-weight-loss diets and never yo-yo diet? (Not eating enough, so you're not supplying the body with ample fuel, is a common cause of fatigue.)

8. Do you take time each day to relax and enjoy life?

9. Do you include moderate exercise in your daily routine?

10. Do you get enough restful sleep each night?

hematocrit, screen only for anemia, which is a late stage of iron deficiency," says Robert Labbe, Ph.D., professor emeritus in the Department of Laboratory Medicine at the University of Seattle in Washington.

For months, years, even decades before the onset of anemia, tissue stores of iron might be depleted.

"Iron deficiency can affect enzymes in the mitochondria [the energy powerhouses within the cells] that are primarily responsible for generating tissue energy," says Labbe. The result is fatigue, poor exercise and athletic performance, and a host of energy-related problems. How do you know if you're low in iron? A blood test that includes a serum ferritin test is the most sensitive indicator of tissue iron levels. A serum ferritin value below 20 mcg/L is a red flag for iron deficiency. (See "Anemia," which begins on page 69, for details on dealing with iron deficiency.)

percent of active and 20 percent of premenopausal women in general are iron deficient.

"Pre-anemic iron deficiency goes unnoticed in many cases because routine blood tests, such as the hemoglobin and

If a blood test shows that you are low in iron, your doctor will advise you on how to deal with the problem. He or she might recommend an iron supplement.

Eat for iron. A moderate-dose iron supplement and iron-rich foods will boost lagging iron stores. Also add a vitamin-C-rich food to each meal, such as orange juice.

Combine small amounts of lean meat with plant foods, such as spaghetti with meatballs or split pea soup with ham. Cook in cast iron and avoid drinking tea and coffee with meals, since these beverages contain tannins that reduce iron absorption.

🍎 **Get enough nutrients.** Iron doesn't work alone. Poor dietary intake of several vitamins and minerals, including the B vitamins, vitamin C, magnesium, potassium, and zinc, can cause fatigue. You can avoid these pitfalls by including in the daily diet at least five servings of fresh fruits and vegetables, five servings of whole grains, three servings of low-fat or nonfat milk products, and two servings of extra-lean meat, chicken, fish, or legumes. On the days you don't eat perfectly, consider taking a moderate-dose, multiple vitamin and mineral supplement.

Where to Start

It's okay to feel tired once in a while, but there is no need to put up with fatigue when it lingers or interferes with your life. Learn to recognize the mental or physical symptoms of fatigue and notice what time of day they usually occur. Are you a morning lark or a night owl?

Keep a journal to identify when you are most energized and most tired, or in the best and worst moods. What precedes your high and low energy levels? Include sleep, stress, diet, and exercise patterns. Then develop a plan that works with your natural energy cycles and combats the blahs. Remember, fatigue can be a symptom of something more serious, so always consult a physician if tiredness persists.

healing diet

PROBLEM FOODS	GOOD FOODS
Coffee	A balanced diet featuring whole
Sugary snacks	grains, fruits, and vegetables
	Protein foods as part of lunch

BEST ADVICE: Always eat breakfast. See your doctor if fatigue persists.

fibrocystic breasts

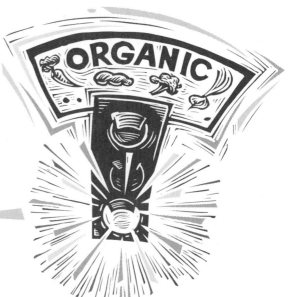

The diagnosis of fibrocystic breasts sounds pretty scary, but what does it really mean? Doctors have used the term "fibrocystic breasts" to label everything from cysts and benign (noncancerous) fatty tumors to microscopic cell changes, breast pain, and nipple discharge. Only since the 1980s have most doctors adopted guidelines that give specific names to each symptom. They've also started using the term "condition" instead of fibrocystic breast "disease" to describe normal changes.

Most women—estimates range from 50 to 90 percent—find lumps in their breasts at some point in their lives. And many women worry about them.

Breasts are normally lumpy, but understandably, given the risk of cancer, lumps still put terror into women's minds, says Dixie Mills, M.D., a breast surgeon at Women to Women, a holistic health center in Yarmouth, Maine.

What to do? You simply have to know your own breasts well enough to develop an intuitive sense of when something feels different. (And whenever you have concerns you should share them with your doctor.)

Some benign disorders, such as infection, polyps in the milk ducts, or nipple discharge, may require medical attention. These kinds of problems can't be prevented or treated by changes in your diet. But other benign changes result from the normal ebb and flow of your monthly hormonal cycle.

These can be influenced by the food you eat and include premenstrual breast pain, general lumpiness, or what doctors call dominant lumps, which are actually cysts, enlarged glands, or benign fatty tumors.

The Food-Hormone Connection

Your breasts are made up of fatty tissue and glands supported by a network of fibrous tissue made mostly of collagen (as are your tendons and ligaments). So where do the lumps come in? Your milk glands and milk ducts, which look like dense clouds on your mammograms, as well as the fibrous connective tissue, can all feel lumpy when you examine your breasts.

As your menstrual cycle prepares your body for a potential pregnancy each month, your breasts swell. They may feel tender, perhaps even painful to the touch.

If you press against the skin, you may feel hard lumps, or nodes. The exact role of each hormone in governing these changes in your breasts is poorly understood, but researchers think that several factors may affect them. These include the ratio of estrogen to progesterone, the presence of other hormones secreted during stress, and the sensitivity of your breast tissue to your own hormones.

What you eat can affect your body's hormone levels. Researchers are not sure which components in which foods have the most effect or exactly how high levels of estrogen affect your breasts, but some evidence links an excess of estrogen to both harmless and malignant changes in the breasts. There are, however, a number of changes you can make to your diet that may prove helpful.

The Role of Fats

Reducing the fats in your diet may alter your hormone levels and diminish premenstrual breast lumps and pain, says Norman Boyd, M.D., head of the Division of Epidemiology and Statistics and professor of medicine at the University of Toronto. Dr. Boyd and his colleagues were the first to demonstrate scientifically that dietary fat alters breast tissues. In one study they looked at effects of a low-fat, high-carbohydrate diet on premenstrual breast symptoms. Twenty-one women who complained of severe, persistent

premenstrual breast pain were divided into an experimental group and a control group. The experimental group was told to reduce their fat intake to 15 percent of total calories and increase their carbohydrates to 65 percent of total calories. The control group got general guidelines about healthy eating. After six months, 60 percent of the experimental group experienced reduced breast swelling, tenderness, and lumpiness.

The researchers also found that extensive areas of dense tissue seen on mammograms are associated with an increased risk of cyclical (premenstrual) breast pain and breast cancer, says Dr. Boyd. In another study, Dr. Boyd and his colleagues examined mammograms of women who followed instructions to eat less fat and more carbohydrates and found that they actually reduced their breast density.

Large-scale studies are currently under way in Canada and the United States to further investigate the role of fats in breast health, but the data won't be complete until the next decade.

Some fats may actually be good for your breasts, however. Among them are olive oil; omega-3 fatty acids, found in cold-water fish like salmon and tuna as well as in flaxseed oil and evening primrose oil; and conjugated linolenic acid (CLA), an omega-6 fatty acid, also found in flaxseed oil, borage oil, and black currant oil.

All of these fats probably help diminish premenstrual breast pain and lumpiness in part by regulating estrogen metabolism.

While the researchers are still sorting all these factors out, here are a few things you can try now:

● **Reduce fat.** No one knows exactly how dietary fats help or harm the breasts, but some experts speculate that since body fat stores estrogen, the less fat you pack on your frame, the less chance you have of promoting harmful changes in your breasts.

Women in cultures that eat a low-fat diet have fewer breast complaints than those who eat high-fat diets. Try sticking to getting less than 30 percent of your total calories from fat—or no more than 60 grams of fat on a 1,800-calorie daily diet. Dr. Boyd advocates sticking to even lower levels, close to 15 percent.

● **Watch your weight.** You store estrogen in body fat, so losing excess weight can help minimize this hormone's contribution to your discomfort.

Excess calories contribute to body fat, which adds estrogen to your body.

● **Go organic.** Animals fed growth hormones and feed containing pesticides and other pollutants store these toxins in their own body fat. Such animal fat is thought to promote breast tumors (and cancer) in the women who eat it. (Here's yet another reason to reduce the amount of meat in your diet.)

Eating unpeeled fruit can also be dicey. When possible, buy organic produce and meats to avoid the toxic effects of herbicides, pesticides, antibiotics, and pollutants. If you are buying nonorganic produce, be scrupulous about cleaning it thoroughly before you eat it.

● **Learn to love olive oil.** Many of the fats and oils that are so prevalent in our American diet have been implicated in fibrocystic breast conditions. Aside from cutting down on fats in general, it may prove helpful to make olive oil your mainstay. Olive oil is what is known as a monosaturated oil, a type of oil that seems to cause fewer problems.

Fiber to the Rescue

Your body loses a certain amount of estrogen every time you move your bowels. That's why a high-fiber diet is good for your breasts. (Finnish women have half the breast cancer rates of Americans, despite high levels of dietary fat found in some of their favorite foods— butter, cheeses, and meats. Investigators believe that's because Finns typically eat 30 grams of fiber daily, compared to 11 grams in the typical American diet.)

David Rose, M.D., a top researcher at the American Health Foundation, measured the estrogen in the blood of women who ate 30 grams a day of wheat bran. He found that they had significantly less estrogen in their bloodstream than women who ate the same amount of corn or oat bran.

● **Add fiber.** Experts have come to believe that eating more fiber can help prevent painful, lumpy breasts. Choose whole-grain cereals and breads. Pick brown rice over white. Eat high-fiber vegetables, such as beans, peas, cabbage, and carrots. High-fiber fruits include raisins and dried apricots. Eat unpeeled apples, pears, and peaches.

Is Caffeine a Culprit?

Some scientists charge that the spate of studies in the 1980s connecting caffeine with breast disorders were riddled with problems. They dispute the claim that caffeine causes breast problems. In fact, some doctors say that since coffee is a diuretic, it may help eliminate excess fluid, thereby helping to reduce premenstrual breast tenderness and swelling.

But other doctors and researchers say that caffeine and related compounds, called methylxanthines, may stimulate the production of fibrous tissue and cyst fluid. These compounds are found in coffee, tea, chocolate, and colas. Methylxanthines affect breast tissue indirectly by activating chemicals involved in your nervous system's response to stress, according to Dr. Mills. Some women may have a genetic sensitivity to these chemicals and caffeine.

Bruce Drukker, M.D., at Michigan State University in East Lansing, is among those who have found that eliminating caffeine from the diet can be helpful. In his practice, he says he's found that at least 60 to 65 percent of the women who rigorously avoid caffeine notice some improvement in symptoms of premenstrual breast pain and other fibrocystic changes.

Dr. Mills observes that abstaining from foods containing methylxanthines helps with PMS swelling and pain, though not with lumpiness, in a good proportion of her patients. The discomfort from caffeine withdrawal may offset the gain in comfort, she notes. Some of her patients compromise by mixing decaf with regular coffee or drink coffee less often and endure a little pain in order to enjoy their morning java.

What's the bottom line here, since doctors don't really agree on whether cutting caffeine can be helpful?

🍎 **Try cutting out caffeine.** It certainly can't hurt to try eliminating all caffeine from your diet to see whether it helps. If you can't do without coffee, tea, or colas, at least switch to decaf versions or save the high test for special occasions. And remember that chocolate and certain over-the-counter medications may contain caffeine, too.

Phytoestrogens To the Rescue

Phytoestrogens are plant chemicals with a molecular structure similar to that of human estrogen. When you consume plants containing phytoestrogens, your brain mistakes these plant chemicals for human hormones and instructs your ovaries to cut back on their production of estrogen, keeping it at a more healthful level. And this, in turn, may help minimize fibrocystic breast changes.

Just as there are good and bad forms of cholesterol, there may be good and bad forms of estrogen. The bad form promotes potentially painful changes in cells and tissues, Dr. Mills explains. Phytoestrogens act like good estrogens, protecting the body from these cell changes.

One form of plant estrogen, called indoles, is found in the cruciferous family of vegetables (cabbage, broccoli, brussels sprouts, cauliflower, and Savoy cabbage). Indoles exert a protective effect. In a 1994 study, one group of women took indole capsules equal to the amount in a head of cabbage; another group drank extra fiber mixed with fruit juice; the third group got placebo (medically inactive, look-alike) capsules. At the end of the first month, all but three women in the indole group had increased levels of a safe form of estrogen; the other groups showed no change.

More studies are being conducted to find out whether lower amounts of indoles will be effective.

Sulforaphane, another plant estrogen that is found in cruciferous vegetables, helps your body get rid of potentially harmful excess estrogens.

Still other kinds of phytoestrogens are found in a variety of fruits and vegetables, beans, seeds, and legumes—including apples, barley, carrots, cherries, coffee, flaxseed oil, fennel, garlic, oats, parsley, potatoes, rye, sesame seed, soy, split peas, spinach, sprouts, and wheat.

How much of all these foods should you eat?

Take five. Experts recommend eating at least five servings of fruits and vegetables a day. If you follow the "strive for five" rule, you'll be getting healthy amounts not only of phytoestrogens but also fiber. Eating a variety of these foods provides good insurance against lumpy, painful breasts.

Eat soy. Women in societies where diet is high in soy tend to have fewer breast problems. Soy foods contain isoflavones, natural substances that can block certain effects of estrogen in the body.

Eating for Healthy Breasts

In addition to the other dietary changes outlined in this section, here are a few other things to be aware of.

Get plenty of vitamin B6. Vitamin B6 deficiency has been linked to PMS symptoms and tender, lumpy breasts.

Good sources of vitamin B6 include bananas, raw cruciferous veggies, nuts (especially walnuts), potatoes, red peppers, and wheat germ.

Cut salt. If you find that you tend to retain water and your breasts become swollen and tender, watching your salt intake should help.

Limit alcohol. Researchers have found that drinking alcoholic beverages raises estrogen levels.

Try natural diuretics. Excess fluid can play a role in premenstrual swelling and tenderness. So it follows that keeping the fluid buildup to a minimum can help control pain.

Natural diuretics, such as herbal teas brewed from chamomile, corn silk, buchu, and uva ursi can flush out some of the fluid that causes breast discomfort. You'll find them at many health-food stores. Apples, asparagus, beets, celery, cucumbers, grapes, parsley, pineapples, strawberries, and watercress also help your body flush out excess water.

healing diet

PROBLEM FOODS	GOOD FOODS
Fatty red meat	Apples
Full-fat dairy products	Asparagus
Fried foods	Barley
Coffee, tea, colas, or chocolate	Beets
Salt	Broccoli
	Brussels sprouts
	Cabbage
	Carrots
	Cauliflower
	Celery
	Cherries
	Flaxseed oil or ground flaxseeds
	Garlic
	Oats
	Organic fruits and vegetables
	Organic lean meats, fish, and poultry
	Parsley
	Potatoes
	Sesame seed
	Soybeans, tofu, and other soy products
	Split peas
	Spinach
	Sprouts
	Whole-grain bread and cereals, especially wheat bran

BEST ADVICE: Eat a high-fiber diet, high in complex carbohydrates and soy foods and low in animal fats and empty calories, to maintain a healthy weight. Avoid foods treated with hormones and pesticides. Go easy on salt and caffeine.

flatulence

If a person could die of embarrassment, flatulence might rank with the world's deadliest diseases. Fortunately, the condition rarely signals a serious health problem. And often just a few simple changes in your diet will keep it under control.

Throughout the day all of us pass intestinal gas or flatus, to use the Latin term. Where does it come from? Many foods and beverages are chock-full of gas. Apples and pears, for example, consist of 20 percent gas. And think of all the gas-charged carbonated drinks you consume. Whipped toppings also contain lots of trapped gases.

But the great majority of flatulence is produced by bacteria in the large intestine. That's right, bacteria. Few realize it, but vast colonies of bacteria live out their lives inside people's large intestines. These bacteria are helpful for the most part, since they feast on foods your own digestive system can't break down on its own—everything from the artificial sweetener in that low-cal dessert you devoured last night to fibers from fruits, vegetables, beans, and grains.

Inevitably, when intestinal bacteria digest these foods, they produce methane as a byproduct. You already know the name of the process: fermentation. The same bacterial reaction creates those tiny bubbles in beer and wine.

Just how much gas these intestinal bacteria produce depends on what you've eaten lately, of course. If you've wolfed down a couple of bean burritos, the intestinal bacteria will enjoy a feast. However, if you ate a juicy salmon steak, the same bacteria will most certainly go hungry.

What's the difference? The fiber in the burritos can't be digested by your own system. So the task gets delegated to your intestinal bacteria. On the other hand, most people readily digest the fats and proteins in salmon.

Turning Off the Gasworks

Relatively little was known about just how much flatulence could be considered normal until a study came out in the June 1991 issue of the medical journal, *Gut*. People in the study were fed a diet of beans. Then the amount of gas they produced was measured. It totaled about a quart a day on average. Since then, other studies have shown that people pass gas about 14 times during the course of a day.

Some people pass gas far more frequently. In fact, 30 percent of Americans experience excess intestinal gas, according

how about those beans?

Of all the gas-causing foods that make up our diet, beans are probably the most notorious. Don't blame the beans themselves, says Steven Peikin, M.D., professor of gastroenterology at the Robert Wood Johnson Medical School at Camden, in New Jersey. Beans are an excellent source of protein. Instead, blame it on the bean skins, which contain carbohydrates your stomach is unable to digest.

Your intestinal bacteria are only too happy to do the job. They break down these carbohydrates into sugars. And that process produces the foul-smelling gas beans are so renowned for.

One way to enjoy beans—at least the dried variety—while avoiding the gas is to soak them in water for 12 to 24 hours. Soaking helps break down the carbohydrate skins. Be sure to rinse the beans thoroughly before cooking them.

Beano, available in pharmacies and health-food stores, contains the enzyme alpha-galactosidase which digests bean skins before your intestinal bacteria get to them. Unfortunately, alpha-galactosidase is destroyed by heat, so it can't be added to recipes that require cooking or baking. Instead, spoon a couple of drops of Beano, which is flavorless, onto each serving of beans.

to Steven Peikin, M.D., professor of gastroenterology at the Robert Wood Johnson Medical School at Camden, in New Jersey. Dr. Peikin has designed special diets to treat intestinal ailments. The consequences—besides embarrassment—include pain and bloating. As a cure, Dr. Peikin suggests cutting out some of the more common gas-producing foods from your diet and changing the way you cook or serve certain foods. As you'll see, these flatus-producing foods fall into some wide-ranging categories.

Consider food additives. Olestra and other fat substitutes cut down on calories because your body can't digest them. The same goes for artificial sweeteners such as

sorbitol. Once again, the job goes to the intestinal bacteria. If either artifical fats or artifical sweeteners give you a problem, consider eliminating them from your diet.

Don't let milk get you. Do you feel bloated and gassy hours after you've had a cup of milk or a double cheese pizza? You may have lactose intolerance—meaning that your body just can't digest the sugary substance called lactose found in all dairy products. Fortunately, plenty of lactose-free dairy products are available in supermarkets and health-food stores, and other products such as Lactaid contain the enzyme needed to fully digest lactose and let you enjoy dairy without discomfort. (See "Lactose Intolerance," which begins on page 225, for ways you can modify your diet.)

🍎 **Deal with wheat.** About six in 10,000 people have difficulty digesting gluten, a protein found in wheat products. Gas is just one symptom. Consult a physician if you believe you have a gluten intolerance. (See "Celiac Disease," which begins on page 95, for more details on this condition.)

🍎 **Review your vegetables.** Prime culprits in the veggie category include: broccoli, brussels sprouts, cabbage, cauliflower, kale, onions, peas, radishes, and turnips. All contain indigestible fibers, which the lower intestinal bacteria love to feast on. These same vegetables also contain sulfur. And sulfur mixed with methane causes odor problems. Cooking draws out some of the sulfur. If raw versions of some of these vegetables cause problems, opt for cooked dishes instead. Also try using garlic, ginger, or nutmeg in cooking. The spices break down gas-causing ingredients.

🍎 **Eat fruit first.** Certain fruits—particularly apples, apricots, bananas, blueberries, and pears—contain pectin, a fiber that intestinal bacteria love. Instead of serving fruit for dessert, start off the meal with fruit as an appetizer. That way, the pectin will be diluted by the other foods you eat.

Dealing with Fiber

Call it an ironic fact of nature, that beans, fruits, and vegetables—all foods that are most certainly good for you—should also create intestinal gas. You don't want to give them up. But you may want to control your portions, advises Dr. Peikin, especially when you know that certain foods are apt to cause problems. Still another way to fight gas is to eat more fiber—especially foods like whole wheat breads and pastas, oat bran cereals, and, yes, vegetables and fruits. Wait a minute, don't these high-fiber foods cause gas? The answer is yes, but a diet consistently high in fiber adds bulk to the undigested foods passed to the large intestine. And that makes the large intestine quick to void these foods as waste. Since the food matter doesn't hang around for long, the intestinal bacteria have less time to do their gas-causing work.

The key is to eat fiber consistently, Dr. Peikin explains. If you suddenly boost the fiber content of your diet from say 10 grams per day to 50 or more grams, your intestinal bacteria could become completely overwhelmed. Opt instead for the generally recommended amount between 20 and 35 grams per day.

healing diet

PROBLEM FOODS	GOOD FOODS
Apples	Bran and other fibrous grains
Apricots	Rice
Bananas	Skinned potato
Beans and legumes	
Blueberries	
Broccoli	
Brussels sprouts	
Cabbage	
Cauliflower	
Dairy products	
Food additives	
Kale	
Olestra and other fat substitutes	
Onions	
Pears	
Peas	
Radishes	
Turnips	

BEST ADVICE: Eat limited amounts of especially troublesome foods and maintain a consistent diet of 20 to 35 grams of fiber per day. Painful gas that persists for more than 24 hours or recurring bouts of gas can be a sign of a more serious problem; see your physician for diagnosis and treatment.

food allergies

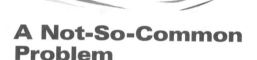

Your toddler gets a rash after eating a peanut butter sandwich. You may be tempted to shrug it off as insignificant. Don't. Because some allergies can cause anaphylaxis—a potentially fatal allergic reaction—you could inadvertently be risking your child's life. That, in brief, is how serious food allergies can be.

"If you have a child that has a mild reaction to a food, say she eats a walnut and has a couple of hives, a parent might think, 'Oh that's nothing,'" says Dean Metcalfe, M.D., chief of the laboratory of allergic diseases in the National Institute of Allergy and Infectious Diseases in Bethesda, Maryland. "But the next reaction to eating a walnut might be serious trouble breathing."

Or perhaps because your child has had a stomach upset or diarrhea after eating milk, eggs, cheese, or wheat, you've carefully cut any one of these foods out of your child's diet. But what you thought was a reaction to food may have been caused by something else—and by needlessly restricting your child's diet, you may be restricting his or her growth.

Of course, adults can have allergic reactions to foods, too, but it's appropriate to begin an examination of this topic with children, because food allergies can be so critical in the first few years.

A Not-So-Common Problem

Many people believe that food allergies are common—but they aren't. A poll of 5,000 households conducted by the Food Allergy Center of Lynbrook, New York, found that someone in nearly one-third of them thought he or she was allergic to milk. In one-fourth someone reported an allergy to fruit. Nearly 16 percent of the households reported that at least one family member had a food allergy, particularly to milk and chocolate. In fact, medical researchers know that only one or two people out of 100 is allergic to any food.

Believing that a child is allergic to a food group when, in fact, no allergy exists often leads to unnecessary and potentially harmful dietary restriction. Here's an example of how that can work: Parents of 11 children referred to the National Jewish Center for Immunology and Respiratory

Medicine in Denver for evaluation of food allergies had systematically cut an average of eight foods from the children's diets because of supposed allergies. Because of their limited diet, the children had dangerously low growth rates and weight gains—and it turned out that only two of the children had any allergies at all.

"It's an unintentional form of child abuse," says Dr. Metcalfe. "The parent is so

what happens during an
allergic reaction?

Normally, your immune system works to keep you healthy. When all is going well, this complex system helps fight off problems, such as colds or infections. But sometimes it can go a bit haywire. If you have an allergy, your immune system mistakenly decides that a certain substance is a dangerous invader and reacts violently to try to get rid of it, just as it would if confronted with bacteria or a virus. In hay fever, for instance, your immune system goes to battle against a harmless pollen. The result is that your nose and eyes run seemingly endlessly.

In food allergies, the response is similar, but it can be much more serious. Your immune system reacts to a specific protein in nuts or shellfish or some other food. It forms antibodies to fight off the protein, and these antibodies release chemicals such as histamine that cause allergy symptoms. With each exposure to the food, the body reacts more strongly, producing more antibodies.

When enough antibodies build up, the food may cause itching or swelling in your mouth, then nausea or other intestinal woes when it reaches your gut. When the substance reaches your skin, itching or eczema may result. But the reaction can be still more serious, even deadly.

Because allergic reactions vary, some people assume that allergies are only a mild inconvenience at most, says Dan Atkins, M.D., director of ambulatory pediatrics at the National Jewish Center for Immunology and Respiratory Medicine in Denver.

"People don't understand that for some kids it can be very severe—for them a little bit of exposure is enough," says Dr. Atkins. "There's such a difference in degree of sensitivity: Johnny gets a hive from eating peanuts, but if Jill gets a bit of peanut she has an anaphylactic reaction."

In anaphylactic shock, blood vessels leak, causing a drop in blood pressure and inhibiting blood and oxygen from reaching the brain. Within a few seconds or minutes after eating, the airways tighten and the tongue and throat swell, and the person begins to have difficulty breathing. This must be treated immediately with an injection of a drug called epinephrine, which shrinks the blood vessels and relaxes the airways.

extraordinarily restrictive of the diet that sometimes the children become malnourished." Parents even sometimes keep their children out of school or away from friends because of their fear of the offending food, he says.

In fact, multiple food allergies aren't at all common. "Only rarely is a person allergic to more than a few foods," says Metcalfe. Of people who are allergic, an estimated 60 percent react to just one food and another 30 percent to two or three foods. And although some allergies can indeed be life-threatening, doctors agree they can be managed successfully without secluding a child from normal life.

Allergy Basics

So how do you know whether you're truly allergic? If you suspect an allergy—or if you're allergic and you fear that your children might be as well—your first step is a visit to a doctor, preferably an allergist. Symptoms of food allergy, which may result within a few minutes or a few hours of eating the food, can include:
● itching
● hives or rash
● sneezing and runny nose
● swollen lips
● swollen hands or feet
● nausea or vomiting
● diarrhea

Adults are most often allergic to shellfish (such as shrimp, crab, and lobster), peanuts, nuts, fish, and eggs. (Peanuts are actually a legume, not a nut.) Children are

most often allergic to eggs, milk, and peanuts. Although children are more likely to be allergic than adults—possibly because of an immature immune system or gastrointestinal tract—you can become allergic at any age.

But you can eat a food several times with no problem before your body produces enough antibodies to react.

And allergies take a while to develop to a dangerous level. "For someone—whether an infant, child, or adult—to develop a food allergy, they must be exposed, often repeatedly," explains Dr. Metcalfe.

Oddly enough, recurrent ear infections in children may also be an indication of food allergy. Researchers at the Georgetown University School of Medicine in Washington, D.C., found that among allergic children, ear problems disappeared when the allergy-causing food was removed. When the foods were reintroduced, the ear infections returned.

To diagnose a food allergy, your doctor will ask questions about your reactions and when they occurred, and may ask you to keep a diet diary. He or she may try an elimination diet, during which you stop eating one or more specific foods. Your doctor may use a skin prick test, during which an extract from the food is placed on the skin and lightly scratched. Reliability of skin tests varies, however. You can have a positive skin test (indicating a problem) and never have an adverse food reaction. One study found the accuracy of skin tests to be less than 50 percent.

That is why a skin test just serves as an indication that there may be a problem with a particular food. "We don't remove foods from a diet based on skin tests," says Dan Atkins, M.D., director of ambulatory pediatrics at the National Jewish Center for Immunology and Respiratory Medicine. And doctors prefer to avoid skin testing if there is a chance of anaphylaxis.

Other tests that might be used in diagnosis include blood tests called RAST (radioallergosorbent test) and ELISA (enzyme-linked immunosorbent assay test) or a food challenge that involves placing food in capsules to be swallowed.

Once you know for sure you or your child has an allergy, your doctor will help you plan a strategy for avoiding the offending food and coping with any reactions that may develop.

Living with Food Allergies

There is currently no treatment for food allergies. All you can do is avoid the food you're allergic to. And most allergies are permanent.

Avoiding a food isn't always simple. Of six youngsters who died of anaphylaxis from food in a 14-month period, all knew they were allergic to that food, but ate it accidentally in cookies, cake, or candy, often in a restaurant or school cafeteria.

Because peanuts or peanut oil are used in many foods where you wouldn't expect, such as puddings or pies, avoiding peanuts can be particularly difficult. And some people can react just by touching or smelling the food, even through an exhaust fan. Here are ways experts advise to cope:

Keep up with the news. Finding "hidden" ingredients in some products can be difficult, especially as they can be called by unfamiliar names. An excellent source of information, says Dr. Atkins, is the Food Allergy Network, a nonprofit organization with a newsletter and a web site. You can reach the network at 800/929-4040 or 703/691-3179, or www.foodallergy.org

Pack it along. Allergic people need to carry a portable dose of epinephrine in either a syringe called Ana-Kit or an applicator called EpiPen. You may want to buy your child a special fanny pack just for the EpiPen, suggests Anne Munoz-Furlong, founder of the Food Allergy Network. Putting the medicine pack on in the morning should be part of getting dressed, just like putting on your shoes.

Start 'em young. One mother trained her peanut-allergic toddlers with "flash cards" she made of pictures of foods cut from advertisements. Long before they could read, her sons knew that Reese's Pieces could make them sick and require a trip to the hospital.

Beware cross-contamination. Scrupulous household habits are also essential. "Cross-contamination can easily happen, even when you're being careful," says Dr. Atkins. "Things such as using the peanut butter knife in the jelly jar or not adequately washing off the ice cream scoop can cause reactions." You may choose not to allow the allergy-causing food in the house at all. But if you do, take special care in washing and rinsing.

Meet with all caregivers. Before the start of a school year, meet with your child's teachers, principal, nurse, counselor, and cafeteria workers, suggests Munoz-Furlong.

They need to understand the seriousness of your child's allergy and what to do if the child has a reaction.

🍎 **Take special care when eating out.**
Servers in restaurants seldom know exactly how a food is prepared, and even cooks may not think it important to mention that a sauce contains egg or peanuts. Your best bet is plain foods. Baked goods often contain problem ingredients, so you're better off giving them a pass.

🍎 **Choose a special formula.** Infants who are unable to breast-feed and who are allergic to milk can sometimes tolerate formula based on lamb meat, soy, or specially treated milk. If a formula is labeled hypoallergic, the Committee on Nutrition of the American Academy of Pediatrics says 90 percent of milk-allergic babies should tolerate it. But you should clear all products with your doctor.

🍎 **Wear a warning.** Children and adults alike should wear a medic alert bracelet or necklace that identifies them as allergic to specific foods and lists their doctor's name.

Allergy Prevention

People tend to get allergies to foods they eat often. "You see a lot of potato allergy in Germany and rice allergy in Japan," notes Dr. Atkins.

What do our kids eat a lot of? Peanut butter. And peanut and nut allergies are apparently on the rise.

On an English island, 15 percent of more than 1,000 children were sensitive to peanuts or nuts. Another study of 622 people with peanut allergy found that the numbers of allergic people within families had increased significantly in three generations. Parents were less likely to be allergic than the children, and grandparents even less likely. The researchers also found that peanut allergies are occurring at younger ages, perhaps because children are exposed to peanuts earlier.

How can you help prevent allergies in your children?

Researchers suggest that early exposure to certain foods can trigger allergies. "Ready availability and early introduction of highly allergenic foods, such as peanuts and nuts, into the diet will only increase the number of people with food allergies," notes Hugh A. Sampson, M.D., a pediatric allergy specialist at the Johns Hopkins University School of Medicine in Baltimore.

Although no one advocates keeping all children away from peanuts forever—it'd be just about impossible, says Dr. Metcalfe—experts agree that it's a good idea to avoid peanuts and other highly allergic foods the first few years. "The first 18 months are the most critical," says Dr. Metcalfe. He advises breast-feeding for at least six months then carefully following pediatric guidelines for the introduction of foods.

"What you're trying to do is avoid problems in early life that will affect growth," he says. "You don't want a child to be sick when really young. You want to get infants over that critical first year or two."

Another advantage of delaying allergies is that it's easier for older children to police what they eat, says Dr. Atkins, and to let adults know when a reaction is occurring. And there's a chance you may be able to avoid allergies completely.

what food allergies aren't

Think you have a food allergy? Maybe you do. Then again, maybe you don't. When allergy specialist Dan Atkins, M.D., first examines people, he sits down and talks with them about the definition of a food allergy.

"Food allergy means a lot of different things to different people," he says. Some people mistake other problems as allergic reactions. If you find yourself bloating after drinking several glasses of milk or getting a headache after drinking wine or eating Chinese food, that doesn't spell food allergy, he says. Instead, you may be unable to digest or be sensitive to something in that food.

Here's a look at food reactions that aren't allergies.

● **Food intolerance.** When you don't digest a food well, the result can be unpleasant symptoms such as bloating or diarrhea. Some people, for instance, cannot digest the sugar in milk or the gluten in wheat.

● **Food sensitivity.** Certain substances in foods seem to cause headaches in some people. Some of these substances occur naturally, such as chemicals in cheese and chocolate, and caffeine in coffee. Others have been added, such as sulfites, a preservative in wine and seafood; monosodium glutamate (MSG), commonly added to Oriental food; and yellow dye number 5.

● **Unrelated problems.** While the symptoms you have may occur after eating certain foods, they may be caused by something else altogether—such as a gastrointestinal problem called irritable bowel syndrome, a hernia, gallbladder problems, or even food poisoning. "If you eat, say, a tuna fillet that was spoiled in a restaurant, you have a reaction that looks like anaphylaxis," points out Dean Metcalfe, M.D., of the National Institute of Allergy and Infectious Diseases. "You can have hives, itching, headache, increased heart rate, and flushing." And reactions such as runny nose, itching, vomiting, or diarrhea are relatively common with childhood illnesses. Fatigue, tingling, or problems sleeping could indicate a thyroid problem, lupus, or Lyme disease.

● **The ick factor.** Finally, there's such a thing as a subjective reaction to food. If you once had a violent illness after eating chicken casserole, you may become nauseated every time chicken casserole passes your lips—even if your initial reaction was caused by a virus or food poisoning. In some cases, a nonallergic person can break out in hives after eating a food they believe they are allergic to, even when in fact they aren't.

"Delaying the introduction of a potentially sensitizing food such as peanuts or fish—to which the allergy is often life-long—can allow the child's gastrointestinal tract and immune system to mature," says Dr. Atkins. "While this doesn't guarantee that the child doesn't become allergic, it may possibly prevent sensitization."

In an at-risk child—one with eczema or a family history of allergy—you may want to be even more careful. If you and your spouse have allergies, that doesn't mean that your children will become allergic, but they will have a tendency to be allergic if exposed to specific foods. "We suggest delaying introduction of foods such as peanuts and nuts to three to four years old," says Dr. Atkins.

One of the best ways to avoid reactions to milk is to breast-feed infants and limit exposure to milk the first year, doctors agree. Nursing mothers may also want to limit their own diets. Eating potential allergens, such as nuts, peanuts, and shellfish while nursing, exposes the infant to the food through breast milk, says Dr. Atkins.

Sometimes children "outgrow" food allergies as their immune systems and gastrointestinal tracts mature. "Milk allergy in a two-month-old is quite different from milk allergy in an eight-year-old," points out Dr. Metcalfe. Infants up to three months or so can have temporary allergies, perhaps caused by an immature immune system, that can cause prolonged diarrhea and vomiting. "These babies often have negative skin tests to the offending food, which is usually milk or soy, but it can be other foods," says Dr. Atkins. However, peanut and nut allergies, which are the most likely to cause anaphylaxis, are usually permanent.

healing diet

PROBLEM FOODS	GOOD FOODS
Chocolate	
Eggs	
Fish	
Milk	
Nuts	
Peanuts	
Shellfish	

BEST ADVICE: If you suspect you or your child has a food allergy, see a doctor for diagnosis and advice on how to deal with the problem. Do not try elimination diets on your child without seeking advice from a health professional.

gallstones

For years, Helen blamed her Sunday afternoon bouts of indigestion on the eggs Benedict her husband made her for breakfast. The recipe was heavenly, but by 1 o'clock Helen would feel anything but. She'd develop a sharp pain in the upper right side of her abdomen, but because the pain rarely lasted more than an hour or so, she never thought to consult her doctor. Until, that is, one Sunday when things got a bit more severe.

Helen's pain radiated up into her right shoulder and became so intense in the area of her abdomen that she vomited. So it was off to the hospital.

Helen was given an ultrasound (a diagnostic technique that uses high-frequency sound waves to detect abnormalities of the intestinal tract) and the verdict was clear: gallstones, three of them, each averaging approximately ¼ of an inch in diameter. Helen, who was 46, was surprised to learn from her doctor that she probably had been harboring her little gems for years.

Silent Until Summoned

Gallstones are actually quite common, developing in approximately one-third of women and one-fifth of all men by the age of 75, reports the National Institutes of Health. The good news, however, is that only about 20 percent of these people ever experience symptoms; the reasons why are not entirely understood.

Also in question is exactly what causes gallstones to develop in the first place, says Steven Peiken, M.D., a professor of medicine at the Robert Wood Johnson Medical School at Camden, in New Jersey. "We have, however, identified certain factors that appear to make their formation more likely," he adds.

Some of these factors are beyond our control—heredity, for example, gender (women are twice as prone as men), and race (African Americans are twice as susceptible as whites). But the other suspected causes of gallstones clearly are within our power to control—first and foremost being the amount of excess body fat we carry, studies show. "Exceeding one's ideal weight by as little as 20 to 30 percent can increase risks by as much as

the problem of
too much and too little

To understand why an underused gallbladder can cause problems, one needs to understand the gallbladder itself. This bit of tissue is a small (3 to 4 inches) pear-shaped gland attached to both the liver and the small intestine by a series of ducts. The gland stores bile produced by the liver for the digestion of dietary fats.

When a meal is eaten, especially one high in fat, the gallbladder contracts, forcing bile into the small intestine to do its digestive duties.

"When people go on crash diets, however, and especially diets extremely low in fat, the gallbladder is not made to contract frequently enough," says gastroenterology expert Steven Peiken, M.D. The result can be a buildup of bile within the gallbladder that in time can begin to thicken and crystallize into the stonelike nuggets that are the root of most gallbladder problems.

Gallstones also can form, however, for just the opposite reason—namely too much eating and the weight gain that tends to go with it.

"In people who are overweight, the composition of the bile itself is adversely affected in a way that makes gallstone formation more likely," Dr. Peiken explains. "We used to think that dietary fat was to blame for this, but the most recent research suggests that it's the obesity that usually results from eating too much fat that's more directly to blame."

Then, too, there is the problem in obese people that the gallbladder actually increases in size to a point where it does not contract completely. "This can leave small residues of bile which in time can grow stagnant and crystallize into stones," says Dr. Pieken.

100 percent, and risks become considerably greater as weight increases beyond that," Dr. Peiken says.

Paradoxically, however, rapid weight loss also has shown evidence of being a gallstone instigator, so anyone looking to reduce gallstone risks by slimming down should be careful not to be in too much of a hurry, Dr. Peiken says. "Studies show that a safe pace seems to be the loss of about 1 percent of one's body weight per week, or approximately a pound and a half for someone weighing 150. The danger in losing weight faster than that is that the gallbladder can begin to suffer by having too little to do."

Understanding The Pain

As Helen learned, gallstones can be present for years before causing any problems, but once an attack does occur, chances of future attacks increase dramatically. "Most gallbladder attacks are the result of a stone getting lodged in the small duct leading from the gallbladder to the small intestine," Dr. Peiken explains. The result usually is intense pain felt in the upper right quadrant of the abdomen (sometimes radiating up into the area of the right shoulder) as pressure within the gallbladder begins to build in response to this blockage. If the stone becomes dislodged, which in most cases it does, the pain passes. But if it does not and appropriate treatment is not sought, the result can be fever, jaundice, liver complications, and sometimes even death if the gallbladder bursts, spilling its toxic contents into the bloodstream.

A gallstone does not have to work its way into such a precarious spot for pain to occur, however. Sometimes just the presence of one or more gallstones within the gallbladder can cause inflammation within the gland that can cause pain when the gallbladder is called into action after meals, and especially after meals containing a lot of fat. "It's the gallbladder's job to release bile into the stomach for fat digestion, so the more fat that's consumed, the more active and hence susceptible to pain an inflamed gallbladder is going to be," Dr. Peiken says.

Steps to Avoid Stones

Although obesity may be the number one controllable risk for gallstones, it's not the only one, points out Henry Pitt, M.D., a professor of surgery and chairman of the department of surgery at the Medical College of Wisconsin in Milwaukee. "More and more, we're discovering that diet and other lifestyle factors may influence gallstone development, and while some of these findings are preliminary, they offer promising new directions for further research," he says. Based on the more intriguing of these discoveries, the following strategies are certainly worth adopting to reduce your gallstone risks, Dr. Pitt says.

Eat foods rich in iron. Working with the knowledge that women of child-bearing age are highly susceptible to gallstones—and are at risk for iron-deficiency as well—researchers from Johns Hopkins Hospital in Baltimore conducted an experiment in which they restricted the iron intake of laboratory animals. Sure enough, early stages of gallstone development were observed within just several weeks.

Consider boosting your consumption of iron-rich foods (lean cuts of beef, clams, leafy green vegetables, and iron-fortified breakfast cereals) with that in mind. You might also ask your doctor about taking an iron supplement. The current RDA for iron is 15 milligrams daily for women and 10 milligrams daily for men.

◗ **Eat more fish.** The fish-gallbladder connection was first discovered by researchers from Johns Hopkins in studies using laboratory animals then a study replicated with humans. Seventeen people with gallstones took fish oil capsules containing 960 milligrams of omega-3 fatty acids three times a day. Within 14 days, signs of gallstone formation in these people slowed. "What's encouraging is that the amount of fish oil used was not unreasonable," Dr. Pitt says. "We suspect that eating fish two or three times a week would work just as well." (Fish highest in omega-3 fatty acids are cold-water species, such as salmon, herring, mackerel, bluefin tuna, anchovies, and sardines.)

◗ **Restrict dietary fat and cholesterol.** Although some experts still feel the link may be only secondary—in other words, dietary fat promotes gallstones only by promoting obesity—Dr. Pitt and an increasing number of other researchers feel the connection is more direct. "Studies using laboratory animals have shown a direct connection, and epidemiological studies also are now beginning to show a link," Dr. Pitt says. (Epidemiological studies look at populations and their activities.) One epidemiological study found that a group of people with gallstones were including significantly more fat and cholesterol in

their diets than a control group that was gallstone-free.

◗ **Get enough fiber.** "Again, the exact mechanism hasn't been identified, but evidence points in the direction of a protective effect," says Dr. Pitt, regarding the role of fiber in the gallstone battle. A National Institutes of Health study of the diets of 4,730 women, as an example, found that diets rich in fiber did, in fact, exert a small though discernible protective effect. "At the very least, eating more fruits, vegetables, and whole-grain foods rich in fiber is a good defense against obesity, which we do know increases gallstone risks," says Dr. Pitt.

◗ **Eat more fruits and vegetables high in vitamin C.** Spurred by evidence that humans and laboratory animals alike are more prone to developing gallstones when they're deficient in vitamin C, Swedish researchers found a gallstone-limiting effect when they gave people 500 milligrams of vitamin C four times a day for two weeks prior to their gallstone surgery.

"Our findings indicate that vitamin C supplementation may influence conditions for gallstone development," they concluded in their 1997 report.

◗ **Don't skip meals.** Skipping meals increases risks of gallstone development by allowing bile within the gallbladder to become more concentrated as it sits unused, explains Dr. Pitt. He advises making it a point to eat at least three meals a day—and preferably four or five smaller ones—with that in mind.

● **Go slow when losing weight.** Rapid weight-loss programs invite gallstones in two ways, Peiken explains. First, such weight loss makes it more likely that unused bile within the gallbladder will thicken and crystallize as it in a sense goes "stale."

Second, the weight loss makes the liver increase its cholesterol output, thereby encouraging greater concentrations of cholesterol within the bile. Based on a study by researchers at the VA Medical Center in Minneapolis, calories should not be restricted to fewer than approximately 900 a day as a bare minimum. (And let's face it. No one should be going on a diet that low in calories anyway, unless it's under a doctor's strict supervision.)

"Another way dieters can protect themselves is to be sure to eat at least one meal a day that contains at least 10 grams of fat," Dr. Peiken says. "For most people, this is enough fat to assure that the gallbladder will undergo contractions capable of emptying it sufficiently to prevent a bile buildup."

healing diet

PROBLEM FOODS	GOOD FOODS
Foods high in fat and cholesterol	Fish
	Fruits, vegetables, and other foods high in fiber

BEST ADVICE: If you experience a gallstone attack, see your doctor. Untreated gallstone problems (assuming you can stand the pain) can lead to serious complications. If you're overweight, lose the excess, but don't let your weight come off too fast. (Typically, 1 pound a week or less is appropriate.)

164

headaches

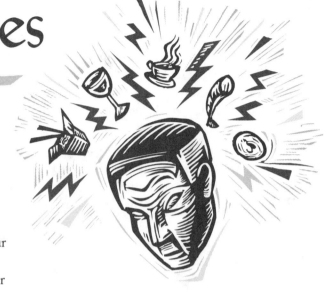

If you've recently found yourself, eyes closed, massaging your temples to ease away waves of throbbing pain, you're in good company. At any given moment, 2 million Americans suffer from a headache, more than 75 percent of them women.

Headaches are the most common ailment a family doctor treats, says Seymour Diamond, M.D., executive director of the National Headache Foundation and director of the Diamond Headache Clinic. Surveys show that between 50 and 90 percent of all people complain to their doctor about headaches at one time or another. And studies show that chronic headaches pose an even greater threat to normal functioning than almost any other chronic condition, including diabetes, arthritis, and depression.

Not all headaches are the same, says Fred D. Sheftell, M.D., co-founder and co-director of The New England Center for Headache in Stamford, Connecticut, and national president of the American Council for Headache Education (ACHE). He puts headaches into two categories: those that are a symptom of a disorder (headaches can be a symptom of more than 300 illnesses, including brain tumors, infections, dental problems, and eye problems) and those that are themselves a disorder. More than 90 percent of people with recurrent headaches have headaches that fall into this second category. This group has a genetic susceptibility to migraine, cluster, and/or tension-type headaches.

Headache Basics

Tension-type headaches are the common, garden-variety headache you get after sitting too long in a cramped position, straining your eyes, staying out in the sun too long, or dealing with a stubborn nuisance. Dr. Sheftell estimates that 75 percent of all headaches fall into this group and about 90 percent of the population gets one from time to time.

We used to think that these headaches were due simply to muscle tension or emotional stress, but today the distinction between tension-type headaches and migraines is less clear-cut and more controversial, says Dr. Sheftell. American researchers believe the two types have a similar mechanism as they develop in the body. European researchers believe they are separate disorders with separate mechanisms. In any case, your body's chemistry, not just tense muscles, is at least partly to blame for tension-type headaches.

Cluster headaches are rare, and their cause is unknown. They occur far more often in men than in women. They consist of intense pain behind or around one eye. Unlike migraines, there is no nausea or light sensitivity associated with cluster headaches. These headaches occur in clusters of one to four a day for weeks or months at a time (thus the name) then disappear completely for months or years.

Most people who suffer from frequent headaches have what doctors term mixed-headache syndrome. That means that sometimes they have tension-type headaches and other times they have migraines, usually characterized by pain on one side of the head, throbbing, nausea, and sensitivity to light or sound.

No matter what kind of headache you've had, the pain may function as a warning signal. A headache may be your body's way of telling you to modify certain behaviors that are harmful to you, says Dr. Diamond. Unhealthy habits like skipping meals, going without sleep, and exposure to prolonged physical or emotional stress predispose you to headaches.

Where Food Comes In

Genetics, stress, hormone fluctuations, and certain weather conditions can bring on headaches, but eating habits can also play a role. In fact, they can either provoke or prevent headaches. Leading headache specialists estimate that between 10 and 40 percent of their patients have clear food-related triggers for headaches. Dr. Diamond finds that 40 percent of his patients say that dietary changes have successfully reduced the frequency, severity, and duration of their headaches. Foods may trigger headaches in children more often than in adults, since kids tend to eat bigger portions of common trigger foods, such as hot dogs, peanut butter, pizza, and chocolate.

Studies have turned up inconsistent findings on the relationship between food and headaches. Some experts claim that many of the studies on the diet-headache link have been poorly designed and executed. They explain that because this line of research is less lucrative than drug research, for example, it is not as hotly pursued as it might be, so we are left with a great deal of confusion and disagreement over the possible relationship between food and headaches.

Still, there is plenty of hope and help for headache sufferers in terms of diet. Clinical results from top headache centers around the country offer a number of usable guidelines. There's a lot to try.

What, when, and how much you eat and drink affect each kind of headache differently. For example, Dr. Sheftell points out that sinus headaches may be provoked by milk, cheese, and foods containing milk products, which foods increase mucus production in people who are sensitive to dairy products. Tension-type headaches may be set off by drinking too much coffee. And migraines can be triggered by a whole host of substances commonly found in our daily diet. But if your headache is caused by eyestrain or by the set of your jaw (as in temporomandibular jaw syndrome, better known as TMJ), it won't matter what you eat—your headache is simply not food related and dietary changes won't help.

People prone to headaches should not only watch what they eat, they should watch when they eat, too. Skipping meals or fasting can bring on headaches.

How Food Can Hurt

Migraines and tension-type headaches are caused by a complex series of biochemical events. Some of these reactions inflame the nerves next to blood vessels in the head and make those blood vessels constrict then dilate. The coursing flow of blood through the dilated veins and arteries in your head causes the pounding throb of headache pain. The inflammation of tissues in your circulatory and central nervous systems only adds to the ouch.

Researchers offer several hypotheses about how food could set off these changes. These include directly constricting or dilating the brain's blood vessels or altering the body's chemistry in ways that indirectly affect the blood vessels and nerves in the head. A food might cause a drop in blood sugar and insulin levels, for example, creating a shortage of magnesium in the brain or otherwise mimicking the effects of severe stress on the body.

As a rule, foods don't directly cause headaches, but they may provoke chemical changes in your brain that do cause headaches. That's why doctors call food a trigger, rather than a cause of headaches.

Headache-prone people are unusually sensitive to certain chemicals in food. Some researchers believe that this sensitivity is partly due to a deficiency of the enzymes that break down these chemicals. So while some people may think that their headaches are due to an allergy to certain foods, that's not necessarily so. Allergic reactions involve the immune system; this enzyme deficiency does not.

Food rarely acts alone in bringing on a headache. Usually two or more factors are involved. For instance, chocolate might give you a headache only right before your period. The combination of your body's hormonal responses and its biochemical response to food creates a kind of short-circuit, bringing on the pounding pain. That's why a certain food might trigger a headache one time but not another. Your odds go up if you drink red wine and eat blue cheese while you are under a good deal of stress, for example.

How much food you eat counts, too, as well as whether you eat it on an empty stomach (risky) or with other foods. The same kind of food or drink also can have widely varying chemical makeup, making your body's reaction much less predictable.

Given that headaches may come on as a delayed reaction, starting anywhere from three to 36 hours after eating or drinking, all these factors complicate how clearly you can pinpoint the cause of your pain.

Many doctors finger the three Cs as the most common troublemakers: chocolate, cheese, and citrus fruits. But tracking down food triggers is more complicated than this short list might suggest.

Keep a food diary. Write down what you eat and when you eat it. Review your entries, checking for common triggers listed in this chapter. Note whether you get a headache within several hours of eating a certain food.

🍎 **Pace your meals.** Since low blood sugar can trigger a headache, keep your blood sugar steady with small, frequent meals containing protein. Eat at regularly scheduled times.

🍎 **Try an elimination diet.** If you can't pin down a given food as your culprit, try eliminating each potential food trigger for a few weeks or until your headaches are under better control. Then reintroduce them one at a time, starting with the foods you think are the least likely triggers.

If you're wondering where to start tracking down your headache triggers, there are a number of specific foods likely to either help or hurt you. Check out the food groups that follow and see whether any of them relate to your personal experience.

Coffee as Culprit?

The caffeine in coffee, tea, colas, and even chocolate may be the number one instigator of tension-type headaches. It's also a key troublemaker in migraines. But for those who are susceptible to headaches, caffeine can also prevent or abort a headache.

Caffeine prevents headaches by constricting your blood vessels. Since headache pain results from your blood vessels opening wide enough to allow a pounding, throbbing flow of blood, caffeine can effectively abort a headache even before it gets underway.

🍎 **Try a quick fix.** A single cup of strong coffee can serve as first aid for a migraine. Dr. Sheftell suggests that at the first sign of an aura or a pain, you might drink a cup of strong coffee or a cola, take two aspirin, and lie down and relax in a dark, quiet room. The episode may pass within an hour or so.

🍎 **Don't overdo it.** Experts draw a clear distinction between dietary and medicinal caffeine. Adding caffeine to aspirin and/or acetaminophen enhances pain relief for acute headaches. Caffeine's painkilling power can equal that of acetaminophen, according to tests by Nicholas Ward, M.D., a psychiatrist at the University of Washington in Seattle. Still, using too much caffeine or discontinuing it abruptly can sabotage your efforts. Your body may start to depend on caffeine to keep its blood vessels tight. After awhile, a rebound effect sets in. The blood vessels swell up again, causing an even worse withdrawal headache.

🍎 **Don't discount caffeine.** Caffeine withdrawal headaches may be more common than once believed, and just among constant coffee sippers. Withdrawal headaches can hit those who average only a cup or two a day. Tests at Johns Hopkins University School of Medicine in Baltimore, Maryland, showed that caffeine withdrawal can strike those who drink as little as a single cup of strongly brewed coffee or three caffeinated soft drinks per day. Symptoms (which may include flulike feelings) can start about 12 to 24 hours after you stop caffeine and may last as long as a week.

You can have a caffeine withdrawal headache without even knowing the cause. If you often wake up in the morning with a headache, it could be due to overnight caffeine withdrawal. One medical journal ran an article stating that caffeine withdrawal should officially be declared a form of mental disorder because it's so severe and disturbing.

🍎 **Try cutting caffeine.** Occasionally using caffeine to avert headaches works best if you cut it out from the rest of your diet and don't use it on a daily basis, doctors say. Experts at Tufts University in Medford, Massachusetts, suggest a program to reduce your dependence on coffee. The idea is to taper off over a couple of weeks. Don't just quit suddenly. Cut back by one cup every few days until you feel comfortable. Or mix regular and decaf to dilute the amount of caffeine and gradually increase the ratio of decaf to caffeine. Cut back on other sources. Avoid colas and Mountain Dew, the biggest sources. Smokers metabolize or use up caffeine in the blood more quickly than nonsmokers, so if you quit smoking, you should also cut back on caffeine. Dr. Sheftell recommends limiting caffeine to one 5-ounce cup of brewed coffee a day.

Alcohol Can Be Mean-Spirited

Alcohol is the number one headache trigger, according to Dr. Sheftell. Dr. Diamond concurs. He notes that it is the most common factor reported in patients' food diaries at his clinic. Between 40 and 60 percent of patients at the Diamond Clinic say alcohol causes their headaches. (And that's not even counting hangover headaches!)

Alcohol affects your system in many ways that can set the stage for a headache. It can make your blood sugar plummet. It can also dehydrate you. Many alcoholic beverages may also contain amines,

substances that constrict the blood vessels. Or it may be "congeners" in the beverages rather than the alcohol that cause the headaches. Congeners, impurities introduced during fermentation that give liquor or wine their taste, are mainly found in dark beverages, such as red wine, brandy, scotch, and bourbon. Alcohol also affects the liver in ways that promote headaches.

🍎 **Think light and white.** If you must drink it, stick to white wine, gin, or vodka, diluted with lots of water, seltzer, or juice. A dry white wine spritzer is your safest bet. White wine has 10 to 13 percent alcohol and very little sugar.

🍎 **Time your drinking.** Liquor's effects become even worse just before or during your period, so consider eliminating it during your premenstrual and early menstrual week.

Amines: What You Need to Know

What do smoked salmon, aged cheese, and red wine have in common (aside from deliciousness)? They can all trigger headaches because they contain amines.

Amines are chemicals manufactured in your body and present in certain foods. They are thought to play an important role in regulating your moods, blood pressure, heart rate, and sleep patterns—and in causing migraines.

The most commonly consumed amine implicated in migraines is tyramine. Tyramine probably does its dirty work by causing release of natural amines in the body. Tyramine is produced in food from the natural breakdown of the amino acid tyrosine. When food is aged, fermented, or stored for long periods, its tyramine levels increase. So the longer you store foods high in tyrosine, such as aged cheeses and sour cream, the more headache-causing chemicals will be present in them.

 Avoid amines. Amines have been targeted as one of the main dietary headache triggers, so if you suspect that you're sensitive to them, stay away from the foods they're found in.

Researchers have identified at least five amines common in our daily diets:

Dopamine: in legumes such as peanuts, peas, broad beans, and soy

Histamine: in cold-water fish, such as salmon and tuna

Octopamine and synephrine: in citrus fruits

Phenylethylamine: in chocolate

Tryptamine: in tomatoes and pineapple

Tyramine: in cheese, yogurt, buttermilk, sourdough bread, wine, and dried or pickled meat and fish.

 Forgo the doggie bag. Don't eat leftovers more than one day old, especially high-protein foods. These form the dreaded amines that are common headache triggers.

The Problem with Chocolate

Chocolate ranks high on the Most Wanted list (in both senses of the phrase) of headache triggers for two reasons. It's so popular and so potent. Surveys show that chocolate sits at the top of most women's cravings for sweets, and it

has been accused of being one of the most powerful headache triggers. It may pack a triple whammy for people who get migraines. Its sugar and cacao (the seeds that make it dark) can wreak havoc with your blood sugar, and its caffeine and amines can constrict your blood vessels and release pain-causing chemicals in your brain.

One study done at the University of Pittsburgh Medical Center, however, may sweeten chocolate's bad reputation to some degree. Sixty-three women who suffered recurrent migraines or tension-type headaches followed a diet restricting foods high in amines, including chocolate. (They also avoided certain other known headache triggers.) In four separate visits to the lab, the women ate chocolate bars twice and carob bars twice, all disguised with mint flavoring. Half the women got no headaches at all. Of those who did, three got a headache within 12 hours of eating chocolate. Another got headaches after eating carob but not chocolate. Six got headaches after eating both.

Even though almost 20 percent of the women who got headaches thought chocolate was responsible, the researchers concluded that chocolate may trigger headaches only when combined with other suspect foods. They speculated that chocolate might fulfill cravings provoked by stress or premenstrual syndrome, which would have caused a headache whether or not they ate the chocolate. So if you are a headachy chocolate lover, there is hope that you might find a way to have your chocolate without the bitter consequences. You'll just need to watch your responses to chocolate very carefully.

Other Food Triggers

Aside from the biggies, there are several other foods and additives that cause problems for some people. Here are some strategies to consider.

🍎 **Walk away from dogs.** Ever been felled by headache pain after eating a hot dog? The culprit is nitrites. Nitrites are chemicals used to preserve foods, prevent botulism, flavor meat, and turn it pink or red.

Nitrites also can make your blood vessels expand, causing a dull, throbbing pain in the temples, usually within 30 minutes of eating nitrite-treated food, says Dr. Sheftell. Nitrites are often found in canned ham, corned beef, smoked fish, salami, bologna, sausage, pepperoni, summer sausage, bacon and, of course, hot dogs.

🍎 **Watch out for MSG.** Monosodium glutamate (MSG) is chemically related to certain chemicals in your brain, called neurotransmitters. Neurotransmitters make brain cells fire, and too many can set off a sort of fireworks display of pain in your brain, if you're one of the 10 to 25 percent of the population who don't metabolize it well.

Dr. Sheftell describes an MSG headache as a band of tightness around the forehead along with pounding pain in the temples. This kind of headache usually occurs within 15 minutes after eating large quantities of MSG on an empty stomach.

MSG is commonly added to Chinese cuisine. But Dr. Sheftell cautions that it's also added to frozen meals; self-basting turkeys; instant gravy; processed meats; canned and dry soups; dry-roasted nuts; some potato chips; prepared tomato and barbecue sauces; salad dressings; and tenderizers and seasonings, including Accent and Lawry's Seasoned Salt. Read your labels! Watch out for ingredients such as hydrolyzed vegetable protein (HVP), hydrolyzed plant protein (HPP), and Kombu extract. All of these contain MSG.

🍎 **Try avoiding aspartame.** Aspartame apparently triggers swift, severe headaches in some people. About 8 percent of people who get headaches link this artificial sweetener to headache pain, according to Dr. Diamond. Clinical trials of aspartame have proved inconclusive; however, Dr. Diamond cautions those who think they might be sensitive to aspartame to avoid it.

🍎 **Consider dairy products.** Dairy products may make some people produce more phlegm and mucus, blocking their sinuses, according to Dr. Sheftell. While this doesn't cause headaches, it does magnify the discomfort of a headache. Dr. Sheftell also thinks that allergies to dairy products may trigger headache pain in some people. Possible problem foods include milk or anything made from milk, such as cheese, cream cheese, sour cream, and yogurt.

Sheftell suggests reducing or eliminating dairy products if you think you are sensitive to them. You can experiment with cutting down or cutting back around the time of your period, in damp, rainy weather, or during stress, and note whether your discomfort improves. (Women should make sure they're getting adequate calcium through other foods in their diet, including salmon and sardines, dark green leafy vegetables, nuts, grains, and fortified orange juice, if necessary.)

🍎 **Don't blame ice cream.** By the way, so-called ice cream headaches, which are somewhat common, are probably due more to the cold hitting the roof of your mouth than from allergy to the milk content. (Plenty of people who are not allergic to dairy products get these headaches.)

🍎 **Watch that salt.** Salt may trigger headaches mainly in children, though no one knows why. If you suspect salt as a trigger in your child's diet, Dr. Sheftell

recommends cutting down on all foods that you haven't prepared yourself, since salt is so common in processed foods.

🍎 **Personalize your antiheadache diet.** Diet is extremely interactive, says Dr. Sheftell. Each individual's response to food is unique. Your personal response to a given food may vary with the rest of your diet, how much exercise you get, where you are in your hormonal cycle, and what emotional state you're in. So no matter how much information you have, the final decisions about your diet are up to you.

healing diet

PROBLEM FOODS

Aged cheese and yellow cheeses colored with annatto (including cheddar, blue, and Brie)
Alcoholic beverages, especially red wine
Aspartame
Bananas
Chicken livers
Chocolate
Citrus fruits (in large quantities)
Coffee, colas, and teas containing caffeine
Dairy products, especially cream, sour cream, and yogurt
Flavor enhancers, such as MSG
Pickled, marinated, and fermented foods
Pizza
Shellfish
Smoked and cured, aged, and packaged meats containing nitrites (including bacon, bologna, corned beef, cold cuts, ham, hot dogs, pepperoni, salami, sausage, and smoked fish)
Sourdough bread
Vinegar
Yeast bread and cakes (doughnuts, coffee cakes, and especially hot, fresh bread)

GOOD FOODS

Fresh or frozen fruits
Whole, unleavened grains

BEST ADVICE: Stick to a natural foods diet, with whole, unprocessed foods you prepare yourself. Keep a diet diary to pinpoint which foods are possible headache triggers for you.

heart disease & stroke

It's America's number one killer. But it shouldn't be. It doesn't deserve to be. Heart disease kills more men and women in this country than any other cause, but many of us can effectively escape its deadly clutch. How? Careful attention to lifestyle. Don't smoke—or quit if you do. Get physical— not only to strengthen your heart and arteries but to reduce stress, which also contributes to heart disease. And eat foods that are rich—not in fat—but in vitamins, minerals, fiber, and complex carbohydrates.

Getting Clogged

The primary cause of coronary heart disease and stroke, according to the American Heart Association (AHA), is atherosclerosis. This is a process that takes place when cholesterol and other debris in the blood collect in damaged spots in the lining of the arteries. As these deposits (called plaque) enlarge, the arteries narrow and can eventually close completely. When the arteries of the heart become blocked, oxygen and nutrients can not get to the heart tissue and it begins to starve. A heart attack occurs when blood flow cannot be restored and the tissue dies. When the arteries of the brain become clogged, the result is a stroke—the third leading cause of death in this country and the number one

cause of disability. Heart attacks and strokes can also occur when an artery is blocked by a piece of plaque or a blood clot that has traveled from some distant part of the circulatory system.

The most notorious artery-clogger is cholesterol, specifically low-density lipoprotein (LDL). LDLs not used up by your body or removed from your blood by your liver can become oxidized. When they do, they get gobbled up by scavenger cells called macrophages. When a macrophage becomes full of oxidized LDLs, it's called a foam cell. Foam cells collect in the lining of damaged areas of an artery wall, eventually forming a nasty hunk of plaque.

Many factors besides LDL help create atherosclerosis and heart disease, however, including high blood pressure (which damages artery walls), obesity, triglycerides (the chemical name for fat), and low levels of HDLs (high-density lipoproteins, the "good" cholesterol, which helps remove the "bad" cholesterol from your body). Usually it's a combination of factors that puts a person at risk for heart disease.

"Someone with high cholesterol and high triglycerides has the greatest risk," says Ronald Krauss, M.D., head of molecular medicine at Lawrence Berkeley National Laboratory at the University of California at Berkeley and chairman of the nutrition committee for the AHA.

What's high? When total blood cholesterol is more than 200 milligrams/deciliter (mg/dL), it's moving into the undesirable range according to the AHA. At 240 mg/dL, your risk of a heart attack doubles. More than 300 mg/dL, and you have a six- to eight-fold chance of heart attack, says Dr. Krauss. More important than the total, however, is the amount of HDL versus LDL cholesterol. Optimum levels as defined by the AHA are a total cholesterol level less than 160 mg/dL, an LDL of 100 mg/dL, and an HDL of 35 mg/dL or greater. A high triglyceride level is viewed with particular concern. Fortunately, diet can help keep all this risky business at bay.

Healing with Diet

A heart-healthy diet can help you maintain an appropriate weight, control blood pressure, lower cholesterol, and prevent diabetes—another contributing factor for heart disease and

here's to your health

Should you toast to your heart's health with a glass of wine at dinner? Several studies suggest that moderate alcohol consumption (no more than one drink a day for women and two for men) can raise the levels of HDL cholesterol (the good kind) and lower LDL cholesterol (the bad kind). It can also prevent blood clots from forming, which is what happens during a heart attack. Nonetheless, the American Heart Association points out that the risks of regular drinking outweigh the possible benefits. Of specific relevance to the heart, heavy drinking can lead to high blood pressure and obesity.

If you don't drink, but still want to get the benefits of wine, lift a glass of purple grape juice instead. In a study conducted at the University of Wisconsin, people who drank a 5-ounce glass of purple grape juice every morning and evening for a week, showed a 60 percent lower tendency to develop blood clots. The magic ingredient? Flavonoids, which are also found in red wine and black tea. So, instead of that after-dinner cup of coffee, sip a cup of tea.

stroke. "Eat plenty of vegetables, fruits, and whole grains and reduce your intake of fat—especially saturated fat—and cholesterol," advises Dr. Krauss. Fruits, vegetables, and whole grains provide lots of nutrients, little fat, and few calories, hence their importance in weight and blood pressure management. In addition, their high fiber content keeps you feeling full so that you don't overeat, slows the release of sugar into the blood (a preventive measure for diabetes), and can lower cholesterol in many people.

But there's even more reason to fill up on fruits and veggies. Many contain antioxidants—vitamins E, C, and beta-carotene—which may prevent the oxidation of LDL. Remember, once LDL becomes oxidized, it's primed to become plaque on your artery walls.

Furthermore, fruits, vegetables, and grains contain phytochemicals—micronutrients, such as flavonoids, that have health-giving properties. Scientists suspect that there are many phytochemicals in foods that have yet to be discovered. So it's wise to get the nutrients you need by eating a variety of whole foods rather than by simply popping supplements.

The AHA makes the following general dietary recommendations for the prevention of heart disease and stroke. They call this the Step 1 diet:

- Keep total fat intake under 30 percent of calories. Of that total, no more than 10 percent should come from saturated fats, no more than 10 percent from polyunsaturated fats, and 10 to 15 percent from monounsaturated fats.
- Eat five or more servings of fruits and vegetables a day.
- Eat six or more servings of grains or grain products (bread, cereal, pasta) a day.
- Consume three to four servings of low-fat dairy products daily.
- Eat no more than 6 ounces of meat a day from low-fat sources such as fish, skinless poultry, and lean meat.
- Egg whites are okay but limit egg yolks to three or four a week.

- Total cholesterol intake should be no more than 300 milligrams a day.
- Sodium intake should stop at 2,400 milligrams a day.

Such is the foundation of a diet that can help keep most of our hearts healthy. Those who have known risks for heart disease—high cholesterol or high blood pressure, for example—would be wise to follow a more aggressive plan. You'll find details later in this section. All of us, however, can take these general recommendations and fine-tune our food choices for maximum prevention of heart disease and stroke.

How Low Should You Go?

Several studies have shown that lowering the amount of fat in your diet can lower your blood cholesterol and triglyceride levels and help with weight control. The average American consumes 34 percent of calories from fat. For someone who eats 2,000 calories a day, that's 680 calories or 75 grams. The AHA wants us to cut back to 30 percent. For that same 2,000-calorie-a-day diet, that's 600 calories or 66 grams of fat. More important than the total amount of fat, however, is the type of fat we eat: saturated (found in meats, eggs, dairy products, and tropical oils), polyunsaturated fats (those in vegetable oils such as corn, safflower, sesame, and soybean), and monounsaturated fats (from olive, canola, and nut oils). Saturated fats can raise cholesterol levels. Polyunsaturates can help lower cholesterol but tend to lower both LDL and HDL. Monounsaturates lower LDL cholesterol but not HDL.

"For some people, diet has a big effect on cholesterol, and for others it has no effect," says Paul Thompson, M.D., director of preventive cardiology at Hartford Hospital in Connecticut. Whether or not a specific diet will work can be determined in two to four weeks. No cheating though.

"You need to be strict 13 out of 14 days," explains Dr. Thompson. "If you cheat a little every day, you undermine the diet." He advises that if you have high cholesterol levels that do not respond to diet, you should talk to your doctor about the possible benefits of drug therapy.

Here's a look at how dietary changes might help you prevent and deal with heart disease and stroke.

Vegetable Power

If I had heart disease, you can bet your bottom dollar I'd be a vegetarian," says Thompson. "If you have to have some meat, eat fish. Don't like fish? Choose defatted, deskinned poultry. If you must have red meat, eat only very lean meats like venison."

🍎 **Max out on fruits and veggies.** Most fruits and vegetables contain very little fat and with very few exceptions (coconut) zero saturated fat. But as Thompson points out, you don't have to be a vegetarian to have a low-fat diet, just choose low-fat options among the other food groups.

🍎 **With milk, think "lite."** When doing dairy, select skim or 1% milk and nonfat or low-fat yogurts, cheeses, and frozen desserts.

🍎 **Buy only lean meats.** Among meats, choose fish first, then skinless poultry, game meats such as venison, low-fat cuts of beef (buy choice or select grades rather than prime and choose from round, sirloin, or loin), lean pork (tenderloin), and lean ham (beware the high salt content though).

🍎 **Let cows live.** Replace a 6-ounce beef burger with the veggie version, and you'll save yourself 20 grams of saturated fat and 150 milligrams of cholesterol, and get instead plenty of fiber and other nutrients.

🍎 **Beware of processed and packaged food products.** Many items, such as frozen dinners, soups, and spaghetti in a can, are high in fat and sodium.

🍎 **Say no to dietary cholesterol.** Cholesterol only comes from animal products and tends to be higher in meats than dairy products. Those foods that pack a heart-stopping punch include organ meats (liver, kidneys, brains) and egg yolks. One egg yolk contains 213 milligrams of cholesterol, and a 3-ounce serving of chicken liver delivers 536 milligrams.

🍎 **Hold the mayo.** More often it's not the fat in our foods but the fat we put on our foods that adds up to excess. Just 1 tablespoon of mayonnaise contains 99 calories, almost all of them from fat. That's 11 grams of fat, one-sixth of a day's total recommended fat intake based on a 2,000-calorie-a-day diet. Use mustard or catsup instead, or if you must have mayo, buy low-fat or nonfat versions.

🍎 **Dump the dips.** Salad dressings, dips for chips and veggies, gravies, and butter and cream sauces—all those silky smooth food coatings will end up coating your arteries, too. There are low-fat options, but the best choice for your health is to flavor foods with

the newfangled fats

There's a relatively new kind of fat on the dietary scene—trans fats. These fats do not occur naturally in foods. We created them. Why? Saturated fats are solid and provide a texture to prepared foods that simply can't be had with liquid oils. So scientists found a way to take polyunsaturated oils and make them more solid through a process called hydrogenation. This chemical process creates what are known as trans-fatty acids. The more solid a hydrogenated fat is, the more trans fats it contains. For example, stick margarine is higher in trans fats than softer tub margarine. Unfortunately, not only are trans fats more solid, they are also more harmful to our health than all other fats, including saturated fats.

Results from the Nurses' Health Study showed that a 5 percent dietary increase in calories from saturated fat versus carbohydrates raised risk of coronary disease by 17 percent. However, just a 2 percent increase in calories from trans fats compared with carbohydrates raised risk by 93 percent. Does this mean butter is better than fat? No, says the American Heart Association. There's far more saturated fat in butter than trans fat in margarine, plus butter contains cholesterol. But do choose soft tub margarine over sticks.

Better yet, don't choose either one. Use olive oil or canola oil in place of margarine whenever you can.

Trans fats can be a little tricky to uncover in foods. You won't find them listed on nutrition labels. Instead look for hydrogenated oils in the ingredients list, particularly of baked goods such as cookies and crackers. And avoid fried foods.

vinegars (balsamic or fruit-flavored) or juices such as lemon, orange, and apple.

● **Go for the fresh.** If you buy foods as fresh as possible and are careful not to overcook them, their natural flavors will need little enhancing. And when it comes to cooking, steam, bake, broil, and poach or sauté in stock or juices, rather than fry food in butter or oil.

● **Count your calories.** Eating low-fat foods doesn't mean you can eat all you want. Consuming too many calories, no matter where they come from, can lead to obesity (defined as a weight 20 percent higher than an individual's ideal weight).

"Now that we've learned how to lower cholesterol and triglycerides, we're seeing obesity emerge as a major risk factor for heart disease," says Dr. Krauss. Obesity by itself puts a person at risk, he says. And research from the Nurses' Health Study, an ongoing look at the effects of various lifestyle factors on the health of 80,000 women, shows that weight gain and obesity significantly raise a woman's risk of stroke caused by a blocked blood vessel in the brain. (For details on achieving and maintaining a healthy weight, see "Overweight," which begins on page 256.)

Be Complex About Carbohydrates

As you decrease the fat in your diet in an effort to lower your cholesterol level, you'll probably increase the amount of carbohydrates you consume. Ironically, carbohydrates tend to raise triglyceride levels in the blood. However, you can offset this effect by eating foods high in complex carbohydrates and fiber—whole grains, beans, legumes, vegetables, and fruits—and limiting consumption of simple carbohydrates— sugars and foods high in sugar. In addition, whole grains and vegetables digest more slowly, which makes them gentle on your blood sugar levels. Plus, they'll keep you satiated longer, so you're less likely to overeat and become overweight.

 Go for whole foods. Reach for whole grains and whole-grain cereals and breads rather than refined carbohydrate products like white bread and baked goods made from flours that have had all the fiber stripped from them.

 Don't be fooled. Check the ingredients list when buying foods labeled "whole wheat" or "seven-grain." Many of them are made from a mixture of flours and contain very small amounts of bran and fiber.

 Crunch, don't sip. Eat whole fruits and vegetables rather than juices. While juices do give you phytochemicals and vitamins, they contain very little fiber.

Fiber Power

Speaking of fiber, the AHA recommends increasing your intake to 25 to 30 grams daily. Most of us consume a mere 10 to 15 grams. And one-quarter to one-third of that fiber should be the soluble form. Soluble fiber is the kind that seems to hold onto cholesterol and fat in the intestines, preventing them from being absorbed into your bloodstream. Scientists aren't sure exactly how soluble fiber works, but they are sure that it can help lower blood cholesterol in some people.

Oat bran has been the poster food for soluble fiber, delivering 2 grams in every 1/3 cup, but psyllium seems to be getting a lot of attention these days, too. Psyllium comes from the seeds of the psyllium plant and is the main ingredient in Metamucil. One tablespoon contains the same amount of soluble fiber as 14 tablespoons of oat bran. But psyllium has no other nutrient value, whereas oat bran contains decent amounts of thiamine, magnesium, and iron. Most of us would do best to simply get our fiber from the foods we eat, although psyllium might be helpful if you have high blood cholesterol. (Taking a psyllium supplement is something to discuss with your doctor.)

Keep in mind that fiber can interfere with absorption of minerals and cause gastrointestinal problems. So don't overdo it. To avoid GI distress as you increase your fiber intake, go gradually and drink at least six to eight glasses of water a day.

Foods high in soluble fiber include beans (especially kidney, pinto, and navy), brussels sprouts, broccoli, prunes, apples, oranges, grapefruit, oatmeal, and oat bran.

These also contain plenty of insoluble fiber, which keeps your colon humming and helps prevent cancer.

Up the Ante on Antioxidants

W e don't have all the data in on antioxidants yet," says Paula Johnson, M.D., M.P.H., cardiologist at Brigham and Women's Hospital in Boston. "But the research thus far is highly suggestive that individuals who are at risk of heart disease may benefit from increasing their intake of antioxidants."

So, what exactly is an antioxidant? The most famous of the antioxidants are vitamins E, C, and beta-carotene (precursor of vitamin A). Exactly how antioxidants prevent cardiovascular disease, scientists aren't yet sure. We know they inhibit oxidation—the chemical process that turns LDL cholesterol "bad," causing it to collect on artery walls and stir up other trouble like encouraging the formation of blood clots. But antioxidants may act on their own to prevent clot formation and plaque buildup.

Like Dr. Johnson, most experts aren't yet willing to come right out and say for certain that antioxidants directly prevent heart disease and stroke. But they do agree that evidence continues to mount in favor of the protective effect of vitamin E.

"The evidence for vitamin E is the strongest and then for vitamin C," says Dr. Thompson. "It's less clear that vitamin A or selenium is beneficial."

Lycopene, an antioxidant found in tomatoes, also shows promise as a protector of the cardiovascular system. A study done in 1997 found that men who consumed a high amount of lycopene in their diets had half the risk of heart disease compared with those who consumed the least amount.

● **Enjoy those fruits and veggies.** Scientific studies aside, most doctors recommend including lots of antioxidant-rich fruits and vegetables in your diet. Along with many important vitamins, you'll get phytochemicals—micronutrients that may have heart-protective properties. Fruits and vegetables are also good sources of magnesium and potassium, which may have a role in preventing heart disease and stroke.

● **Stock up often.** To get maximum nutrient content, try to shop for fresh fruits and veggies at least two times a week, advises Katherine Sherif, M.D., assistant professor of medicine at the Institute for Women's Health at Allegheny University in Philadelphia. "As produce sits around, it loses nutrients," she points out. Steam or microwave vegetables to hold onto nutrients and flavor.

● **Get more vitamin E.** You can find this vital nutrient in wheat germ oil, safflower oil, fortified cereal, sunflower seeds, hazelnuts (filberts), wheat germ, soybeans, and cereal. Unfortunately, you'd have to eat a lot of any of these foods to achieve the amounts of vitamin E found to be most protective against heart disease (100 to 600 international units). Those who wish to increase their intake to such levels may want to take a supplement.

● **Seek C.** Foods high in vitamin C include sweet peppers, broccoli, papaya, kiwifruit,

homocysteine and B vitamins

Bet you thought cholesterol was the nastiest culprit for clogging up arteries. Well, here's another potential heart-stopper—homocysteine, an amino acid that's formed during protein metabolism.

Not only does homocysteine damage artery walls, creating spots where plaque can build up, it also stimulates growth of certain cells that form plaque, assists cholesterol in collecting on artery walls, and seems to encourage blood clotting. Several studies have linked high levels of homocysteine in the blood to incidence of heart disease and stroke.

There are various chemical processes that convert homocysteine into a harmless amino acid. Those chemical processes involve certain enzymes and vitamins, specifically folic acid and vitamins B6 and B12. People who have genetically defective enzymes and those who are deficient in folic acid, B6, and B12 can't process homocysteine. It just builds up in the blood and carries out a relentless attack on the arteries.

You can't do anything to fix your enzymes, but several studies show that individuals with high homocysteine levels who are also deficient in these B vitamins can lower their homocysteine levels by increasing their vitamin intake. The Nurses' Health Study, an ongoing look at the effects of lifestyle factors on the health of more than 80,000 women, found that the women who had the highest intake of folic acid and vitamin B6 had the lowest risk for heart disease.

"B vitamins can clearly lower levels of homocysteine in individuals who are vitamin B deficient, and studies show that higher intakes have reduced the risk of heart disease, but we still don't know for sure whether they are connected," says Ronald Krauss, M.D., head of molecular medicine at Lawrence Berkeley National Laboratory in Berkeley, California, and chairman of the nutrition committee for the American Heart Association.

Though more research is being done to determine definitively that B vitamins can help prevent heart disease and stroke, you don't have to wait for results to make sure you are getting the RDA for B6 (1.6 milligrams a day for women; 2.0 milligrams for men) and B12 (2.0 milligrams a day for both women and men). And it's appropriate to aim for 400 micrograms of folate every day, says Dr. Krauss. You don't want to get any more than that though, because excess folate can mask a serious condition called pernicious anemia.

Foods high in folate: fortified cereal, orange juice, lentils, most beans, spinach, wheat germ, romaine lettuce, asparagus, and broccoli

Foods high in vitamin B6: fortified cereal, potatoes, bananas, chickpeas, chicken breast, beef, tuna, and white turkey meat

Foods high in vitamin B12: fortified cereal, steamed clams, mackerel, tuna, salmon, and beef

citrus fruits, watermelon, strawberries, and cantaloupe.

🍎 **Eat foods rich in beta-carotene.** These include pumpkin, sweet potatoes, carrots, spinach, winter squash, red peppers, romaine lettuce, broccoli, mangoes, and cantaloupe.

🍎 **Learn to love lycopene.** This beneficial phytochemical is found in rich supply in tomato sauce, raw and cooked tomatoes (cooking seems to make lycopene more available), tomato juice, watermelon, catsup, guava, and pink grapefruit.

Soybeans for a Better Heart

A low-growing legume, soybeans are achieving pretty tall status among doctors and nutritionists. Researchers are discovering numerous health benefits of a diet high in soy foods, including protection from heart disease and stroke. It appears that consuming soy foods reduces blood levels of LDL cholesterol and triglycerides without lowering HDL cholesterol. In 1997 the Harvard Women's Health Watch reported that an analysis of 38 studies of the effect of soy on cholesterol levels found that total cholesterol was reduced by 23.3 points, LDL by 21.7, and triglycerides by 13.3. And research at Wake Forest University Baptist Medical Center in Winston-Salem, North Carolina, found that soy protein was just as effective as hormone replacement therapy in preventing stroke among postmenopausal women.

Soybeans contain phytoestrogens called isoflavones. We've long known that estrogen protects women from heart disease by keeping cholesterol in control. When estrogen production stops with menopause, cholesterol rises and so does a woman's risk of heart disease. Apparently, the phytoestrogens in soy offer a protective effect similar to estrogen. Researchers also speculate that soy may prevent the growth of certain cells on the lining of arteries that lead to the buildup of plaque and may help keep blood vessels flexible.

How much soy do you need to eat to reap its benefits? Experts recommend between 30 to 50 milligrams a day.

🍎 **Get to know soybeans.** The amount that experts recommend is not really a lot of soybeans. But then again, most of us simply aren't used to eating soybeans on a regular basis. It will help to get acquainted with as many sources for soybeans as you possibly can and start incorporating some into your diet. Sources include green soybeans, dried soybeans (often called soy nuts), soybean sprouts, tofu, powered soy protein, and soy milk.

🍎 **Use soybeans as a veggie.** Finding honest-to-goodness green soybeans isn't easy (in this country), but they're beginning to appear mixed with other veggies in the frozen food aisle.

🍎 **Try powder.** Consider buying powdered soy protein and mixing it into fruit juice or fruit smoothies.

Looking After Your Heart

There are several other dietary strategies for dealing with heart disease and stroke that you should be aware of.

👄 **Go for garlic.** Not everyone's a believer, but several studies suggest that eating garlic regularly can lower cholesterol levels and may keep blood clots from forming as well.

One medical review of several studies on the effect of garlic consumption on cholesterol levels concluded that: "The best available evidence suggests that garlic, in an amount approximating one half to one clove per day, decreased total serum cholesterol levels by about 9 percent in the groups of patients studied."

👄 **Make a milk mustache.** Dietary calcium has been shown to moderately reduce total cholesterol and LDL according to the AHA. Aim for a good 800 to 1,200 milligrams of calcium a day, equivalent to three to four servings of low-fat or nonfat milk or yogurt. Foods high in calcium include low-fat and nonfat yogurt and milk; fortified orange juice; low-fat cheeses; and dark-green leafy vegetables such as kale, turnip greens, and broccoli rabe.

healing diet

PROBLEM FOODS	GOOD FOODS
Egg yolks	Beans
Meat	Fish
Whole milk, butter, and other full-fat dairy products	Foods high in fiber
	Foods low in fat
	Fruits
	Oat bran
	Olive oil
	Poultry without the skin
	Soybeans
	Vegetables
	Whole grains

BEST ADVICE: If you have heart disease or have experienced a stroke, you should be under a doctor's care.

heartburn

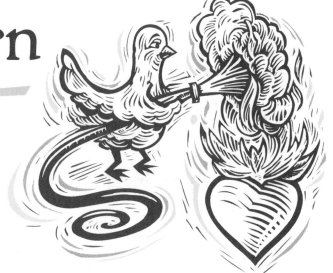

Heartburn is as common, not coincidentally, as our love for those "two all-beef patties, special sauce, lettuce, cheese, pickles, and onions on a sesame seed bun." And those "all you can eat" spaghetti nights at the local fire hall. Even our on-the-run breakfasts of doughnuts and coffee—especially when followed by more coffee—can bring on "the burn."

"It's not our stomachs that are to blame for heartburn as much as it is what we put in them," explains Henry D. Janowitz, M.D., clinical professor of medicine, emeritus, at the Mount Sinai School of Medicine in New York and author of *Good Food for Bad Stomachs*.

Dr. Janowitz estimates that approximately half the adult population experiences heartburn at least once a month, and that another 20 percent suffer at least weekly.

What's the cause, other than our diets, of this all-too-ubiquitous gripe that bubbles up an estimated $1.2 billion in sales of over-the-counter remedies every year?

Heartburn has nothing to do with the heart, first of all. Its searing pain usually is felt in the area of the heart—although it can radiate into the back and up into the jaw in extreme cases. But it's the esophagus, in fact, that's getting "burned." Heartburn is actually a symptom of a disorder doctors call gastroesophageal reflux disease (GERD), which, despite its complicated name, is actually a fairly simple—and correctable—problem.

Heartburn, an Inside Look

To understand heartburn, you need to understand the digestive tract," says Dr. Janowitz. At the bottom end of the esophagus, which is the tube leading from the mouth to the stomach, is a small valve called the lower esophageal sphincter (LES). The LES is supposed to keep the contents of the stomach in their place. In response to certain dietary or other lifestyle infractions, however, this valve can malfunction by relaxing and allowing the highly acidic contents of the stomach to back up into the esophagus, causing considerable pain to its sensitive linings.

If frequent, such backups (clinically known as refluxes) can inflame the esophagus, leading to a condition called esophagitis, in which event just the act of swallowing becomes painful. If untreated, this condition can lead to ulcers within the

could it be a heart attack?

Back in 1923, when heart attack victim President Warren Harding died of what was diagnosed as "acute indigestion," doctors thought heart attacks were heartburn. Clearly, the conditions can mimic one another closely. Here are key differences to look for, lest a misdiagnosis as tragic as President Harding's should happen to you.

● The pain of a heart attack generally is more severe than heartburn and commonly is experienced as a very uncomfortable feeling of tightness or squeezing in the chest as opposed to simply a burning.
● The chest pain of a heart attack may be accompanied by pain radiating into the left arm, back, neck, or jaw, and may produce dizziness, sweating, nausea, and shortness of breath as well.
● The pain of a heart attack will not subside in 10 or 15 minutes, as is usually the case with heartburn, nor will it be relieved by an antacid. (If your pain does subside in 15 minutes or so, it still could indicate a heart problem known as angina, in which the heart muscle becomes starved for oxygen temporarily following physical exertion or emotional excitement.)

Any chest pain exhibiting any of the above symptoms *definitely* should send you as quickly as possible to the nearest hospital or your doctor. In fact, if you have any doubts at all about whether your chest pain is heartburn or something more serious, call your doctor.

esophagus, bleeding, and eventually a buildup of scar tissue that can make swallowing not just uncomfortable, but, in extreme cases, difficult to accomplish at all.

"This is why it's important to get heartburn under control," says Dr. Janowitz. "It can seem like a relatively benign condition at the outset, but if left untreated, it can lead to serious complications, indeed. Anyone who experiences heartburn more than three or four times a week, or is awakened by it at night, or vomits blood, or has trouble swallowing definitely should seek medical advice."

Foods that Can Stoke the Fire

Why are some of us bothered by heartburn more than others? "We're not sure why some people are more susceptible to reflux problems, but we do know that there's definitely a dietary connection," Dr. Janowitz says. Some foods tend to have a relaxing effect on the LES, thus increasing chances of reflux. Other foods tend to encourage heartburn by causing the stomach to put out excessive amounts of acid in the first place. There also are foods—fatty foods, for example—that can encourage heartburn simply by being slow to digest. The longer any food remains in the stomach, the more acid it's going to produce, and hence the greater the chances are going to be that an acidic "spill" can occur, Dr. Janowitz explains.

Then, too, there are foods spicy or acidic enough to irritate the esophagus directly—even before they reach the stomach—and these, too, should be avoided by the heartburn-prone, Dr. Janowitz says.

Worst of all for people who get heartburn, however, are the "multiple offenders," those foods that can be guilty of more than one of the above crimes simultaneously. Coffee and chocolate, for example, not only tend to produce excess stomach acid, they also have a relaxing effect on the LES, thus increasing the likelihood that this acid will bubble its way into trouble. Foods high in fat also can produce a double whammy, by relaxing the LES while also delaying gastric emptying.

If heartburn is a problem for you, the problem foods listed on page 186 under "Healing Diet" are the ones you should be most careful to avoid. No two people with heartburn are exactly alike, however, Dr. Janowitz stresses. There may be certain foods that are troublesome for you that are not on these lists, so let your personal experience be your guide.

Foods that Soothe

Just as there are foods that can ignite heartburn, there are foods that can help put out the flames. Studies show that some foods not only can help neutralize excess acid in the stomach, in much the same way as an antacid would, but they also help keep the muscles of the esophageal sphincter in an appropriately contracted state. Best of these gastric peacekeepers seems to be nonfat milk, but other high-protein foods low in fat (such as fish, very lean meats, and skinless chicken and turkey) also are acid neutralizers, Dr. Janowitz says. Regular milk, traditionally thought to help ease heartburn, actually has been shown to have the opposite effect due to its high fat content.

Other foods well-suited for the heartburn-prone are steamed or boiled vegetables, rice, pasta, baked or boiled potatoes, gelatin, puddings, and noncitrus fruits such as apples, peaches, and pears, Dr. Janowitz says.

Dousing the Flames

Your best dietary strategy for getting a handle on heartburn is to learn to avoid the foods that offend and eat more of those that can help you mend. It's not the only tactic for achieving greater digestive peace, however. Making certain changes in your lifestyle also can have a powerful impact on controlling heartburn, says Steven Peikin, M.D., a professor of medicine at the Robert Wood Johnson Medical School and head of gastroenterology at the Cooper University Medical School at Camden, in New Jersey. For example:

🍎 **Trim down if you're overweight.** This is especially true if your extra pounds are in the area of your waist. Excess abdominal fat (and also pregnancy) can make acid reflux more likely by increasing pressure on the stomach. People who get heartburn should avoid wearing tight-fitting clothing around their waists for the same reason.

🍎 **Don't overeat.** The commercial of several years ago featuring the heartburn sufferer incredulous for having eaten "the whole thing" was right on target. The fuller the stomach gets, the more acid it produces, and the easier it is for this acid to overflow into the esophagus. People who get heartburn should eat lightly with this in mind. Better to have four or five small meals a day than two or three feasts.

🍎 **Remain upright after eating.** You want to keep gravity on your side, so avoid lying down for at least three hours after eating. By lying down, you put your stomach on the same plane as your esophageal sphincter, thus making reflux that much more likely.

🍎 **Don't drink.** Alcohol is both a stomach-acid instigator and a tissue irritant, so it can

drug alert!

Certain medications also can promote heartburn or stomach upset, either by having a relaxing effect on the esophageal sphincter or irritating the stomach directly. They include most over-the-counter and prescription painkillers (such as aspirin and ibuprofen), certain heart medications (calcium channel blockers, beta blockers, and nitrates), drugs to treat angina and high blood pressure, some antibiotics, and medications for asthma and spastic colon. If you regularly take medications for a health problem, check with your doctor to be sure it's not contributing to your digestive woes.

cause trouble both as it's going down (by irritating the esophagus) and once it gets there (by producing excess acid for the stomach to spew into the esophagus). Beer or alcohol mixed with carbonated beverages (acid producers in their own right) can be especially troublesome.

🍎 **Reduce stress.** "Stress seems to stimulate the production of chemicals that in turn promote excessive stomach acid in some people," says Dr. Peikin.

Given that stress also can lead to erratic and less than healthful eating habits, alcohol consumption, and smoking (which also contributes to heartburn), it's no wonder that heartburn is much more common in the harried.

healing diet

PROBLEM FOODS

Category I:
Foods that Produce Excess Stomach Acid
Beverages containing caffeine
Carbonated beverages
Chocolate
Decaffeinated coffee
Milk and cream

Category II:
Foods that Relax the Lower Esophageal Sphincter
Beverages containing caffeine
(including coffee, soft drinks, cocoa, and tea)
Butter, margarine, and mayonnaise
Chocolate
Fatty cuts of beef and pork, and poultry with skin
Fatty or greasy foods, especially those that have been deep-fried
Foods or mints containing spearmint or peppermint
Nuts
Onions and garlic
Pastries and rich desserts
Salad dressings
Whole-milk dairy products and cream

Category III:
Foods that Irritate the Esophagus
Alcohol
Black pepper
Chili powder
Citrus juices, including lemon, orange, and grapefruit
Tomatoes

Category IV:
Foods that Delay Gastric Emptying
Foods high in fat, including meats and fried foods
Full-fat dairy products, including butter and margarine
Cooking oils
Rich desserts
Salad dressings

GOOD FOODS
Baked or boiled potatoes
Fish
Gelatin
Noncitrus fruits such as apples, peaches, and pears
Nonfat milk
Pasta
Puddings
Rice
Skinless chicken and turkey
Steamed or boiled vegetables
Very lean meat

BEST ADVICE: Although heartburn is by far the most common cause of digestive discomfort, it is not the only one. Other potentially more serious conditions can mimic some of heartburn's symptoms, so it's important to rule these conditions out before assuming that heartburn is your problem. If you're at all in doubt about the cause of your digestive woes, play it safe and see your doctor.

high blood pressure

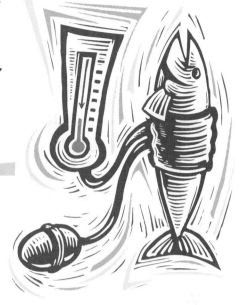

They call it the silent killer. And for good reason. Unless you regularly check for it, you won't know you have high blood pressure until something bad happens—a heart attack, stroke, kidney failure, eye damage. Fifty million Americans have high blood pressure, and of those, more than one third (35 percent, or 17.5 million) don't know they have it.

Though people with high blood pressure may be unaware of anything going on, throughout the entire network of their cardiovascular systems, blood is continuously slamming away at artery walls, doing damage. High blood pressure (also called hypertension) was directly responsible for almost 40,000 deaths in 1995 (the most recent year for which statistics are available) and was an accomplice in an additional 190,000 fatalities.

For African Americans especially, high blood pressure poses an enormous health risk. The prevalence of hypertension in African Americans is among the highest in the world. African Americans develop hypertension earlier in life than whites and on average have higher blood pressures, pushing the rate of death from heart disease 50 percent higher, the rate of death from stroke 80 percent higher, and the rate of hypertension-related kidney disease 320 percent higher than rates for the general population. The good news in this bleak picture is that adequate treatment

effectively lowers blood pressure in African Americans as in the rest of the population.

And adequate treatment begins at home with changes in lifestyle. Though doctors don't know what causes high blood pressure in 90 to 95 percent of cases, they do know that obesity, smoking, heavy drinking, and lack of physical activity can make it considerably worse. Healthy habits and a healthful diet can both prevent high blood pressure and lower it. In some cases diet and exercise are all that are needed.

Blood Pressure Basics

Blood pressure is the amount of force your blood exerts against your artery walls. It's defined by two measurements. The systolic pressure is caused when the heart contracts and pumps blood out through the arteries. This is the higher of the two numbers. Diastolic pressure is the pressure of your blood when the heart is at rest. The total measurement is given as a combined systolic/diastolic number—135/85, for example. The higher the pressure, the harder it is for blood to flow through your blood vessels.

What's High?

A systolic pressure over 140 accompanied by a diastolic pressure over 90 is considered high. Ideally, say the medical experts, you would like to have a blood pressure reading of 120/80 or lower.

Though blood pressure readings up to 130/85 are considered normal, the National Institutes of Health (NIH) urges everyone to strive for the ideal. Why? There's risk of a stroke or a heart attack even in someone with normal blood pressure. And the higher your blood pressure rises over optimal, the higher your risk of associated disease. Even if your blood pressure is optimal, it tends to rise with age. The entire population should seek to have the best possible diet to prevent a rise in blood pressure.

Fortunately, for most of us, hypertension is highly preventable and controllable. Even those whose blood pressure has crept up to 159/99 can effectively knock it back with changes in lifestyle (although people with a history of diabetes, stroke, artery disease, signs of heart disease, or kidney disease may need medication in addition).

A Dash Will Do It

What kind of diet does it take to lower blood pressure? Experts point to the DASH diet as a likely solution. The DASH diet was nicknamed for the study that defined it. This diet, rich in fruits, vegetables, low-fat

Classification	Systolic	Diastolic
Optimal	under 120	under 80
Normal	under 130	under 85
High normal	130-139	85-89
Stage 1: mild hypertension	140-159	90-99
Stage 2: moderate	160-179	100-109
Stage 3: severe	180-209	110-119
Stage 4: very severe	over 209	over 119

dairy products, and other low-fat foods, significantly reduces blood pressure in people with mild hypertension and those with normal blood pressure.

The Dietary Approaches to Stop Hypertension (DASH) study was conducted to test the effectiveness of overall diet rather than isolated vitamins or minerals in lowering hypertension. Researchers around the country worked with a total of 459 people (59 percent were African Americans and 49 percent were women). Of those, 133 had mild hypertension and 326 had normal blood pressure. They were randomly divided into three groups, and each group was asked to follow one of three diets:
- A typical American diet low in fruits, vegetables, and dairy products, and higher in fat than it should be
- A typical American diet but rich in fruits and vegetables
- A combination diet rich in fruits and vegetables, low-fat dairy products, and other low-fat foods

And the winner was? The combination diet. After eight weeks, those on the typical American diet showed little change in blood pressure. Those on the high fruit and vegetable diet showed some change in their systolic pressure but none in diastolic. The combination diet successfully lowered both systolic and diastolic pressure. The most dramatic decline occurred among those with high blood pressure, who saw their systolic pressure drop by 11.4 points and their diastolic by 5.5 points. But even those who entered the study with normal readings saw reductions of 3.5 in systolic pressure and 2.1 in diastolic pressure. Though this might not sound like much, a 2- to 3-point drop in blood pressure can reduce risk of cardiovascular disease by 5 to 10 percent.

The results showed the diet to be as effective as drug therapy for individuals with mild hypertension, says Laura Svetkey, M.D., associate professor of medicine at Duke University in Durham, North Carolina. Dr. Svetkey is a principal investigator for the DASH and upcoming DASH2 studies. The diet worked for men and women of all ethnicities, actually lowering blood pressure further among African Americans than the rest of the population.

We don't know exactly why this diet works, explains Dr. Svetkey. It could be a combination of nutrients or perhaps some unknown nutrients.

Will it work for individuals with more severe hypertension?

"We're hopeful that it will," she says. "We don't know. It did have a greater effect in those with higher blood pressure than those in the normal range, but it's possible that the effectiveness would plateau after a certain point."

Making the DASH diet even more effective is how easy it is to stick to. "We wanted to create a diet that we could propose as a feasible way of eating," says Dr. Svetkey. And they succeeded. Although most diets leave you feeling deprived, this one allows you to eat a variety of foods from peanuts to pasta and, yes, even a little red meat. The specific daily dietary guidelines for someone who consumes 2,000 calories a day are as follows:

● seven to eight servings of grains or grain products, such as breads and pastas
● four to five servings of vegetables
● four to five servings of fruit
● two to three servings of low-fat or nonfat dairy products
● one to two servings of red meat, poultry, or fish (a serving is 3 ounces)
● one serving of nuts or legumes

For more detailed information on this diet, including serving adjustments based on your daily calorie needs, check out the DASH study web site at http://dash.bwh.harvard.edu or call 800/575-WELL.

Lowering Blood Pressure

In addition to the DASH diet, there are a number of strategies that can help get those numbers down.

Think vegetarian. Prefer not to eat meat? Although the DASH diet effectively lowers blood pressure, so does a vegetarian diet. Vegetarians as a whole have lower blood pressure than meat eaters. And researchers have found that when meat eaters go on a vegetarian diet, their blood pressure drops, and when vegetarians go on a meat diet, blood pressure rises, says Dr. Svetkey. Which is better, the DASH diet or a vegetarian one? "My guess is that they would be comparable," says Dr. Svetkey. Though the DASH diet wasn't tested against a vegetarian diet, it's similar in its content of fruits, vegetables, and grains.

🍎 **Go bananas.** These fruits are high in potassium, which causes your body to excrete sodium through your urine, thereby possibly helping to control blood pressure. There is clear evidence that potassium is beneficial to the prevention and control of hypertension, says Dr. Svetkey. Researchers at Johns Hopkins University pooled the results of several studies and found that low potassium intake was associated with the development of high blood pressure, and that increasing potassium lowered systolic pressure by about 3 points and diastolic pressure by 2 points.

The recommendation for daily potassium intake is 3,500 milligrams based on a 2,000-calorie diet. You can accomplish this easily through the foods you eat. Foods high in potassium include apricots, peaches, prunes, oranges, cantaloupe, potatoes, lima beans, stewed tomatoes, sweet potatoes, spinach, winter squash, catfish, lean pork, lean veal, cod, flounder, trout, skim milk, and yogurt.

🍎 **Mind your minerals.** Several studies have suggested that diets low in calcium and magnesium may be related to hypertension and that increasing intake of these minerals may lower blood pressure, but experts say the evidence isn't very strong. Although some studies do indicate that magnesium lowers blood pressure, other research in which magnesium supplements were given to individuals with high blood pressure found no effect, says Eva Obarzanek, Ph.D.,

a research nutritionist with the National Heart, Lung, and Blood Institute.

The evidence is a little stronger for calcium, but researchers have seen only a small effect on systolic pressure and not enough to recommend taking supplements, says Dr. Obarzanek.

Nonetheless, doctors and nutritionists emphasize that you should get your daily requirement of both of these important minerals through your diet. Whether or not calcium lowers blood pressure, it builds strong bones and can help prevent osteoporosis. Experts recommend consuming 1,200 milligrams daily from such foods as low-fat dairy products.

You can get the recommended 350 milligrams of magnesium a day through a well-balanced diet. Magnesium-rich foods include wheat germ, fortified cereals, sunflower seeds, halibut, mackerel, spinach, swiss chard, and most nuts. Not surprisingly, the DASH diet fulfills requirements for both of these minerals, providing 1,200 milligrams of calcium and 484 milligrams of magnesium on the 2,000-calorie-a-day plan.

🍎 **Eat more fish.** The research on the benefits of fish oils is a bit wishy-washy, too, with some studies suggesting that large amounts of omega-3 fatty acids (the kind found in cold-water fish like salmon) lower hypertension and others finding no effect. Regardless, consuming large quantities of fish oil, which requires supplements, can produce abdominal discomfort as well as other unpleasant side effects. It can't hurt, however, to eat fish a couple times a week, and it's even recommended for its possible role in reducing blood clotting and lowering cholesterol.

Fish high in omega-3s include Atlantic herring, salmon, bluefin tuna, Atlantic mackerel, swordfish, eastern oysters, and rainbow trout.

🍎 **Watch that drinking.** Down too many beers, and you'll push up your blood pressure. Going above and beyond moderation in your alcohol intake not only can contribute to hypertension but can interfere with efforts to lower blood pressure. Drinking is a risk factor for stroke, according to the National Heart, Lung, and Blood Institute.

Though moderate drinking appears to have some protective effect against heart disease, do keep it moderate. This means no more than 1 ounce of alcohol per day for men, the amount in 24 ounces of beer, 10 ounces of wine, or one mixed drink. Halve that for women, due to lower body weight and slower alcohol metabolism.

🍎 **Watch your weight.** As your waistline expands, blood pressure rises. In fact, according to the NHLBI, being overweight makes you up to six times more likely to develop high blood pressure than if your weight were optimal, especially if you put on pounds around the waist.

But what goes up, can come down. As you lose weight, both blood pressure and weight drop simultaneously. Some studies show that blood pressure comes down almost 1 point for every pound lost, says Dr. Svetkey. And you don't have to get down to your ideal weight. For someone 30 pounds overweight, losing just 10 pounds can have

a significant impact on blood pressure. (For full details on losing weight, see page 256.)

The Salt Connection

The sodium controversy rages on as the blood pressure of those who consume lots of salty foods rockets upward. Some studies have concluded that a low-sodium diet has no effect on lowering blood pressure. Others have suggested that low-sodium diets may even increase risk of heart disease. But in many of these studies the data wasn't carefully analyzed, says Dr. Svetkey. She points out that research published in support of sodium has been funded by the salt industry.

We have 40 years of evidence—trials, observational studies, meta-analysis—showing that high sodium intake causes high blood pressure, says Dr. Obarzanek. There's no question that cutting back on salt in the diet works in reducing hypertension, says Dr. Svetkey.

But will it work for everyone? Isn't it true that some people are salt-sensitive and others are not? Researchers do know that African Americans tend to be more salt sensitive, but Dr. Obarzanek points out there's a range of responsiveness in the population to every nutrient and every dietary change. Take the case of cholesterol. For some individuals, lowering dietary fat significantly reduces cholesterol levels. Others may find little effect, but doctors still recommend a low-fat diet to anyone with high cholesterol and risk of heart disease. The same goes for sodium and high blood pressure. Experts recommend that everyone limit sodium intake to 2,400 milligrams a day. That's not easy given all the salt that's added to processed foods, says Dr. Obarzanek. And to go below that you need to cook from scratch.

Becoming a Salt Sleuth

According to the AHA, about 75 percent of the sodium in our diets comes from processed foods and baked goods. Salt is also found in some surprising places, such as processed cookies, candy, soft drinks, and cereal, which don't taste salty at all. Beware of breads and rolls, too. Other foods high in sodium include canned soups, stews, frozen dinners, cured meats, chips, dips, pretzels, popcorn, olives, and pickles. Read the nutrition information on all packaged foods before buying.

healing diet

PROBLEM FOODS	GOOD FOODS
Alcohol	Fish
Fatty foods	Fruit
Meat	Low-fat dairy products
Salty foods	Low-fat foods in general
	Vegetables

BEST ADVICE: If you have high blood pressure, it is vital that it be controlled. If dietary measures do not bring your blood pressure down, be sure to follow your doctor's other recommendations for treatment.

high cholesterol

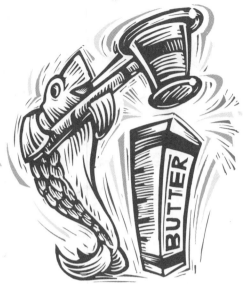

Once upon a time the only thing we knew about fat was that it made food taste good. We happily sat down to a dinner of pan-fried steak, a baked potato topped with a dollop of butter, and a small side salad. And when someone had a heart attack, we thought it "just happened."

Today, we know better. Eating a diet high in fat—especially saturated fat—and cholesterol raises blood cholesterol levels in most people. And leading health authorities all agree on one thing—high blood cholesterol levels increase the risk of heart disease and stroke.

In fact, high blood cholesterol is a leading risk factor for developing cardiovascular disease, says Gerald Fletcher, M.D., member of the American Heart Association Task Force on Cardiac Risk Reduction, and professor of Medicine at Mayo Medical School in Jacksonville, Florida. "When a person has too much cholesterol circulating in the blood, it can slowly build up within the walls of the arteries feeding the heart and brain," he explains. "This can form plaque, thick, hard deposits that can clog those arteries, causing atherosclerosis." This condition is also known as coronary artery disease.

And coronary artery disease is the number one killer of American men and women. About every 29 seconds, someone in this country suffers a coronary event, and about every minute someone dies from one.

The formation of a clot in the region of this plaque can block the flow of blood to part of the heart muscle and cause a heart attack. If a clot blocks the flow of blood to part of the brain, the result is a stroke.

Stroke is the third leading cause of death behind heart disease and cancer, according to the National Center for Health Statistics. In addition, stroke is the leading cause of serious, long-term disability in the United States.

"Keeping blood cholesterol levels in check is crucial because heart disease is the number one killer of both men and women in the United States," says Dr. Fletcher.

The good news in this rather grim picture is that there are plenty of steps you can take right now to cut your cholesterol, thereby lowering your risk of heart disease and stroke. But first, it's crucial to

translating the numbers

When you visit the doctor and have your cholesterol tested, you get a report in the form of some numbers. What do those numbers actually mean?

Your main cholesterol "number" refers to the total amount of cholesterol in your blood.

Cholesterol is measured in milligrams per deciliter (mg/dL) of blood. (A deciliter is a tenth of a liter.)

A reading of less than 200 mg/dL is desirable; a reading of 200 to 239 mg/dL is viewed as borderline high, and 240 mg/dL and above is considered high cholesterol.

Besides total cholesterol, measurement of HDL cholesterol should also be done. A healthy person who is not at high risk for heart disease and whose total cholesterol level is in the normal range should have an HDL-cholesterol level of more than 35 mg/dL. An LDL- cholesterol level of less than 130 mg/dL is "desirable" to minimize the risk of heart disease.

If you are aged 20 or older, you should have your blood cholesterol level checked at least once every five years, according to the American Heart Association.

understand the terms that doctors use when they discuss fat and cholesterol in your blood and in your diet.

Cholesterol Defined

All the cholesterol your body needs—and it does need some— is made by your liver (about 1,000 milligrams a day). It is used to build cell membranes and brain and nerve tissues. Cholesterol also helps your body make hormones and bile acids that are needed for digestion. When doctors talk about serum cholesterol or blood cholesterol, they're talking about the amount of this fatty substance that is in your blood.

Dietary cholesterol is in the foods you eat. It is found only in animal products. Examples include egg yolks, liver, meat, some shellfish, and whole-milk dairy products. The American Heart Association (AHA) recommends that you limit your average daily cholesterol intake to less than 300 milligrams.

Types of Cholesterol

The two main types of blood cholesterol are low-density lipoprotein (LDL) and high-density lipoprotein (HDL).

LDL—heart disease culprit. "Low-density lipoproteins tend to deposit cholesterol in the arteries," says Basil Rifkind, M.D., senior scientific advisor of the Vascular Research Program at the National Heart, Lung, and Blood Institute.

The higher your LDL level, the higher your heart-disease risk. That is why LDL is often called the "bad" cholesterol.

HDL—the good guy. About one-third to one-fourth of blood cholesterol is carried by high-density lipoprotein. "This type of lipoprotein carries cholesterol away from the arteries and back to the liver, where it is passed from the body," explains Dr. Rifkind. "High-density lipoprotein also removes excess cholesterol from atherosclerotic plaques, slowing their growth."

The higher your HDL level, the lower your heart-disease risk. That's why it's called the "good" cholesterol. "We know that HDL protects against heart disease, especially heart attack," confirms Dr. Rifkind. "Exercise can raise your HDL and triglyceride levels." (Triglycerides are another type of blood fat.)

Controlling Those Numbers

What exactly affects blood cholesterol levels? Diet and a lot of other things as well. Here's a look at the big picture, starting with diet.

What You Eat

The saturated fat and cholesterol in the foods you eat raise total and LDL cholesterol levels.

The type of fat you eat is important. There are three types of dietary fat— saturated, monounsaturated, and polyunsaturated. The distinction between these fats is a chemical one, but that chemistry means everything when it comes to the impact it has on your cholesterol levels. Simply put, all fat is made of mostly carbon and hydrogen atoms.

Saturated fats have the maximum possible number of hydrogen atoms attached to every carbon atom. It is "saturated" with hydrogen atoms. Saturated fats tend to raise levels of LDL-cholesterol in the blood. Saturated fats are mostly found in foods of animal origin, including butter and lard.

Monounsaturated fats are missing one pair of hydrogen atoms in the middle of the molecule. This gap is called an "unsaturation," and the fat is said to be "monounsaturated" because it has one gap. Monounsaturated fats tend to lower levels of LDL-cholesterol in the blood. Olive oil and canola oil are monounsaturated fats.

Polyunsaturated fats are missing more than one pair of hydrogen atoms. Polyunsaturated fats tend to lower levels of both HDL-cholesterol and LDL-cholesterol in the blood. Safflower oil and corn oil are polyunsaturated fats.

Body Weight

Being overweight can make your LDL level go up and your HDL level go down. If you are overweight, losing even a small amount of weight—5 to 10 pounds—can improve your blood cholesterol levels. But don't go on a crash diet to see how quickly you can lose those pounds. The healthiest and longest-lasting weight loss happens when

protect your kids from
heart disease

How old do kids have to be before you have to start worrying about protecting them from heart disease? Would you believe age 2? Medical research is indicating that having high blood cholesterol levels at a young age may lead to atherosclerosis (heart disease) later in life. In this condition, cholesterol combines with other substances to form plaque—a thick, hard deposit that can clog the arteries feeding the heart and brain.

There is compelling evidence that this damaging process begins in childhood and progresses slowly into adulthood. Then it often leads to coronary heart disease, which is the number one killer of American men and women. Check out these facts:
• About 37 percent of American youth age 19 and younger have blood cholesterol levels of 170 mg/dL or higher. (In adolescents this is considered high, comparable to a 200 mg/dL level in adults.)
• About 42 percent of the people discharged from hospitals for coronary heart disease are younger than 65 years. Many of these adults have children who may have coronary heart-disease risk factors that need attention.

high blood pressure.) Aerobic exercise—the kind that uses oxygen to provide energy to large muscles and raises your heart and breathing rates—is what you want. Examples of aerobic exercise include walking, jogging, and swimming. Bonus: Aerobic exercise will also condition your heart and lungs.

Heredity

Your genes influence how your body makes and handles cholesterol. If high cholesterol runs in your family, you may want to consider consulting your doctor to get tested for high-cholesterol conditions. One of the most common of these diseases is familial hypercholesterolemia. "If your parents have the abnormal gene for familial hypercholesterolemia, you have a one in two chance of inheriting that gene," notes Dr. Rifkind.

Age and Gender

you take it slowly, losing ½ to 1 pound a week. Diets don't work—you need to alter your eating patterns to reflect a healthy lifestyle change for the rest of your life.

Exercise

Besides losing weight, increased exercise and physical activity helps raise HDLs. (Exercise can also help control diabetes and

Blood cholesterol levels in both men and women begin to go up at about age 20. Premenopausal women have levels that are lower than men of the same age. After menopause, a woman's LDL-cholesterol level goes up—and at the same time so does her risk for heart disease.

"Research is showing us that postmenopausal women who take hormone replacement therapy have far fewer heart attacks," notes Dr. Rifkind. "Their HDL level is up to 15 percent higher, and their LDL level is about 10 percent lower. However, more research is needed to confirm this because women who take estrogen are different from those who do not. Women on hormone replacement therapy are of a different socioeconomic group, they are not as heavy, and they smoke less. So there may be other factors here leading to a lower risk of heart disease."

The Healthy Children Program

There is a lot you can do to help reduce your children's risk of developing heart disease later in life. Follow these guidelines from the AHA for children ages 2 to 19:
- Serve your children a wide variety of foods.
- Set a heart-healthy example. Select, prepare, and eat foods low in saturated fat, total fat, and cholesterol.
- Keep their saturated fat to less than 10 percent of total calories.
- Total fat should be an average of no more than 30 percent of total calories.
- Limit their dietary cholesterol to less than 300 milligrams per day.
- Encourage physical activity, such as running, swimming, and dancing.
- Plan a fitness vacation. Instead of lying on the beach, spend your days hiking, biking, or exploring by canoe.
- Play basketball or softball with your kids as often as possible.

testing
kids' cholesterol

Pediatricians don't always check children's cholesterol levels. But sometimes maybe they should.
"If you have a history of early-onset heart disease in your family, including heart attack, or if you or your husband has high cholesterol, talk to your doctor about having your child's cholesterol level tested at an early age," says Basil Rifkind, M.D., senior scientific advisor for the National Heart, Lung, and Blood Institute's Vascular Research Program. "It's important to note that whether or not your children have high cholesterol, they ought to be on a low-fat, heart-healthy diet."

Getting Your Cholesterol Down

Once you have your cholesterol number in hand, if it's high, you know you have some work ahead of you to get it down where it belongs. Follow these practical tips to lower it. *Note:* If you have been diagnosed with high cholesterol and are taking cholesterol-lowering medication, it's important to continue taking your medicine in addition to following these tips.
 Lose foods high in saturated fat.
"Saturated fat raises your blood cholesterol more than anything else you eat," says Dr. Fletcher. "Saturated fat interferes with the

way the liver breaks down cholesterol. Eating foods low in saturated fat is the best way to lower your cholesterol level."

Foods high in saturated fat include red meats, whole milk, cheese, butter, cream, cocoa butter (watch that chocolate!), palm oil, coconut oil, and palm kernel oil. Some of these oils are used freely in processed baked goods. It's a good idea to develop a habit of reading labels as you shop.

Choose foods for wellness. "Aim for a plant-based diet high in fruits, vegetables, and whole-grain foods that are naturally low in fat and high in starch and fiber," advises Dr. Fletcher. Follow these AHA Guidelines to keep high blood cholesterol at bay:

● Keep your total fat intake to less than 30 percent of daily calories.

● Limit saturated fat to less than 10 percent of total calories.

● Limit your cholesterol intake to no more than 300 milligrams per day.

● Consume foods containing 20 to 30 grams of fiber each day. (Currently, the average American is eating only about 10 to 15 grams of fiber daily.)

Choose foods low in total fat. Since many foods high in total fat are also high in saturated fat, eating foods low in total fat will help you eat less saturated fat. When you do eat fat, have unsaturated fat instead of saturated fat. Unsaturated fat is usually liquid at room temperature and can be either monounsaturated or polyunsaturated. Foods high in monounsaturated fat include olive and canola oils. Foods high in polyunsaturated fat include safflower, sunflower, corn, and soybean oils.

Get those calories down. Any type of fat is a rich source of calories, so eating foods low in fat will also help you eat fewer calories. Eating fewer calories can help you lose weight—an important part of lowering your blood cholesterol.

Eat more foods that are high in starch and fiber. These include vegetables, fruits, breads, and cereals instead of high-fat foods. High-fiber foods not only keep your cholesterol in check, but they also help you feel more full, so you're not as hungry. And don't forget to pare down the amount of food you eat—smaller portions mean smaller waistlines.

Choose foods low in cholesterol. Dietary cholesterol also can raise your blood cholesterol level, although usually not as much as saturated fat. Dietary cholesterol is found only in foods that come from animal sources. Many of these foods are also high in saturated fat. Foods from plant sources do not have cholesterol but can contain saturated fat.

Munch on a Macintosh. Or Granny Smiths, for that matter—apples are a great source of fiber.

When eaten regularly as part of a low-fat, low-cholesterol diet, soluble fiber (the kind found in apples) has been shown to help lower blood cholesterol. "Soluble fiber binds to cholesterol and helps to excrete it out of the body," says registered dietitian Connie Diekman, spokesperson for the American Dietetic Association.

"The key high-fiber foods that give you maximum benefits are oats, hot and cold oat breakfast cereal, oat bran, and all beans," says Diekman. "Fruits and vegetables are also good sources, especially apples, oranges, grapefruit, broccoli, and sweet peppers. And don't forget grains, such as rice, barley, bulgur, and couscous."

It's important to note that many commercial oat bran and wheat bran products (muffins, chips, waffles) actually contain very little bran. They may also be high in sodium and fat.

Get grainy. Choose whole-grain breads and rolls as often as possible. "Grains are rich in starch and soluble fiber, and low in fat and calories," says Diekman. "For lunch, fill a whole-wheat pita with ½ cup of nonfat cottage cheese, then top with veggies, sprouts, and low-fat Catalina salad dressing."

Broaden your horizons. "There are other grains besides oatmeal and rice," says Diekman. "Most of us eat the same foods over and over again. Try some new grain side dishes to get more fiber in your diet, such as couscous, bulgur, wehani rice, barley grits, rye berries, millet, triticale, and kasha."

Sneak in that fiber. "Try to incorporate high-fiber plant foods in every meal in your eating plan," says Diekman. "For example, beans and barley make a base for great soups, casseroles, and stews. Use beans as a topping for baked potatoes and incorporate them into pasta dishes. I serve my family broiled pork chops with apple slices. They're a real hit!"

Grab some grapes. "Grapes are a good source of pectin, a type of soluble fiber," explains Diekman. "Eating grapes, and drinking grape juice, is an easy and convenient way to get more fiber in your diet. Pack grapes in your lunch bag—and the kids' lunch, too." (For more information on how to lower your children's cholesterol levels, turn to "Protect Your Kids From Heart Disease" on page 196.)

Nosh on breakfast cereals—anytime. Like to nibble between meals? Replace high-fat snacks such as chips and cookies with a bowl of cereal. Breakfast cereals are generally high in starch and fiber, and low in saturated fat and calories. They also have no cholesterol. Fill a bowl with cereal, skim milk, and fruit any time of the day or night. "Be sure to check the label," advises Diekman. "If fiber is not in the top three ingredients, keep looking. All-Bran is the highest source of fiber in one serving."

Stock up on nonstick cooking spray. Nonstick vegetable oil cooking spray should be a staple in the kitchen of every heart-healthy cook. Bake, roast, or microwave cook with it instead of shortening, butter, or margarine. Spray it on pans, griddles, and baking dishes. A spritz of cooking spray has zero fat or cholesterol, compared to a tablespoon of butter which has 6.8 grams of saturated fat, and 28 grams of cholesterol.

Fish for health. The Inuit, or Eskimo, people of Alaska and Greenland are relatively free of heart disease despite a high-fat, high-cholesterol diet. The staple food in their diet is cold-water fish rich in omega-3 polyunsaturated fatty acids.

Research indicates that people who eat fish regularly have lower rates of heart disease. One possible reason is that the omega-3 fatty acids in fish appear to slow down the process of blood clotting. While more research is needed on the possible health benefits of omega-3 fatty acids, it's a good idea to include fish in some of your meals each week. And simply replacing

cholesterol-cutting kitchen tips

Once you've been told that you need to get your cholesterol level down, you have to pay attention to every food that passes your lips. While you're getting used to reading labels and making sure everything you eat passes the low-cholesterol, low-fat rules, you might want to start forming some healthy food preparation habits. If you incorporate these 10 tips into your daily meal preparation, you'll go a long way toward slashing those numbers.

- **Forget about frying.** Instead, steam, boil, bake, or microwave vegetables. Or for a change, stir-fry in just a small amount of vegetable oil.
- **Toss your frying pan.** Roast, bake, broil, or simmer meat, poultry, or fish rather than frying.
- **Learn that for everything there is a season.** Try flavoring vegetables with herbs and spices instead of fatty sauces, butter, or margarine.
- **Try a little un-dressing.** Think of using flavored vinegars or lemon juice on your salads rather than dressings. Or use smaller servings of oil-based or low-fat salad dressings.
- **Liquify.** Use vegetable oil in place of solid shortening, margarine, and butter whenever possible.
- **Don't throw away the flavor.** Try whole-grain flours to enhance flavors of baked goods made with less fat and cholesterol-containing ingredients.
- **Lighten up.** Replace whole milk with low-fat or skim milk in puddings, soups, and baked products.
- **Hold the mayo.** Substitute plain low-fat yogurt or blender-whipped low-fat cottage cheese for sour cream or mayonnaise.
- **Lose the fat.** Choose lean cuts of meat and trim fat from meat before and/or after cooking. Remove skin from poultry before or after cooking.
- **Do a little substitution.** Use egg whites in recipes calling for whole eggs. Use two egg whites in place of each whole egg in muffins, cookies, and puddings.

some of the red meat in your diet will lower your cholesterol.

Regarding fish oil supplements, there is insufficient evidence that they are beneficial, and little is known about their long-term effects. "It's best to stick as close to the real thing as possible, and broil a salmon steak for dinner," notes Dr. Fletcher. "Our biggest concern with fish oil supplements is that we don't know at what point the supplements will make the blood too thin, increasing the risk of hemorrhage."

Grill a soy burger. In a study published in the *New England Journal of Medicine*, people with high cholesterol were able to reduce their total cholesterol by 10 percent when they substituted soy for animal protein. They also decreased their LDL cholesterol by 13 percent. In addition, their HDL cholesterol levels increased by 3 percent. Study participants ate several servings of soy products each day.

In another study, people with high cholesterol substituted soybean protein and oil for milk protein and fat. Study participants had their HDL cholesterol increase by 9 percent and their LDL cholesterol decrease by 14 percent.

Exactly how soy may lower cholesterol is still under investigation. Research scientists suspect that merely replacing animal foods with soy products helps lower cholesterol levels.

Some scientists believe there are certain properties of soy that may affect receptors for cholesterol in the body. Yet others theorize that soy estrogens reduce cholesterol levels. More research is needed to determine exactly why soy helps control cholesterol levels in the body. In the meantime, there's every reason to take advantage of its super cholesterol-lowering abilities. Soy is available in tofu, tempeh, soy milk, soy flour, and soy-protein powder. You can incorporate more soy in your diet by taking these easy steps:

• For breakfast, prepare farina or oatmeal with soy milk. Add a sliced banana and some raisins for flavor and texture.
• Fill your blender with soy milk or tofu, frozen fruit, one banana, orange juice, wheat germ, and some honey. Blend until smooth.
• At your next barbecue, toss a few soy burgers and soy hot dogs on the grill instead of regular hamburgers and hot dogs. (Check the labels for fat and sodium content.)
• Replace chicken or beef with cubed tofu in your next stir-fry.
• Check out the nutritional drinks that contain soy at your local health-food store. "Make sure you check the label to see if soy is in the top three ingredients," cautions Diekman. "Soy has no taste, so many manufacturers add fillers, sweeteners, and fat to make it taste better. You want a beverage that is a good source of soy, but is also low in fat, sugar, and calories."

While you're at the health-food store, look over all the unfamiliar products that contain soy. Be adventurous and try one that you haven't tried before.

Check your oil. "Oils rich in monounsaturated fats, such as olive and canola oil, tend to lower LDL cholesterol without touching HDL levels," notes Diekman. "People living in the Mediterranean regions, such as Greece and Italy, have a high-fat, high-cholesterol diet. And yet, they have a low rate of heart disease. The staple in their food is olive oil. They also eat a plant-based diet rich in fresh fruits and vegetables, especially grains."

Eat right when eating out. For breakfast, choose an omelet made with egg substitute or egg whites, hot or cold cereal, toast with margarine and jam, or an English muffin or bagel with nonfat cream cheese.

For lunch, choose a salad with dressing on the side, regular-size or child-size hamburger (hold the mayo), turkey, chicken, or roast beef sandwich, or a soup that is not cream-based.

For dinner, choose pasta with low-fat marinara sauce, grilled or broiled fish or skinless chicken, lean steak (trimmed of fat), vegetarian entrée, baked potato topped with low-fat yogurt, and vegetables (plain or with a little oil).

Room for dessert? Top off your meal with fresh fruit sorbet, sherbet, ice milk, or nonfat frozen yogurt.

Socialize healthfully. When asked to bring a covered dish to parties, make it low-fat. Scoop out a small head of purple cabbage and fill with a dip made of low-fat cottage cheese and salsa. Surround with precut, prewashed fresh, raw vegetables.

That way, you'll have at least one low-fat item from which to choose, and you'll be able to munch all you want.

Cool down. "Preliminary evidence suggests that emotional stress can up cholesterol levels," says Dr. Fletcher. "Stress causes an increase in the hormone adrenaline, which we suspect may indirectly cause cholesterol levels to go up. We do know that exercise can help you handle stress better." In the meantime, it's a good idea to keep your stress level under control.

healing diet

PROBLEM FOODS	GOOD FOODS
Butter	Bread
Cheese	Cereal
Chocolate	Foods high in fiber
Coconut oil	Foods made with soy
Cream	Fruit
Egg yolks	Vegetables
Foods high in cholesterol or saturated fat	Whole grains
Fried foods	
Palm kernel oil	
Red meat	
Whole milk	

BEST ADVICE: Follow your doctor's advice about lowering your cholesterol. Remember that whether or not you're taking prescription medications to lower your cholesterol, diet is an important part of keeping your cholesterol under control.

immunity

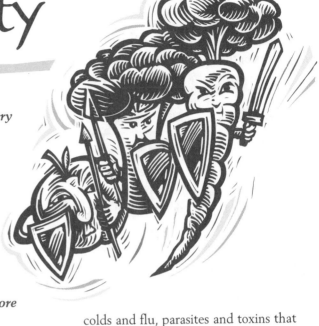

First the bad news: More than 1 million bacteria currently are camped out on every square inch of your newly washed skin.

But now good news: Should any of those bacteria make the mistake of venturing beneath your skin, they would confront the collective wrath of a germ-fighting force numbering in the trillions. Your immune system has the power to produce one type of particularly voracious germ-killer—the neutrophil— at the miraculous rate of more than 80 million in a single minute.

"We tend to take our immune systems for granted, but we'd be dead within just a matter of days without them," says Terry Phillips, Ph.D., D.Sc., a professor of microbiology and immunology and the director of analytic immunochemistry at the George Washington University Medical Center in Washington, D.C. Dr. Phillips also has coauthored a book on immunology titled *Winning the War Within*. "If you think of your body as a country, your immune system is your army, navy, marine corps, CIA, and even sanitation department all wrapped up into one," he says.

An Inside Look at The Enemy

And what exactly is your immune system up against? More than just those bacteria on your forearm, unfortunately. We're bombarded daily by viruses such as those that cause

colds and flu, parasites and toxins that can contaminate our food, and fungi that can come as close to us as our underwear and shoes. Our immune systems also are responsible for protecting us from the pollens that we breathe from various plants and the chemical contaminants that can pollute our water and air. Even if you were to get stuck with a splinter you couldn't entirely remove, your immune system would dispatch specialized cells capable of turning it into a "meal."

"We tend to think of our immune systems as protecting us only from organisms such as bacteria that are alive," says Dr. Phillips, "but they're responsible for guarding us from the myriad of man-made pollutants in our environment as well."

Breathe exhaust fumes from a bus or smoke from a friend's (or your own) cigarette, for example, and it's your immune system that gets the call. Your immune system is responsible even for controlling the proliferation of your body's own cells, such as in the case of cancer where cells begin to divide at a rate than can be lethal.

Heroic, but Still "Human"

Your body may appear to be at peace, in other words, but it's not. It's at war constantly, and the battles it wages are in no way polite, as the names of some of your immune system's more pugnacious participants make clear: You have killer T-cells, which inject toxic chemicals into enemy cells causing them to swell and explode. And you have macrophages ("macro" meaning big and "phage" meaning eater), which literally devour any foreign bodies (such as splinters) deemed a threat to your health. Not only does your immune system have brawn, however, it also has brains. Specialized cells known as B-cells act as your body's CIA, keeping records of all your body's battles so that future skirmishes can more easily be won. You even have cells (called helper T-cells) that act as messengers between the troops and cells (suppressor T-cells) whose job is to signal a cease-fire once victory has been assured.

As spectacular as the human immune system is, however, it's still "human." It can get knocked out of whack whenever you get knocked out of whack, whether by emotional stress, extreme physical fatigue, not getting enough sleep, crash dieting, smoking, or drinking too much alcohol. Some over-the-counter medications (including aspirin, antihistamines, cortisol creams, and decongestants) also can inhibit immune response, as can certain prescription drugs.

"We now know that even just being overweight or getting insufficient exercise can lower immunity," says David C. Neiman, D.H.Sc., director of the Department of Health, Leisure, and Exercise Science at Appalachian State University in Boone, North Carolina. Dr. Neiman's experiments have shown that T-cells don't function as well in people who are overweight (but return to normal when weight is lost) and that a lack of physical activity can cause a similar (but also reversible) effect.

Feeding the Troops

In much the same way as "an army marches on its stomach," as Napoleon said, your immune system marches on what you put into your stomach. "The role of diet in immune function is critical," Dr. Phillips says. "The immune system is like every other system of the body in that it simply cannot function as it was designed if nutritional requirements are not met."

Studies show that malnutrition during infancy, for example, can stunt immune function for life. And history has made all-too clear the problems (scurvy and rickets) that can arise from major deficiencies in such key nutrients as vitamins C and D.

"What we're talking about here, however, are borderline deficiencies, which millions of Americans are guilty of without knowing it," Dr. Phillips says. "People who go on crash diets or who eat erratically often suffer from nutritional deficiencies, and the elderly who tend to limit their food intake also are at risk for being nutritionally deficient."

Even for the rest of us, however, getting all of the key ingredients for a robust immune system can be difficult, especially in our world where so much food is now either "fast," highly processed, or just plain junk from the start.

The Hazards of Excess

But deficiencies aside, a danger also exists in getting too much of certain immune-enhancing nutrients, research shows, so mega-dosers should beware. "Every vitamin and mineral works best within a certain dosage range, and taking too much can be as bad, or even worse, than taking too little," states Stuart M. Berger, M.D., a former researcher at the Harvard School of Public Health and author of *Dr. Berger's Immune Power Diet*.

Too much iron, for example, can be detrimental to the immune system, as can excessive amounts of vitamin E, vitamin A, calcium, and zinc. Even seemingly innocuous water-soluble vitamin C can begin to lose its effectiveness if taken in excess, Dr. Berger says. Then, too, just too much food in general can slow down the immune system, as can excess fat in the diet and, as mentioned, excess fat on our bodies.

"The fatter you are, the worse shape your immune system is going to be in," Dr. Berger says.

Obesity apparently decreases the ability of certain immune cells to mature. It also

reduces their responsiveness when they are confronted with troublemaking virus or bacteria. These problems do, however, correct themselves when normal weight is restored.

Vitamins Germs Hate Most

So are you ready for a roundup of the nutrients that bacteria, viruses, parasites, fungi, and even cancer cells preferred you did not make a regular part of your diet?

Good, because there are plenty of them—vitamins and minerals alike. "What we eat is the single largest area in which we can affect our immunity," Dr. Berger says. "Your immune system can help keep you healthy, alert, energetic, and looking and feeling younger than your years, but only if you feed it what it needs." Or, as Dr. Phillips says, "The incredible complexity of the immune system makes a varied and well-balanced diet essential. Eating for a strong immune system is like putting together a jigsaw puzzle: Without all the pieces, the picture is going to be incomplete." That said, here are the "pieces" you need:

🍎 **Get enough vitamin A.** This vitamin (which exists in plants as its precursor, beta-carotene) is critical for immune function, because in addition to aiding in the production of T-cells, it helps maintain germ-catching moisture within the mucous membranes of the nose, eyes, mouth, and lungs. If these membranes become dry, microbial invaders have an easier time of slipping past what should be their sticky defenses.

Vitamin A also assists the kidneys in removing the debris of immunological warfare (including the cellular remains of vanquished foes) from the bloodstream.

The best food sources for vitamin A or beta-carotene include carrots, pumpkins, sweet potatoes, spinach, kale, winter squash, cantaloupe, mangoes, and apricots.

Pay attention to the Bs. There's barely an aspect of the immune system that these important vitamins do not benefit, research shows. In addition to helping to energize the immune system in general by aiding in the metabolism of carbohydrates and protein, the B vitamins help stimulate the thymus gland (the site of T-cell production) while playing a role in the production of numerous hormones that are essential to immune function.

The best food sources for B vitamins include brewer's yeast, meats, whole grains, milk, eggs, legumes, nuts, and brown rice.

Enjoy foods rich in vitamin C. Most famous for its ability to combat colds, vitamin C, like the B vitamins, is an immune system jack-of-all-trades. It helps maintain the health of the thymus and lymph nodes (the storage cites for T- and B-cells). It also helps regulate levels of interferon, an important immune system messenger. Vitamin C even helps keep the appetite of macrophages appropriately voracious.

Best food sources for vitamin C include oranges and other citrus fruits, red peppers, strawberries, kiwifruit, cantaloupe, broccoli, brussels sprouts, currants, honeydew melon, and kohlrabi.

Make sure you get enough vitamin E. Another key immunity booster, vitamin E, appears to speed the protective activity of T-cells while helping to neutralize free radicals—potentially harmful molecular misfits caused naturally by the process of oxidation within the body, but also unnaturally by such man-made affronts as cigarette smoke and polluted air. As proof of the interaction between immune-enhancing nutrients, vitamin E also assists vitamins A and C in their germ-fighting roles.

Best food sources for vitamin E include sunflower oil, safflower oil, wheat germ, mayonnaise, corn oil, olive oil, mangoes, and blackberries.

Best Immune-Boosting Minerals

Vitamins may be the catalyst for immune-enhancing activities within and between the body's germ-fighting cells, but minerals—by controlling water and levels of acidity within the body—help provide the proper environment for these processes to occur. The immune system, therefore, is as dependent on a proper balance of minerals as it is on vitamins. Here are the most important of these minerals and the best foods in which to find them.

Get enough iron. In addition to being a key component of various proteins and enzymes important to the immune system, iron helps boost immunity by increasing the oxygen-carrying capacity of the blood. Too little iron, and your cellular soldiers simply don't get the air they need to fight with their accustomed vigor. Both T-cells and natural killer cells lack their normal aggressiveness when iron is deficient, and macrophages begin to lose, quite literally, their germ-devouring appetites.

The best food sources for iron include clams, pork, beef, chicken, tofu, oysters, soybeans, whole grains, potatoes, dried fruits, and blackstrap molasses.

Look for magnesium. This mineral is critical to immune function for two reasons—the production of white blood cells (the raw material from which most immune cells originate) and for putting the brakes on immune function so your cellular warriors don't begin attacking friendly cells they should not. Because this mineral can easily be depleted (by certain prescription drugs, alcohol, and even the phosphoric acid used in many carbonated beverages), it's important to get magnesium regularly in your diet.

The best food sources for magnesium include rice, pumpkin seeds, sunflower seeds, tofu, halibut, wheat germ, almonds, mackerel, spinach, and cashew nuts.

Pack in potassium. Known to many fitness buffs as a key electrolyte important for fueling exercise, potassium also helps fuel the immune system by assisting in the release of energy from fats and carbohydrates. It also participates in the synthesis of proteins from amino acids and helps energize the lymph system, which is responsible for producing as well as storing most of the cells (lymphocytes) of the immune system.

The best sources for potassium include potatoes, oranges, avocados, clams, nonfat yogurt, raisins, rainbow trout, dried apricots, cantaloupe, lima beans, bananas, skim milk, and yams.

Catch enough copper. This mineral, like most of the other nutrients important for immunity, is made most conspicuous by its absence. Deficiencies have been shown to reduce T-cell activity and decrease the production of a substance known as interleukin-2, which is responsible for helping the cells of the immune system communicate with one another.

The best food sources for copper include cereals, nuts, legumes, meats, shellfish, oysters, and grapes.

Seek out selenium. Like vitamins A, C, and E, selenium is an antioxidant (meaning it helps arrest the harmful activities of reactive molecules within the body known as free radicals). But research shows it also is needed to keep T-cells active. The mineral also seems to make vitamin E more effective in its germ-fighting duties.

The best food sources for selenium include seafood, meats, eggs, whole grains, garlic, and vegetables (depending on the selenium content of their soils).

Don't forget the zinc. This mineral is fast establishing itself as an immune power superstar, and not just for its recently publicized abilities to shorten the length and severity of colds. Zinc is important for maintaining the vitality of the thymus, the gland responsible for the maturation of virus-killing T-cells.

Research shows that natural killer cells (those most adept at arresting cancer) also need adequate zinc to do their best work. So do neutrophils, cells that speedily devour bacteria and other foreign matter in much the same way as your immune system's slower-acting macrophages. Zinc also is a component of more than 100 enzymes important to good health, so it's definitely a mineral that shouldn't be missed.

"All things considered, zinc may be the single most important key to a healthy immune system, and in older people especially," Phillips says.

The best food sources for zinc include oysters, meats, clams, salmon, wheat germ, beans, nonfat yogurt, wild rice, whole grains, and peas.

healing diet

PROBLEM FOODS	GOOD FOODS
Alcohol	Fruits
	Vegetables
	Whole grains

BEST ADVICE: Eat a balanced, varied diet rich in vitamins and minerals. Achieve and maintain an appropriate ideal weight for your body.

insomnia

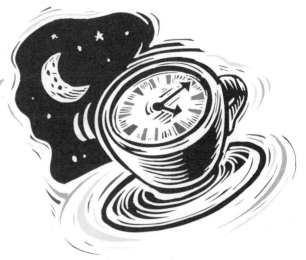

You're tired, but you can't fall asleep. Or you doze for short stretches between tossing and turning all night. Then again, maybe you sleep just fine for awhile, but you're awake and wired at 4 a.m. when you really want to sleep until 7. Do any of these situations describe your sleep pattern? These are all forms of insomnia.

Odds are, you've experienced at least one of these problems at some point in your life. Insomnia is one of the most widespread health problems in our society. According to a 1995 Gallup survey, almost half of U.S. adults suffer from at least occasional insomnia. And a good 20 million people suffer chronic insomnia in this country.

Insomnia is a symptom, not a disease. Causes range from anxiety, depression, and stress to something as obvious as too much partying. In fact, the problem can stem from any of more than 80 different medical disorders, including such diet-related conditions as anorexia, bulimia, and apnea (breathing problems) aggravated by obesity. So while dietary habits may not be the leading cause of your sleepless nights, there is solid evidence that what you eat, when you eat, and how you eat can affect the quality of your sleep.

The good news is that there are any number of dietary measures you can take to help you get a better night's sleep.

Cutting Out Caffeine

The most obvious insomnia instigator is caffeine—the number one pick-me-up and keep-me-up substance in our society. Every sleep specialist advises people with insomnia to monitor their caffeine intake. Because caffeine sensitivity is highly individual, there's no way to say you can drink X amount and no more. Some people can sleep soundly after a cappuccino nightcap; others won't sleep well if they munch so much as a chocolate bar after lunch.

Peter Hauri, Ph.D., author of *No More Sleepless Nights* and director of the Mayo Clinic Insomnia Program in Rochester, Minnesota, reports one study that showed that people experiencing caffeine-induced insomnia had higher concentrations of caffeine in their blood at midnight (eight hours after drinking an afternoon coffee) than did similar people who drank the coffee without experiencing sleep problems. Caffeine sensitivity can heighten with age, according to Dr. Hauri.

The only way to determine how much caffeine you can drink without having it alter your sleep is to monitor your own intake and pay attention to how it affects your sleep. Don't forget that caffeine is found not only in coffee and tea, but also in chocolate and colas (as well as foods containing these flavorings). It is also an ingredient in many over-the-counter and prescription drugs.

Eating Patterns Nix Sleep

Poor diet habits can lead to physical and psychological problems that can ruin your sleep. After all, certain nutrients—calcium, magnesium, copper, iron, and zinc, as well as the B vitamins—are keys to a good night's sleep.

Nutrients that Promote Sleep

To you, sleep probably seems like a fairly simple process—even if you do have insomnia. You get into bed, you close your eyes, and (hopefully) you drift off.

To your body, however, sleep is a far more complex process. No one has ever put together a nutritional formula that is just right for promoting sleep, at least not yet. But scientists are beginning to get a look at just how intricate the chemistry of sleep really is. They already know there are a few things you can do to help the natural process along.

The main minerals that help promote sleep are calcium, magnesium, zinc, iron, and copper.

Calcium acts as a natural sedative and is essential for normal sleep. Researchers at the University of Alabama found that even a minor calcium deficiency can lead to muscle tension and insomnia. You can get calcium from dairy products, salmon, sardines, broccoli, cauliflower, figs, leafy greens, oranges, almonds, tofu, and soybeans.

Magnesium also acts as a natural sedative and can blunt the effects of anxiety. Studies show that tiredness, weakness, and chronic fatigue improve with extra magnesium and potassium. You can find magnesium in meats, seafood, greens, and dairy products. You'll get potassium from apples, dried apricots, avocados, bananas, cantaloupe, citrus fruits, and potatoes.

Zinc deficiency has been linked to frequent nighttime waking and crying in infants. You might ask your pediatrician about using a formula that contains zinc. Adults can get their zinc from oysters, meats, yogurt, and fortified cereals.

Studies on trace minerals done at the USDA Agricultural Research Services Human Nutrition Research Center in Grand Forks, North Dakota, found that deficiencies in iron and copper and overabundance of aluminum disrupted sleep patterns. (Regular antacid users can easily get 1,000 milligrams of aluminum a day. You might consider switching to an antacid that does not contain aluminum.) Sea vegetables such as dulse and kelp rank among the richest food sources of minerals and trace elements. Get your copper from oysters, chickpeas, Brazil nuts, cashews, and prunes. Meats, fish, poultry, beets, dried beans, fortified cereals, and leafy green vegetables are high in iron.

The B vitamins are also key to a good night's sleep. B vitamins regulate your body's use of tryptophan and other amino acids. Paradoxically, B vitamins can also act as energizers, causing overstimulation and sleeplessness. But cigarette smoking, alcohol, stress, and birth-control pills may deplete your body's supply of B vitamins. Pyridoxine (vitamin B6) also helps your body maintain proper levels of magnesium in the blood. Meats, whole grains, brewer's yeast, bananas, and potatoes are high in pyridoxine.

Niacin (vitamin B3) has sometimes been used to relieve insomnia caused by mild depression. Studies done at the University of Alabama Department of Neurosciences showed that niacin prolonged REM (dream) sleep and decreased time awake in people suffering from insomnia. You get niacin from peanuts, sunflower seeds, red hot peppers, tomatoes, kelp, lean meats, poultry, and fish.

Vitamin B12 and folic acid also help some people sleep better. B12 is found in bean sprouts, dulse, fish, dairy products, eggs, beef, and pork. For foods high in folic acid, look to avocados, broccoli and other cruciferous vegetables, legumes, yeast, and many raw vegetables.

The amino acid tryptophan may also help induce sleep. Although its effects are mild, about 50 percent of people with insomnia are helped by dietary increases of tryptophan. Tryptophan occurs naturally in protein-rich foods. The average person eats 1 to 2 grams of tryptophan daily. Synthetic tryptophan was taken off the market in 1989 because contaminants introduced during manufacture cause side effects ranging from aching muscles and joints to fatigue, skin rash, and blood disorders. It is currently available only by prescription.

Most of the clinical research depended on nutrients supplied from supplements other than from food. But don't try supplementing in high doses (much above the Recommended Dietary Allowance) without consulting a nutrition professional.

Eating Too Much or Too Little

It's also possible to create a poor night's sleep by eating too little...or too much. People on diets (and people with anorexia) sleep poorly and tend to wake up frequently in the second half of the night. But even a simple case of hunger pangs can wake you up and send you scurrying to the fridge. For some people, getting up in the middle of the night to satisfy hunger becomes a chronic sleep problem. Dr. Hauri calls this disorder The Dagwood Syndrome.

Some dieters manage to create a particular kind of sleep disorder by eating too few calories during the day, according to Gary Zammit, Ph.D., director of the Sleep Disorders Institute at St. Lukes-Roosevelt Hospital in New York City. After dieting all day, their appetite rebounds at night, and they wake up with cravings that drive them to binge. He has seen patients who will eat a pound of butter or a whole jar of mayo during that wee-hour visit to the refrigerator. Unfortunately, these people feel so guilty the next day that they cut way back on calories again, setting up a vicious cycle.

Although cases like this are extreme, many people do inadvertently train themselves to wake up for snacks during the night. Dr. Zammit says that one of his patients used to buy a loaf of French bread on her way home from work each night. She'd slice it up and keep it by her bed so she could nibble on it throughout the night.

Eating too much can wreak as much havoc with your sleeping habits as eating too little. You may feel sleepy right after a rich five-course spread, but ultimately it will more likely keep you up than help you sleep. Heavy meals tax your digestive system and may cause indigestion and heartburn. Heartburn regularly disrupts the sleep of 30 million adults, according to Dr. Zammit. Heartburn, also known as GERD (gastroesophageal reflux disease), happens when you lie down and gravity washes your stomach acid up into your esophagus. Heavy people are more likely to experience this problem. Extra weight pressing down on the stomach contents aggravates the condition. (For details on dealing with this problem, see "Heartburn" on page 182.)

Detecting Food Allergies

Another dietary sleep stealer may lurk in your immune system if you're at all sensitive to any of the foods you've eaten. The symptoms of food allergies are subtler than those of respiratory allergies, so you might not realize that something you ate for dinner may be what is keeping you up at night.

In infants, milk allergies can provoke colic or middle-of-the-night crying jags. In children and adults, researchers have found that the most common food allergies are to chocolate, corn, red and yellow dyes, egg whites, milk, nuts, seafood, wheat, and yeast. Suspect the relatives of these foods, too. If you are allergic to corn, you'll also need to avoid cornstarch, sorbitol, mannitol, corn syrup, dextrose, caramel color, corn oil, and corn bran. Avoiding any foods that you're allergic to should help restore normal sleep.

Add monosodium glutamate (MSG) to the list of possible sleep disrupters in your diet. Often used in meat tenderizers, flavor-enhancers, and Chinese food, MSG can overstimulate the nervous system, making you feel wired if you're sensitive to it.

Booze Won't Help You Snooze

Doctors used to recommend a nightcap—a nip of brandy, a glass of wine, or some other alcoholic beverage—at bedtime to help bring on sleep. Today experts agree that even though alcohol does help you fall asleep faster, it's more likely to wreck your sleep than lull you. Alcohol is estimated to cause at least 10 percent of chronic insomnia cases.

Alcohol can cause frequent wakings during the night, and it disrupts the important dream stage of sleep. Paradoxically, alcohol also relaxes the muscles in the throat and can suppress the body's awakening mechanisms, according to Dr. Hauri. This effect can trigger or aggravate a sleep condition known as apnea, which is especially dangerous to people with lung or cardiac disease.

In some people, a habitual nightcap to keep insomnia at bay may trigger a dependency on alcohol, since alcohol's ability to bring on sleep diminishes after three or more consecutive nights. A person using alcohol as a sleep aid needs increasingly more alcohol to fall asleep.

Sleep-Enhancing Foods

I s there anything you can eat that will actually help conduct you to the Land of Nod? Yes, some foods do seem to do the trick, although doctors aren't quite sure why that is. An early theory contended that foods high in tryptophan, an amino acid that the brain converts to a sleep-inducing chemical, serotonin, were good sleep promoters. That would mean that beans, dairy products, fish, meats, peanuts, poultry, and leafy greens would make you sleepy.

Not so, says psychologist James Perl, Ph.D., author of *Sleep Right in Five Nights: A Clear and Effective Guide to Conquering Insomnia.* The amount of tryptophan in these foods is far lower than the amounts of tryptophan found to induce sleep in the laboratory. If a bedtime glass of milk helps you sleep, it may be due to a placebo effect.

Researchers now say that eating carbohydrates is a more effective way to help boost tryptophan's effects on your brain. So complex carbohydrates, like crackers, cereal, bread, or pasta, make better bedtime snacks than protein alone. And you could combine the two, as with cheese and crackers or milk and cereal.

herbs for sleep

Turned off by sleeping pills that leave you groggy the next day?

There are a number of gentle herbal teas that people have used for hundreds of years to bring on sleep. Among the most popular: catnip, chamomile, fennel, hops, melissa, passionflower, primrose, rosemary, skullcap, and valerian. Most of these herbs can be purchased in commercial teabags, and a cup before bedtime might be the most relaxing nightcap you could drink.

That would enhance tryptophan effects even more, according to Dr. Perl.

Eating raises your metabolic rate, the rate at which your body burns fuel. Dr. Zammit theorizes that this metabolic increase, termed the thermic effect, may be what brings on sleep.

Better Sleep, A to ZZZZ

L eading researchers recommend a number of ways to manage food and eating habits for better sleep.

🍎 **Avoid alcohol for at least six hours before bedtime.** Drink sparkling mineral water, seltzer, club soda with a twist of lemon or lime, or herbal tea instead.

🍎 **Balance your diet.** Dr. Hauri advocates the same diet recommended by the major health organizations in this country (and by this book): one containing lots of fresh fruits and vegetables, whole grains, and fiber. Such a diet ensures that you won't shortchange yourself on the key nutrients that aid sleep.

🍎 **Cut back on caffeine.** If you are sensitive to caffeine, or if you suspect you might be, make sure your evening meals and snacks are caffeine-free. If you can't give caffeine up completely, restrict it to more than six hours before bedtime.

🍎 **Eat lightly.** Hard-to-digest foods may cause indigestion, heartburn, gas, or cramping. That means fats and heavily spiced foods.

🍎 **Don't starve yourself.** Hunger pangs are uncomfortable and will keep you up.

🍎 **Try eating a light bedtime snack.** A combination of carbs and protein, such as cheese and crackers or cereal and milk, seems to have a mild sleep-inducing effect for some people.

🍎 **Go light on liquids before you retire.** If the call of nature is disrupting your sleep, try not to drink anything for a half-hour before bedtime. If you limit your fluids and still wake up to urinate, eat something salty, say, a couple of saltines, to help you retain a little more fluid. (Don't try this if you're on a sodium-restricted diet.)

🍎 **Switch milk for colicky babies.** Ask your pediatrician whether you should substitute breast milk or nonmilk formula for cow's milk.

🍎 **Nix the MSG.** Sensitive people may experience stimulant effects from this common food additive. Try ordering Chinese food without the MSG. And be aware that meat tenderizers and flavor-enhancers often contain this ingredient.

🍎 **Time your snacks carefully.** The best time for a bedtime snack, according to Dr. Zammit, is 30 minutes or more before lights-out.

healing diet

PROBLEM FOODS	GOOD FOODS
Alcoholic beverages	Cereal with milk
Beans, cucumbers, and other gas-producing foods	Crackers with cheese
Coffee	Bread with turkey
Colas	Herbal teas (especially
Chocolate	chamomile, hops,
Hot peppers	passionflower, valerian)
MSG-containing foods	
Tea	

BEST ADVICE: Don't go to bed too hungry or too full. Eat a balanced diet of light meals and snacks at regular times, with a light bedtime snack 30 minutes before lights-out.

irritable bowel syndrome

For a condition that rarely presents a serious health risk, irritable bowel syndrome (IBS) sure has a lot of names: spastic colon, spastic colitis, mucous colitis, nervous stomach, nervous diarrhea, and functional bowel disease.

The names reflect the mystery that surrounds IBS. No one is exactly sure what causes it. Fatty foods and certain fruits were once seen as culprits. So was stress. Now researchers generally agree that some foods along with stress can trigger incidents of IBS with people who are predisposed to it. Likewise, changing your eating habits can help minimize its symptoms.

Those who suffer from IBS will tell you their symptoms run the gamut of gastrointestinal complaints: bloating, excess gas, and nausea, as well as periods of constipation followed by bouts of diarrhea. In turn, these symptoms may be accompanied by weight-loss, headache, prolonged fatigue, impaired concentration, anxiety, and depression. By far the most common symptom is abdominal pain, according to Gerard Guillory, M.D., IBS specialist in Denver and author of *IBS: A Doctor's Plan for Chronic Digestive Troubles.* People alternately describe the pain as cramping, burning, or sharp, he says.

If any of the symptoms sound familiar, take heart. You're definitely not alone. By some estimates, IBS symptoms account for roughly half of all gastrointestinal complaints. And overall one in five adults experiences IBS to some degree.

For a long time it was believed that women were more apt to develop IBS than men. Often the first signs occur with women in their 20s, and the condition has been linked with premenstrual syndrome. But Dr. Guillory has a different explanation. Women, at least in this country, are more likely to see a doctor about their symptoms, he says. In India, where men see doctors more often than women, IBS is more common among men.

Getting a Diagnosis

Many people go for years without even realizing they have IBS, says Dr. Guillory. It's easy to understand how. Everyone from time to time experiences excess gas or periods of constipation, he explains. Typically people chalk this up to the double pepperoni pizza they ate the night before. Sometimes IBS symptoms will disappear for years. But they can return with a vengeance and seriously affect your quality of life. It's not uncommon for people who experience serious bouts of IBS to fear eating out, traveling by car, or visiting anyplace without the knowledge that a bathroom is close by.

Often doctors recommend counseling, together with diet and other therapies, to help quell people's fears. But there is one significant silver lining: IBS doesn't cause actual damage to your intestinal tract. Steven Peikin, M.D., professor of gastroenterology at the Robert Wood Johnson Medical School at Camden, in New Jersey, says many of the people he diagnoses with IBS "are happy they don't have a worse disease."

Because it does no physical harm, doctors call IBS a functional disorder versus an organic disorder. With organic disorders, the intestine becomes diseased, inflamed, or infected in some way. Organic intestinal diseases come with symptoms like fever, weight loss, and blood in stools—symptoms people with IBS don't have, says Dr. Guillory.

In fact, doctors won't even make a diagnosis of IBS until tests show that you have no organic intestinal diseases, he says. So when you see a doctor about IBS, you'll likely have blood, urine, and stool samples tested. And for good reason: IBS symptoms can mimic those of more serious conditions.

Abdominal pains, for example, might indicate an ulcer. And difficult-to-pass stools can be a sign of a bowel obstruction, including a tumor.

Pinpointing the Causes

The symptoms of IBS arise for quite different reasons. Technically speaking, with IBS the muscles in the digestive system contract erratically. When they contract too much, they produce diarrhea. And when they contract too little, the result is constipation. Some researchers believe these erratic contractions are similar to what occurs with asthma attacks, says Dr. Guillory. In fact, some physicians have nicknamed IBS "asthma of the gut."

Just as with asthma, IBS has numerous and often little-understood causes. One study showed that young women on crash diets experienced IBS in above average numbers. Another found an above average incidence among runners. There may even be a link between traumatic childhood events and IBS, according to Dr. Guillory. All these things may make a person more likely to develop IBS, he says, and doctors know of three key factors that can trigger the actual symptoms:

● Stress
● Lack of fiber
● An intolerance or sensitivity to certain foods

In many cases all three factors play a role, says Dr. Guillory.

Stress

Even though your digestive system functions without your having to think about it, how you feel definitely affects the way you digest your food. Who hasn't felt butterflies in the stomach right before making an important speech? Well, that reaction is even stronger if you have IBS.

Hours after you've calmed down following a stressful event, the muscles in your digestive system can tighten up or spasm and bring on an IBS episode.

Fiber

Compared to dealing with stress, adding more fiber to your diet should be a snap. Nature makes fiber readily available in such plant foods as vegetables, fruits, grains, and nuts. And doctors recommend that all of us eat 20 to 35 grams of fiber per day. But people with IBS may especially benefit from a high-fiber diet, according to one study done in 1991. When researchers looked at the diets of 72 people with IBS, they found that all of those who ate more than 30 grams of fiber per day showed improvement over the six-month study period.

What makes fiber work so well? By absorbing water—up to 15 times its weight—fiber prevents diarrhea. Also, because all that fibrous plant matter by its very nature takes up lots of space, it prompts the large intestine to quickly void it as waste, thus preventing constipation. And because fiber speeds up the passage of food through the digestive system, it conditions the muscles of the large intestine to work normally. And this, explains

Guillory, helps reduce the spastic attacks that bring on diarrhea. (To learn about how to add the recommended amounts of fiber to your diet, read "Constipation," which begins on page 105.)

Food Sensitivities

Fiber alone may not ward off IBS symptoms completely. In fact, certain high-fiber foods rank among the foods that may actually trigger IBS symptoms—especially if you have a food intolerance. (See the list of Problem Foods at the end of this section to help pinpoint your own sensitivities.)

One thing to be aware of: It's easy to confuse a food intolerance with a food allergy. Allergies to food are actually fairly rare. The Mayo Clinic estimates that only 1 to 2 percent of the population suffer from food allergies. If you're one of them, your body will call up the antibodies of the immune system to actually do battle with foods you're allergic to—just as if those foods were harmful viruses.

By contrast, food intolerances arise when your body doesn't make enough of the necessary enzymes to digest a particular food properly. For anyone with IBS, a food intolerance can wreak havoc with the digestive system, exaggerating minor cramps and creating bad bouts of diarrhea.

Up to 19 percent of Caucasians have a food intolerance, as do 70 percent of African Americans and up to 90 percent of Native Americans and Asians. And the most common food intolerance of all is lactose intolerance. It occurs when you don't produce enough of the enzyme lactase to digest dairy products properly. One study found that all but 17 of 110 participants experienced relief of their IBS symptoms after going on a strict lactose-free diet. (For more details on this condition, see "Lactose Intolerance," which begins on page 225.)

What makes things complicated for anyone with IBS is that there are lots of potential trigger foods. Sometimes your system can withstand small amounts of these foods without going ballistic. Let's say you're intolerant of chocolate. Giving in and enjoying a piece of chocolate cake at a friend's house can make you crampy all the next day. But if you ate just a small amount, you might feel fine. Other times—especially times when you're stressed—your gut runs amok after eating even the slightest morsel of chocolate.

"The biggest IBS culprits are overeating and greasy, fatty foods," says Dr. Peikin. But with so many potential trigger foods, how can you ever discover which ones to stay away from?

Keep a food diary. Just as you would with an ordinary diary, you'll be recording details of your day that you're otherwise liable to forget. But the focus here is on food. Keep the diary simple, Dr. Guillory recommends. Write down what foods you ate and the time you ate them.

Also include the circumstances of the day: Did you wolf down breakfast while rushing to prepare for an important meeting? Or did you savor a late brunch, followed by a Sunday afternoon nap? Next jot down how you feel during the course of the day: bloated, irregular, or relaxed?

Keep up with your diary for about two weeks, Dr. Guillory advises. That way you and your doctor will have plenty of information when you set about designing a diet that works for you.

Making Food Work For You

Since people differ greatly in the foods they can and cannot eat, Dr. Guillory recommends that you let a registered dietitian help you create workable recipes. People think nothing of hiring a personal trainer to help them exercise, he says. If you have IBS, a professional dietitian can likely help you a lot more.

But simply eating the right foods isn't enough, he says. You must learn to eat in a relaxed manner. Just look at the eating habits of many people, and you can understand how digestive disorders develop, says Dr. Guillory. Grabbing meals at crowded fast-food restaurants doesn't help. Neither does eating while working or while the kids are screaming.

Instead, you should make mealtimes the part of the day when you relax, he advises. Call it positive biofeedback. When you relax during meals night after night, the intestinal muscles are gradually conditioned to behave themselves.

Here's some other advice from Dr. Guillory:

Thoroughly chew your foods. Yes, your mother told you to do this. And she was right. Chewing well makes things easier on the rest of your digestive system.

Don't drink liquids when eating. Liquids contribute to bloating and can dilute digestive juices.

🍎 **Think small.** Try eating more frequent, smaller meals each day—as many as six.

🍎 **Take a hike.** A walk after a meal helps you relax and aids digestion.

🍎 **Freeze ahead.** Have mini meals prepared in advance and kept in case bad days leave you not wanting to cook.

🍎 **Try an herbal tea.** Peppermint relaxes the smooth intestinal muscles. Gingerroot settles the stomach.

🍎 **Think ahead.** Take along safe foods when you're traveling. Order low-fat or vegetarian meals on planes by calling at least a day or more in advance.

🍎 **Make excuses.** Make sure friends understand that you have a digestive disorder when visiting—that's all you need to explain. They'll understand that this prevents you from eating certain foods, and they won't be offended if you have to say no.

🍎 **Follow the rules.** Peikin has devised diets to treat a host of digestive disorders, including IBS. His cardinal rules for an anti-IBS diet:
- Increase the fiber
- Lower the fat
- Reduce lactose (found in milk and dairy products)
- Cut down on hot spices
- Limit gas-forming legumes
- Maximize nutrition, minimize calories

healing diet

PROBLEM FOODS	GOOD FOODS
Alcohol	Fish
Bacon	Foods high in fiber
Broccoli	Fruit
Cabbage	Most vegetables
Citrus fruits	Rice
Coffee and other caffeinated beverages	
Cured meats	
Eggs	
Fatty foods	
Milk and dairy products	
Onions	
Sausage	
Wheat	

BEST ADVICE: Mild cases: Stick to a high-fiber, low-fat regimen of about 2,000 calories per day. More severe cases: Develop a nutritious diet with the help of a physician or professional dietitian.

kidney stones

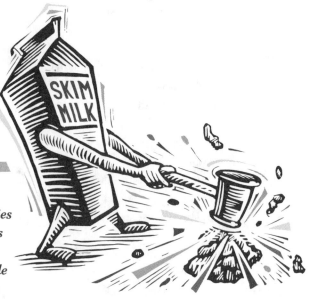

Not only are kidney stones among the oldest maladies known to afflict our species (they've been found in Egyptian mummies more than 7,000 years old), they're also among the most painful. "If you ask people to rate the pain of passing a kidney stone on a scale of one to ten, many will put it at an eleven," says kidney specialist David M. Wilson, M.D., of the Mayo Clinic in Rochester, Minnesota.

Kidney stones also, unfortunately, are quite common, forming in an estimated 10 percent of men and 5 percent of women at some point in their lives. Their incidence, moreover, appears to be on the rise, especially in women, reports the National Institutes of Diabetes and Digestive and Kidney Diseases in Bethesda, Maryland. Research also shows that kidney stones tend to run in families, that Caucasians are more prone than African Americans, that people between the ages of 20 and 40 are at the greatest risk, and that once a person gets one kidney stone, odds increase dramatically that more will follow.

Stones Under The Microscope

What's at the source of these painful intruders that can grow to the size of a golf ball in some cases? Where do they come from?

Doctors aren't sure, but they do know of certain risk factors, and they do know how stones form. They start as tiny crystals that develop within the urine and build up on the inner surfaces of the kidneys—two bean-shaped organs that remove excess water and waste products from the blood in the form of urine.

In most people this process goes smoothly, because urine normally contains chemicals that prevent stones from forming. In folks less fortunate, however, and for reasons not fully understood, these chemicals either are absent or fail to do their job, and stones begin to form.

factors that
increase risks

Some people are predisposed to developing kidney stones due simply to genetics, gender, and/or race. But other factors also are known to come into play—some of which are more within our control than others. "There usually is a balance in the urine between chemicals that promote crystal formation and those that inhibit it, and we know that a number of factors can cause this balance to be upset," says Dr. David M. Wilson, M.D., of the Mayo Clinic in Rochester, Minnesota.

Among the factors less within our control are:
- chronic urinary tract infections
- blockage of the urinary tract
- certain medications (diuretics and calcium-based antacids)
- bed rest for several weeks or more
- various diseases of the metabolism (those affecting kidney function, especially)
- chronic inflammation of the bowel
- surgeries that bypass the intestines

Usually these stones (between 80 and 90 percent) consist of calcium combined with oxalate or phosphate, but other types also can develop. Strive stones, for example, are caused by infection within the kidneys.

The Pain of Passage

If kidney stones stay small enough, they may remain in the kidney pain-free and cause no harm, or they may pass through the urinary tract unnoticed, and they often do. But other times, these stones can grow into jagged masses as large as 1½ inches in diameter before beginning their journey out of the body by way of the narrow ducts (urethras) leading from the kidneys to the bladder and eventually the small tube (urethra) through which we urinate. Because neither of these passageways usually measures more than about ⅛ of an inch in diameter, this journey can be an understandably memorable one.

The pain of passing a kidney stone can indeed be an ordeal, Dr. Wilson says, often starting suddenly in the area of the back or the side just below the edge of the ribs. It then can begin to radiate downward and forward into the groin area as the stone begins to move, and it can cease if the stone comes to rest. This pain of passage also may be accompanied by bloody, cloudy, or especially foul-smelling urine, nausea, and vomiting, an inability to urinate completely, or weakness, fever, and chills (usually signs of an accompanying infection).

Stone Makers vs. Stone Breakers

Kidney stones are not entirely a result of illness or genetic destiny, however, says kidney stone researcher, Gary C. Curhan, M.D., Sc.D., of Massachusetts General Hospital and the Harvard School of Public Health in Cambridge, Massachusetts. "More and more we're finding that diet can affect kidney stone development in some people. Avoidance of certain foods, combined with an increase in the consumption of others, may have a protective effect."

Giving across the board dietary advice for the prevention of kidney stones is difficult, however, because no two stones—or stone sufferers—are exactly alike, Dr. Curhan says. (If you currently have a stone, or have had one in the past, you should see your doctor for urine and blood tests on which dietary recommendations can then be based.) Since more than 80 percent of all stones are of the calcium-oxalate variety, however, the following recommendations can be helpful for most people at risk for stone formation, Dr. Curhan says.

Drink lots of fluids. This is without a doubt the single most valuable piece of advice someone worried about kidney stones can follow, Dr. Curhan says. The reason is simple: The more dilute the urine,

the more difficult it is for stones to form. Your goal should be to drink enough fluids to produce at least 2 quarts of urine daily, Dr. Curhan says. Usually the consumption of approximately eight 8-ounce glasses of liquid a day is sufficient to produce such an output, but excessive sweating due to hot weather or heavy exercise may require more. If in doubt, measure your urine production to be sure and monitor it for color as well. If it's darker than a pale yellow, you need to drink still more.

Give a green light to dairy products rich in calcium. Once thought to encourage kidney stone formation, dairy foods high in calcium (low-fat milk, yogurt, and cheese) now are being found to have a protective effect, Dr. Curhan says. In a study done by Dr. Curhan and other researchers from the Harvard School of Public Health, people with the highest consumption of calcium-rich dairy products were found to reduce their risk of stone formation by as much as 50 percent over people whose calcium intakes were lowest.

Calcium-rich foods appear to decrease the body's absorption—and hence presence in the urine—of potentially troublesome oxalates, Dr. Curhan explains. By contrast, Dr. Curhan's research has found that calcium consumed in the form of supplements, as calcium carbonate, may actually increase kidney stone risks, and especially if taken on an empty stomach. It's best, therefore, to get your calcium in low-fat dairy products, he says, or at least to be sure that if you do take a calcium supplement, you do so at mealtimes only.

🍎 **Give a red light to foods high in oxalate.** "We now feel that urinary oxalate may play an even more important role than urinary calcium in the process of stone formation," Dr. Curhan says. Oxalate is most prevalent in leafy green vegetables such as spinach, collard greens, Swiss chard, dandelion greens, parsley, and rhubarb. These foods should be eaten sparingly by anyone who's already had a calcium oxalate stone or who may for other reasons be at risk, Dr. Curhan says.

Reducing oxalate in the diet need not mean avoiding fruits and vegetables entirely, however, but rather simply choosing varieties whose oxalate content is relatively low. Fruits and vegetables low in oxalate include broccoli, brussels sprouts, lettuce, mushrooms, turnips, cabbage, cauliflower, radishes, and peas in the vegetable family, and such fruits as oranges, grapefruit, peaches, plums, mangoes, melons, nectarines, bananas, cherries, avocados, and pineapple.

🍎 **Limit animal sources of protein.** Though not as pernicious as foods brimming with oxalate, animal sources of protein (meats, poultry, and fish) probably also should be limited by people at risk for kidney stones, Dr. Curhan says. "Intake of animal protein increases the concentration of both calcium and uric acid in the urine, which can contribute to stone formation, while it also decreases concentrations of citrate, which is a natural stone inhibitor," he explains.

This needn't be reason for a total animal flesh embargo, however, but rather just a cutback. Brian Morgan, Ph.D., a research scientist with the Institute of Human Nutrition at Columbia University College of Physicians and Surgeons in New York City, says people at risk for calcium oxalate or uric acid stones probably should limit their intake of animal proteins (meat, cheese, poultry, and fish) to no more than about 6 ounces a day.

🍎 **Cut back on sodium.** "Our research and that of others has found a correlation between high sodium intakes and kidney stone development," Dr. Curhan says. This is not surprising given that sodium has been shown to increase the concentration of calcium in the urine, he adds. As the body attempts to excrete excess sodium, it also excretes calcium, hence the greater urinary concentrations.

Try to keep your sodium intake to less than about 2,400 milligrams a day with this in mind. Table salt, soy sauce, pickled foods, most canned soups, luncheon meats, snack chips, and processed cheese are the most prolific sodium sources.

🍎 **Eat more foods high in potassium.** Dr. Curhan's research also has found a connection between kidney stones and potassium—a protective one. So foods high in this important mineral should be high on your stone-fighting list. Good potassium sources are potatoes, prunes and prune juice, peaches, raisins, currants, cantaloupe, avocados, clams, nonfat yogurt, skim milk, orange juice, bananas, and yams.

🍎 **Walk away from stones.** Last but not least, exercise may help us flex our muscles against kidney stones. Exercise increases the uptake of calcium by the bones. That helps decrease the amount of calcium that ever makes it to the kidneys or the urine in the first place.

healing diet

PROBLEM FOODS	GOOD FOODS
Beans	Avocados
Beets	Bananas
Blueberries	Cantaloupe
Celery	Clams
Cheese	Currants
Chocolate	Low-fat milk and other low-fat
Eggplant	dairy products
Fish	Peaches
Grapes	Potatoes
Leafy green vegetables, such as spinach,	Prunes and prune juice
collard greens, swiss chard, dandelion greens,	Raisins
and parsley	Water and other fluids
Meat	Yams
Meat	
Peanuts	
Poultry	
Rhubarb	
Salty foods	
Strawberries	
Summer squash	
Sweet peppers	

BEST ADVICE: Every kidney stone is different. If you've ever had a stone, you should discuss appropriate dietary measures with your physician. (The tips in this section deal only with the most common types of stones.)

lactose intolerance

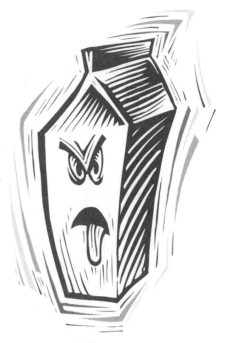

You're troubled by uncomfortable gastrointestinal symptoms—gas, diarrhea, or bloating. The culprit, you decide, must be milk. So you swear off dairy products.

For all but a few people, that's a big, big mistake. For one thing, milk and other dairy products are packed full of important nutrients, including calcium, all in one handy little package. And the fact is, researchers say, milk causes unpleasant symptoms only in a very few people.

Lactose intolerance is "a far overblown problem," says Steven R. Hertzler, Ph.D., R.D., assistant professor of nutrition at Kent State University in Ohio.

This doesn't mean that you positively don't have lactose intolerance. What it does mean is that even if you think you have it, there's a good chance that you don't. So what's going on with your troubled tummy? And, more importantly, what can you do about it?

Lactose Intolerance Basics

Lactose intolerance means having gas or other symptoms specifically because of the inability to break down and digest lactose—the sugar found in milk and other dairy products. Researchers are finding, however, that some people who believe that they are lactose intolerant actually can digest lactose without experiencing any problems. Perhaps more surprisingly, they're also finding that even people with diagnosed lactose intolerance have few or no symptoms after drinking a cup of milk or more.

It is true that plenty of us lack the enzyme lactase, which handily breaks down lactose before it even reaches our small intestines. With rare exception, we're equipped with it as children.

But as we grow up, we begin to lose this enzyme. By age five or six, 70 percent of the world's population—including about 50 million Americans—don't have it, explains Fabrizis L. Suarez, M.D., Ph.D., research associate in the Medical School and instructor in the Department of Food Science and Nutrition at the University of Minnesota in Minneapolis.

The minority of people who retain the enzyme are generally those of northern

European heritage, whose ancestors perhaps depended on dairy foods for sustenance.

Even if you lack the enzyme, however, that doesn't mean you will get symptoms after drinking milk. "The body has other mechanisms to avoid these symptoms, and most of the people we have tested can tolerate 2 cups of milk a day," says Dr. Suarez. He has studied people who have trouble digesting lactose and found that besides the 2 cups of milk, they can eat 8 ounces of yogurt and 2 ounces of cheese daily with only minor symptoms.

And medical studies have found that those who have symptoms can apparently make some minor dietary adjustments that will help their bodies adapt.

How Intolerant Are You?

Some people who think they are severely lactose intolerant, surprisingly enough, still have the enzyme. In one study, Dr. Suarez and other researchers tested 30 people who said they had severe lactose intolerance and always had problems after drinking less than a cup of milk. When these people were tested, however, nine of them turned out to digest lactose just fine.

And even those who were lactose maldigesters—unable to break down lactose—had the same symptoms whether they drank milk or another substance that looked and tasted like milk, even though it didn't have any lactose in it. Apparently, says Dr. Suarez, they were mistaking symptoms of something else for lactose

intolerance. In another study, Dr. Suarez found that lactose maldigesters can tolerate 2 cups of milk a day. Others who thought they were lactose-intolerant did have some flatulence, but it occurred whether or not they had a food or beverage containing lactose.

In one of Dr. Hertzler's studies, aimed at studying the symptoms of lactose intolerance, people with a history of intolerance were given up to $1\frac{1}{2}$ quarts of milk a day. "We were really surprised that with these large doses of lactose, people were having only mild symptoms," he says.

So what's going on?

"Sometimes a person's psychological reaction to a certain food is strong," says Dr. Hertzler. And in some cases, people may have another problem, such as irritable bowel syndrome, that's causing the symptoms.

Milk: The Right Stuff

So, what's the big deal about drinking milk? Those milk ads featuring famous folks with milk mustaches are cute, and they carry a really valid message: Milk is good for you.

It's well known that it's absolutely crucial to get plenty of calcium during childhood and adolescence when your bones are still being formed. "But calcium is also important during the adult years to maintain the bone that has been formed and during later years to reduce the amount of bone lost," says Susan I. Barr, Ph.D., professor of nutrition at the University of British Columbia at Vancouver.

And without ample calcium to build bones and help keep them strong, the result can be osteoporosis, or brittle bones that crumble. "Women are at greater risk than men," notes Dr. Barr, "but men are by no means immune from osteoporosis." (For full details on this condition and what to do about it, see "Osteoporosis," which begins on page 244.)

Other dairy products that are excellent sources of calcium are yogurt and cheese. Although you can get calcium from nondairy sources, the amount of calcium in plant foods is markedly lower than that found in dairy products. For instance, you'd have to eat 14 servings of red beans to get the calcium you do from a cup of milk.

And it's important to remember, points out Dr. Hertzler, that you don't have to digest the lactose in milk in order to absorb the calcium in that milk.

where milk haters
go for calcium

If you simply can't stand milk, cheese, or yogurt, or have severe lactose intolerance—or are a strict vegetarian who refrains from dairy products—you can turn to other foods for your calcium. It just takes a bit of planning.

Perhaps the easiest route is calcium-fortified juices, which can pack as much calcium as milk. Another good source is canned sardines or salmon—as long as you eat the little crunchy bones as well. Other decent sources are tofu that's been set in calcium, turnip and mustard greens, and blackstrap molasses. (About two servings of greens equals a cup of milk.) Lesser amounts of calcium are available in almonds, cabbage, broccoli, white beans, kale, rutabaga, and sesame seed.

Supplements aren't the best source of calcium, but if you are a strict vegetarian, you may want to consider supplementation to boost your calcium intake.

How to Handle Dairy Products

If you experience discomfort after ingesting dairy products, you probably avoid them like the plague. That's the wrong approach, says Dr. Hertzler. Few of us give our intestines much thought, but the fact is they have bacteria whose job is to break down things such as lactose. And with some gentle encouragement—namely, a steady dose of lactose—these bacteria multiply to help handle the job. In a study at Kent State, when people who could not digest lactose received daily doses of lactose, after three days the number of bacteria that help break down lactose had tripled.

At first, the bacteria working on the lactose produce significant gas, but that abates, too. After 10 days of daily doses of lactose, symptoms of gas frequency and severity decreased by half.

"The bacteria in the large intestine get used to lactose over a period of time," says Dr. Hertzler. "The way bacteria ferment lactose changes in favor of less gas production." Apparently, the bacteria that can ferment it the best take over.

This was also shown in a three-week study of 17 African-American teenage girls at Purdue University in Lafayette, Indiana, 14 of whom could not break down lactose. They received a high-calcium, dairy-based diet that gave them 1,300 daily milligrams of calcium, and their symptoms decreased markedly after the three weeks.

Ready to try to pump some dairy into your diet? Here's what to do:

🍎 **Eat more dairy.** Start small, advises Dr. Hertzler. You may want to start with yogurt or hard cheeses, then begin daily doses of half a cup of milk. Then add another half cup later in the day. Remember that everyone is different. Be persistent. It takes a while for your system to adjust to the lactose.

🍎 **Drink milk with meals.** When you drink milk alone, it heads straight to the small intestine, reaching it in about 10 minutes, says Dr. Suarez. "Milk plus food will take around seven hours, which lets the lactose enter the colon slowly," he says. This gives the lactose-chomping bacteria a better chance to break down the lactose without excessive gas production.

🍎 **Time your doses.** It's much better to have a cup of milk with breakfast, and another with dinner, advises Dr. Suarez. This spreads out your doses of lactose so you don't overwhelm those friendly bacteria.

🍎 **Try hard cheeses.** While cheeses such as cheddar and Swiss are good dairy sources of calcium, they contain very little lactose. "The cheese is made from the 'curd' part; the lactose is in the 'whey' part and is removed," says Dr. Barr.

🍎 **Choose yogurt.** It's easier to digest lactose in yogurt with live bacteria than in other dairy foods. (Look for the words "live cultures" on the label.) Eating yogurt with other foods may help digest the lactose in the yogurt, according to a study at the University of Minnesota. Even yogurt with live cultures can vary. One study found that symptoms varied according to the brand of yogurt, so you may want to shop around. In general, however, all yogurt contains less lactose than milk.

🍎 **Reach for acidophilus milk.** Acidophilus milk, with acidophilus bacteria added, can go down easier than regular milk. In a study at the David Grant U.S. Air Force Medical Center in California, children who could not digest lactose experienced fewer symptoms with acidophilus milk or yogurt than with regular milk.

🍎 **For a last resort.** If all else fails, then, says Dr. Hertzler, turn to an over-the-counter digestive aid that contains the enzyme lactase. These digestive-aid products are available at your local pharmacy. You can add it to milk before you drink it or take it with lactose-containing foods. Using it will break down lactose, but it also means that your own bacteria won't gear up to handle milk products. So if you find yourself with no digestive aid on hand, your unprepared gut may not be happy about the sudden appearance of lactose.

healing diet

PROBLEM FOODS	GOOD FOODS
Milk, if drunk on a less than regular basis	Acidophilus milk
	Hard cheeses, such as cheddar and Swiss
	Yogurt with active cultures

BEST ADVICE: Milk and other dairy foods are such good sources of calcium that it's worth the effort to try to develop tolerance to them. If you give it your best shot and still can't learn to enjoy milk, make a point of eating plenty of plant foods that contain calcium and consider taking a calcium supplement.

macular degeneration

Maybe you aren't fond of spinach. Maybe you're even less fond of its cousin, collard greens. Well, maybe you'll want to rethink your dinner options and find a way to like these humble greens. Research suggests that these foods can help protect your vision. B. Randy Hammond, Ph.D., who studies eye disease, is certainly convinced. He eats spinach two or three times a week.

Meet Your Macula

You will probably never know you have a macula until something goes wrong with it. It's the small light-sensitive area in the middle of your retina at the back of your eyeball. These cells take in the image received by the lens and send it to your brain to interpret. Over the years, light can eventually damage the macula, causing small deposits of cellular waste matter to accumulate or small blood vessels under the retina to leak or swell.

The early result of this macular degeneration is difficulty seeing small print and distant objects, and gradual loss of central vision. Macular degeneration is the leading cause of blindness in older Americans, affecting one of three people older than 75.

There are two types of macular degeneration—one with leaking blood vessels that can be treated with laser surgery. Ninety percent of people with macular degeneration, however, have the "dry" type that currently has no effective treatment.

Foods That May Help

Enter the carotenoids. These are the yellow, orange, and red pigments that abound in many fruits and vegetables, giving them their bright colors. Carotenoids supply a number of health benefits. Carrots, for example, are packed with beta-carotene, a carotenoid that's often in the news.

Researchers are now finding that vegetables such as spinach and collard greens may help protect the macula, possibly partly because of two carotenoids in these foods, lutein and zeaxanthin.

The natural pigment found in the macula protects the macula from light damage by filtering out harmful light rays, points out Dr. Hammond, a professor at Arizona State University in Tempe. "The thicker it is, the less light gets through to harm the macula," he says.

Because macular pigment is made up of lutein and zeaxanthin, the very same stuff found in spinach and collard greens, it was logical for scientists to investigate whether eating more of these vegetable pigments would thicken the macular pigment. The Eye Disease Case-Control Study Group at five ophthalmology centers studied 876 people between the ages of 55 and 80. Of this group, 356 had macular degeneration. Researchers found that those who ate the most carotenoids were 43 percent less likely to get macular degeneration—and those who ate spinach and collard greens had the least chance of getting the disease.

Learn to love greens. A leading researcher of the Eye Disease Case-Control Study Group, Johanna M. Seddon, M.D., of the Massachusetts Eye and Ear Infirmary in Boston, concluded that increasing the carotenoid-containing foods you eat, particularly dark green, leafy vegetables, may decrease the risk of serious age-related macular degeneration. Dr. Hammond's studies also support this theory. In one of Dr. Hammond's studies, 13 people ate spinach daily for 15 weeks. Macular pigment density increased in four weeks for most of them and remained high several months after they stopped eating the spinach.

Get more zinc. Some studies suggest that zinc intake may also be related to macular degeneration. When Julie Mares-Perlman, Ph.D., assistant professor of ophthalmology and visual sciences at University of Wisconsin Medical School, in Madison, studied nearly 2,000 people ranging in age from 43 to 86, she found that people with the highest intake of zinc from food had the lowest risk for early macular degeneration. (You can find zinc in beef, crab, oysters, poultry, and milk.)

Eat more fruits and vegetables. Researchers have long suspected that antioxidants, nutrients found in many fruits and vegetables—which combat damage done by unstable "free radical" molecules—may help protect your eyes. A two-year study at Johns Hopkins Hospital in Baltimore, Maryland, involving 976 people found that those with high blood levels of vitamins C and E and beta-carotene were least likely to have macular degeneration.

Stay away from fatty foods. There's also a possibility that the more saturated fat you eat, the higher the risk for macular degeneration. In the Wisconsin survey, signs of macular degeneration were 80 percent more common in the people who ate the most saturated fat and cholesterol.

How could dietary fat affect your eyesight? It could clog arteries or collect in the retina and slow nutrient supply, explains Dr. Mares-Perlman, the study's lead author. She stresses, however, that more research is needed before any definitive link is established. "We don't know whether it was the saturated fat content diet, or other aspects of high-fat diets—perhaps low in antioxidants—that was responsible," she says. However, because decreasing fat and cholesterol intake has plenty of known benefits, it's best in any case to cut back on the butter, cheese, cream sauces, fatty meats, chips, and dips.

● **Switch to wine.** Another possibility comes from a study at Howard University Hospital in Washington, D.C., which involved 3,072 people, ages 45 to 74, with eye changes that might lead to macular degeneration. Researchers found that those who consumed moderate amounts of wine had less chance of developing the eye disease. (Beer or liquor did not show a protective effect.) Again, this is only one study, and the researchers certainly don't suggest that you take up drinking to protect your vision. If you currently drink, however, you may want to consider switching from beer or liquor to wine. Remember the key word "moderate"—which doesn't mean several glasses a day.

To Supplement or Not to Supplement

Maybe you truly hate greens or don't like to take time to cook. Why not just pick up a bottle of supplements under the "Eye" section in your local vitamin store instead?

Supplements offer several problems, says Dr. Hammond. When a study shows that spinach or collard greens helps prevent macular degeneration, it's a good guess that the lutein and zeaxanthin are helping, but they could be working with something else in the food.

"Food contains many beneficial compounds that we cannot measure that may actually be the compound of importance," says Sheila West, Ph.D.,

associate professor of ophthalmology at the Johns Hopkins University School of Medicine in Baltimore, Maryland.

There are two other points to keep in mind. First, studies show that vitamins and minerals alone don't do the job:

● In the Eye Disease Case-Control Study, which showed the benefit of spinach and collard greens, supplementing with vitamin A, E, or C didn't have a significant effect.

● The Johns Hopkins study that linked high blood levels of certain vitamins to less risk of macular degeneration found that using vitamin supplements showed no benefit.

And, second, results of the effects of many nutrients aren't definitive. A Japanese study showed that 35 people with macular degeneration had lower zinc and vitamin E blood levels than 66 people without eye damage, suggesting that low levels of these nutrients are linked with macular degeneration. Conversely, however, a study of 312 people at the Australian National University showed no relation between levels of vitamin E and beta-carotene in the blood and macular degeneration. Another Australian study, from Sydney University, found no link between levels of vitamin E in the blood and rates of macular degeneration, and only a weak suggestion that selenium levels in smokers might be linked to the disease.

What does all this mean? It means no one knows yet exactly what nutrients may help your eyes.

Experts agree that many of us are low in specific nutrients. A large ongoing study at the DVA Medical Center in Chicago showed that people with macular degeneration have a low intake of vitamin E, magnesium, zinc, vitamin B6, and folic acid.

But most experts say that the answer is a diet high in fruits and vegetables—not supplements. "There are lots of other food components that have health benefits," says Dr. Mares-Perlman. "And some nutrients in the form of a supplement aren't very usable by your body."

Dr. Hammond advises people to increase their intake of lutein- and zeaxanthin-containing foods such as spinach and other dark green leafy vegetables.

If, despite your best efforts to pack in nutrients, you're concerned that you're not getting enough, experts agree that it's generally safe to add a multivitamin and mineral supplement. You should never, however, take any other supplement without checking with your doctor.

healing diet

PROBLEM FOODS	GOOD FOODS
Fatty foods	Beef
Foods high in cholesterol	Carrots
	Collard greens
	Crab
	Milk
	Oysters
	Poultry
	Spinach
	Wine in moderation

BEST ADVICE: If you have macular degeneration, you should be under the care of your doctor. Do eat a balanced diet rich in fruits and vegetables and low in fatty foods and cholesterol.

menopause

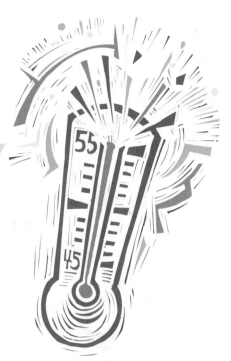

You're at a wedding reception and are being served your favorite part of the meal—coffee and dessert. As you enjoy the wedding cake, you wonder what kind of lives the newlyweds will have, and hope for the best. All of a sudden, you begin to feel warm, very warm. You're sweating, and your husband announces to you and everyone else at the table that your face and neck are flushed. Realizing it's your first hot flash, you can't help but think that both you and the newlyweds are about to begin a new chapter in your lives.

What is menopause anyway? And why does it cause things like hot flashes and other inconvenient, unpleasant symptoms in some women and not others?

Menopause is the point in a woman's life when menstruation stops permanently. This is usually confirmed when a woman has not had a menstrual period for 12 consecutive months, and there is no other obvious biological or physiological cause. Known as the "change of life," menopause is not a disease. Rather, it is a perfectly natural event. It marks the last stage of a gradual biological process in which the ovaries reduce their production of female sex hormones—a process that begins about three to five years before the final menstrual period. This transitional phase is called the climacteric, or perimenopause.

More than one-third of the women in the United States—about 36 million—have been through menopause, according to the North American Menopause Society. With a life expectancy of about 81 years, a 50-year-old woman can expect to live more than one-third of her life after menopause.

The Intricate Dance: How Menopause Works

The ovaries contain structures called follicles that hold the egg cells. You are born with about 500,000 egg cells, and by puberty there are about 75,000 left. Only about 400 to 500 ever mature fully to be released during the menstrual cycle. The rest degenerate through the years. During the reproductive years, a gland in the brain generates hormones that cause a new egg to be released from its follicle every month.

The follicle then produces the sex hormones estrogen and progesterone, which thicken the lining of the uterus. This enriched lining is prepared to receive and nourish a fertilized egg that could develop into a baby. If fertilization does not occur, estrogen and progesterone levels drop, the lining of the uterus breaks down, and menstruation occurs. This more or less regular monthly cycle continues until a woman is in her 30s, which marks the onset of a series of physical changes.

Although doctors aren't really sure why, in her 30s a woman's ovaries begin to produce less estrogen and progesterone. In their late 30s, some women may not ovulate each month.

During the six years or so immediately prior to natural menopause, menopause-related changes start happening in a woman's body.

Irregular Menstrual Patterns

About two years prior to menopause, before menstruation stops completely, most women notice changes in their menstrual cycles. Bleeding may last fewer days than previously, or it may go on for more days.

The blood flow may be lighter or heavier. The time between periods often changes. Often women may go several months without a period, then have it return unexpectedly.

This change in bleeding patterns is typically caused by not ovulating every month, and is normal and natural.

when?
the big question

In the Western world, most women experience natural menopause between the ages of 45 and 55—on average at about age 51. But it can occur as early as in a woman's 30s and, rarely, as late as in her 60s. Although women today begin to menstruate earlier than their forebears, the average age at menopause has not changed much for hundreds of years.

Genetics play an important role in determining the time of menopause. In one British study, researchers asked more than 1,000 women their mother's age at menopause. Premature menopause was defined at younger than age 40, and early menopause was younger than age 45. The researchers found that women in the study were six times as likely to experience premature or early menopause if their mothers also had premature or early menopause. Ask your mother when she became menopausal—it will give you some idea when you might reach it yourself.

Hot Flashes

Hot flashes are the most common symptom of menopause, affecting 60 to 80 percent of menopausal women in the United States. During a hot flash, the face and neck become flushed and warm, with red blotches appearing on the chest, back, and arms. This is often followed by sweating then cold shivering as body temperature readjusts. A hot flash can last a few moments or 30 minutes or longer. Some women experience night sweats, or hot flashes during sleep.

Hot flashes appear to be a direct result of decreasing estrogen levels. If there is no estrogen, your glands release other hormones that dilate blood vessels and destabilize body temperature.

As you get older, hot flashes gradually become less frequent and intense. Most women have hot flashes for two years or less, while a small percentage have them for more than five years.

Vaginal and Urinary Tract Changes

As a woman ages, the walls of the vagina become thinner, dryer, less elastic, and more vulnerable to infection. These changes can make sexual intercourse uncomfortable or even painful.

Tissues in the urinary tract also change with age, sometimes leaving women more susceptible to involuntary loss of urine (incontinence), particularly if certain chronic illnesses or urinary infections are also present. Exercise, coughing, laughing, lifting heavy objects, or similar movements that put pressure on the bladder may cause small amounts of urine to leak.

The Last Hurrah

By the early to mid-50s, periods finally end altogether. However, estrogen production does not completely stop. The ovaries decrease their output significantly, but still may produce a small amount. Also, some estrogen is produced in fat cells with help from the adrenal glands.

Other changes associated with perimenopause and menopause include fatigue (probably from disrupted sleep patterns), mood swings, fluctuations in sexual desire or response, forgetfulness, and difficulty sleeping. Depression, headaches, dizziness, and heart palpitations have not been proved to be related to lowered hormone levels, although many women do report these symptoms.

It's important to note that menopause affects each woman differently. It is truly an individualized experience. Some women notice little difference in their bodies or moods, while others find the change extremely bothersome and disruptive. Estrogen and progesterone affect almost all tissues in the body, but everyone is influenced by them differently. Many disturbances fade over time.

As women move beyond menopause, they are at a higher risk for other conditions which may be related to reduced estrogen levels. These conditions include osteoporosis and heart disease.

In short, there are a number of menopausal-related changes. If you're experiencing these changes, contact your health-care professional to confirm their cause and consider ways to treat them, if needed. There is a wide range of treatment options available to women today, both prescription and nonprescription. Doctors generally prescribe hormone replacement therapy (HRT) to those women who seek symptom relief. However, HRT for menopause is controversial, and its safety and effectiveness from long-term use is still

surgical menopause

If a woman before the age of menopause has both her ovaries removed surgically, she experiences an abrupt menopause. She may be hit harder by menopausal symptoms than those women who experience it gradually and naturally. Her hot flashes may be more severe, more frequent, and longer. She may have a greater risk of heart disease and osteoporosis, and may be more likely to become depressed. The reasons for this are unknown.

When only one ovary is removed, menopause usually occurs naturally. When the uterus is removed (hysterectomy) and the ovaries remain, menstrual periods stop, but other menopausal symptoms (if any) usually occur at the same age that they would naturally. However, some women who have a hysterectomy may experience menopausal symptoms at a younger age, possibly due to a decreased blood supply to the ovaries as a result of surgery.

being investigated. You'll need to discuss the pros and cons with your doctor in order to determine what is appropriate for you.

Fortunately, there are also a number of dietary steps you can take to help you deal with the symptoms of menopause.

Menopause and Nutrition

Doctors do know that good nutrition plays an enormous role in achieving wellness for women of all ages, including menopausal and postmenopausal women," says Sadja Greenwood, M.D., assistant clinical professor in the Department of Obstetrics, Gynecology, and Reproductive Sciences at the University of California at San Francisco, and author of *Menopause, Naturally.* "Think of menopause as a time when you're preparing for the

second half of your life. Take charge of your daily health practices and inform yourself of ways to eat healthy food. Sound nutrition at this time in your life can keep you healthy, energetic, and vital, and prevent the chronic and acute diseases of aging, such as heart disease, diabetes, cancer, and osteoporosis."

Phytoestrogens— What's in a Name?

A menopause treatment that is undergoing intensive research right now is phytoestrogens—natural substances that are found in many plants, herbs, seeds, and beans. Phytoestrogens are chemically similar in structure to human estrogen. They have estrogen-like effects, but without any negative side effects.

There are two basic types of phytoestrogens—isoflavones and lignans. Isoflavones are most commonly found in legumes, with soybeans being the richest source. The lignan type is found in almost all whole grains, cereals, and vegetables, with the highest concentration in the oilseeds, especially flaxseed (also called linseed).

In certain cultures where large amounts of phytoestrogen-containing foods are consumed, women report fewer menopausal symptoms, such as hot flashes. When they do have hot flashes, they don't last as long and are less intense.

Soy's Effect on Hot Flashes

Australian researchers first made the link between soy foods and menopausal symptoms when they noticed a dramatic difference in the incidences of hot flashes across cultures. The scientists noticed that only 14 to 18 percent of the women studied in China and Japan ever experience a hot flash, while up to 80 percent of women studied in the United States and Europe experience them. The study also found that women living in Japan and China add soy to their diets daily and excrete up to 1,000 times more phytoestrogens in their urine than their American and European counterparts.

Studies are currently underway in the United States and elsewhere to clarify soy's effectiveness and the amounts that would be necessary to achieve an effect.

Researchers at the Bowman Gray School of Medicine in Winston-Salem, North Carolina, for example, studied 43 women between the ages of 45 and 55. The women were chosen because they experienced at least one bout of hot flashes or night sweats daily. In addition to their regular diet, researchers gave the women about 2 tablespoons of soy protein powder, which they either added to juice or milk, or sprinkled over cereal. After six weeks, the women had less severe hot flashes and night sweats, along with other health benefits.

Choosing the Right Foods

The right diet, it seems, not only can help treat the symptoms of menopause in many cases, but also help promote vibrant health and wellness. Once past menopause, women are at a higher risk of heart disease, osteoporosis, cancer, diabetes, and obesity. Eating a balanced, nutritious diet helps keep all those conditions at bay. Here's a guide to help you make the right dietary choices.

● **Add soy to your diet.** Follow these easy tips to slip soy into your meals:

• For breakfast, prepare farina or oatmeal with soy milk. Add a sliced banana and some raisins for flavor and texture.

• Fill your blender with either soy milk or tofu, frozen fruit, one banana, orange juice, wheat germ, and honey to taste. Blend the drink until smooth. "Every day, I mix together a drink of soy milk, one date, one banana, and a small amount of sugar-free chocolate powder," says Dr. Greenwood. "I toss all the ingredients into a blender. In the summer, I add an ice cube."

● At your next barbecue, toss a few soy burgers and soy hot dogs on the grill instead of regular hamburgers and hot dogs.

● Replace chicken or beef with cubed tofu in your next stir-fry.

● Check out the nutritional drinks that contain soy at your local health-food store. To get a product high in soy, be sure it is listed in the top three ingredients. Read the label for sugar and fat content.

Know your soy. Soy is available in tofu, tempeh, soy milk, soy flour, and soy-protein powder. Check the labels for soy products that are low-fat or fat-free. Soft tofu is lower in fat than firm tofu because it contains more water (less whey has been drained off). Also check for calcium content—the levels can vary quite a bit.

Reach for flaxseed. These tiny seeds are packed with essential fatty acids, which are important to menopausal women because low levels have been associated with drying of vaginal and bladder tissues (not to mention skin and hair). Your body cannot manufacture essential fatty acids, so they must be supplied by the diet each day. Flaxseeds are rich in omega-3 and omega-6 fatty acids.

"Whole flaxseeds have laxative and anti-inflammatory properties," explains Dr. Greenwood. "Grind up the flaxseeds in a coffee grinder and sprinkle them onto a salad."

You can also combine flaxseed oil with a little vinegar to make a salad dressing. It breaks down very easily, so be sure to refrigerate after use.

Both flaxseeds and flax oil are sold in health food stores.

Fish for heart health. According to the American Heart Association, heart disease is the number one killer of American women. In addition, the incidence of heart attacks increases ten-fold after menopause—between the ages of 55 and 65. Research shows that omega-3 fatty acids may help protect against heart disease and stroke when part of a low-fat diet. Besides flaxseeds, omega-3s are also found in such cold-water fish as salmon, mackerel, and trout.

Warm up to lentil soup. "Legumes, such as lentils, garbanzo beans, kidney beans, lima beans, and black beans are very high in protein and fiber, and are low in fat," says Dr. Greenwood. "Replace some of the meat in your diet with beans. Meat contains animal protein, which can cause you to lose calcium in the urine, promoting osteoporosis. And high-fiber foods have been shown to lower the risk of certain cancers, especially colon cancer."

Go for whole grains. "Whole grains, such as oats, corn, barley, millet, buckwheat, rice, and whole wheat are great sources of fiber, vitamins, and minerals," says Dr. Greenwood. "Menopausal women need these nutrients to help ward off heart disease, cancer, and diabetes."

Researchers suspect a high-fiber, low-fat diet may help regulate estrogen levels. In addition, the high-fiber content of whole grains binds to cholesterol, helping to carry it out of the body.

High-fiber foods can also help you keep weight in check. "Eating a meal of high-fiber foods will stay in your stomach longer and make you feel full, so you won't eat as much," says Dr. Greenwood. Consume foods containing 20 to 30 grams of fiber each day.

(Currently, the average American is eating only about 10 to 15 grams of fiber daily.)

🍎 **Stock up on sweet potatoes.** They're chock-full of beta-carotene, a precursor of vitamin A. "Research is suggesting that vitamin A may protect against breast cancer," says Susan Lark, M.D., author of *The Estrogen Decision* and *The Menopause Self-Help Book*. "Other research suggests that a high intake of plant foods containing beta-carotene protects against heart attacks in high-risk people."

Vegetables high in vitamin A are orange, red, or dark green in color—such as squash, peppers, carrots, kale, and lettuce.

🍎 **Start each day with a glass of juice.** Just one 8-ounce glass of orange juice contains twice the recommended dietary allowance of vitamin C. "Fruits and fruit juices are excellent sources of bioflavonoids and vitamin C, which helps control excessive menstrual flow as well as provide the body with weak plant sources of estrogen," says Dr. Lark. Also, guava, red bell peppers, and papaya are high in vitamin C.

🍎 **Go bananas.** "Bananas are high in potassium, which can help beat menopausal fatigue," says Dr. Lark. Potassium also helps lower high blood pressure and protects against heart disease. It can also decrease bloating and fluid retention. Other good food sources of potassium include potatoes, oranges, grapefruit, berries, peaches, apricots, and melons.

🍎 **Drink milk daily.** One glass of skim milk contains a whopping 38 percent of the RDA for calcium. "Calcium is an important mineral for menopausal women because it helps prevent osteoporosis," explains Dr. Lark. "Dozens of studies have reinforced this point."

In one study, for example, women and men age 65 and older who used both calcium and vitamin D supplements experienced a lower incidence of bone fracture, as well as reduced loss of bone mass in the hip and spine.

Calcium is the most abundant mineral in the body, and 99 percent of it is deposited in the bones and teeth. However, calcium absorption becomes much less efficient by the time women reach their menopausal years due to aging of the digestive tract. Both the National Institutes of Health and the National Osteoporosis Foundation recommend that postmenopausal women take calcium supplements—1,500 milligrams daily—to compensate for calcium loss.

"The average American women takes in 400 to 500 milligrams of calcium each day," says Dr. Lark. "This is about one-third of the RDA for postmenopausal women."

Besides milk and supplements, other sources of calcium include green leafy vegetables, salmon (with bones), nuts, seeds, tofu, and blackstrap molasses.

🍎 **Let the sun shine in.** Vitamin D is a fat-soluble vitamin that can either be ingested in the diet or formed on the skin through exposure to sunlight.

"Vitamin D helps prevent osteoporosis by aiding in the absorption of calcium," says Dr. Lark. "Another advantage of taking calcium and vitamin D was noted in a study of over 35,000 women in which the two nutrients showed a protective effect against colon cancer."

Vitamin D can be found in multivitamins, fish oil supplements, and fortified milk. Dr. Lark recommends that postmenopausal women get 400 international units each day.

🍂 **Cool that flash with vitamin E.** "Early research is beginning to show that vitamin E can be helpful for hot flashes, night sweats, and vaginal dryness," says Dr. Lark.

In one study, researchers found that vitamin E helped hot flashes in 64 percent of women tested.

"To treat hot flashes, I recommend starting with 200 international units. And if that doesn't help, go up to 600 or 800 international units," explains Dr. Lark. "For vaginal atrophy, you can open a capsule of vitamin E and apply the oil directly to your vaginal tissues."

Besides supplements, good food sources of vitamin E include vegetable oils, raw nuts, seeds, fruits, and vegetables.

🍂 **Time it right.** "A common symptom of menopause that food can help manage is insomnia," says Dr. Greenwood. "Some women wake up from night sweats or because they have to urinate. Then, they can't fall back asleep again." If this scenario sounds familiar, follow these tips:

● **Have a light dinner.** "Then, have a bedtime snack of carbohydrates with milk, such as a bowl of cereal with milk and sliced bananas, or yogurt," says Dr. Greenwood. "These foods have an abundance of the amino acid tryptophan, which will help you fall back to sleep. If when you wake up and can't go back to sleep, get up and have the snack then."

● **Watch that booze.** It can disrupt your sleep. Avoid alcoholic drinks two hours before bedtime.

Foods to Limit

Along with all the wonderful and healthy foods that you can add to your diet to help with menopausal symptoms, there are also a few foods you might want to cut back on.

● **Hot, spicy foods.** If you're prone to hot flashes, cut back on hot, spicy foods and hot beverages because they can trigger them. Keep a log: What were you eating or drinking just prior to a hot flash?

● **Caffeine.** Caffeinated foods and beverages such as coffee, black tea, soft drinks (especially cola), and chocolate are stimulants. Also check the label of any over-the-counter medications you take—some contain caffeine.

"Caffeine belongs to a class of chemicals called methylxanthines, which stimulate the central nervous system," explains Dr. Lark. "Many menopausal women reach for these products to combat fatigue. However, high levels of caffeine in the diet have been associated with anxiety, irritability, and mood swings."

Caffeine also acts as a diuretic, leeching not only excess water, but also important nutrients out of the body. These include potassium, zinc, magnesium, vitamin B, and vitamin C. Coffee also reduces the absorption of iron and calcium from food and supplements.

And in one study, researchers found that women at risk who drank more than three cups of coffee per day tripled the risk of hip and spinal fractures.

● **Alcohol.** "Excessive amounts of alcohol can intensify almost every type of menopausal symptom, such as osteoporosis, hot flashes, night sweats, insomnia, depression, and mood swings," explains Dr. Lark. "Alcohol acts as a central nervous system depressant."

Researchers have found that women who consumed more than 7 ounces of alcohol per week nearly tripled their risk of hip fracture. In addition, alcohol is a diuretic and can dehydrate the mucous lining of the vagina and bladder. It can also cause the loss of important minerals, such as calcium, magnesium, and zinc.

Dr. Lark recommends drinking alcohol in moderation, if at all. This would mean imbibing no more than 4 ounces of wine, 10 ounces of beer, or 1 ounce of hard liquor in social settings.

● **Salt.** Condiments and food additives, such as table salt and monosodium glutamate (MSG), can be extremely high in sodium. Sodium helps regulate water balance in the cells. Water tends to accumulate where sodium is prevalent.

Too much sodium can lead to water retention, bloating, and high blood pressure. These problems are very common in menopausal women who are at a higher risk for heart disease. In addition, excess sodium can raise your risk of osteoporosis because it speeds up calcium loss from the body.

Check for salt and sodium in frozen and canned foods, cheeses, potato chips, hamburgers, hot dogs, cured meats, and pizzas. Instead of salt for flavoring, use herbs, such as garlic, basil, and oregano.

● **Fat.** The worst kind of dietary fat is found in meat, cheese and other whole-milk dairy products, and saturated fats (the kind that is hard at room temperature). "When used in excess, these fats contribute to heart disease, cancer, obesity, and arthritis," says Dr. Lark. "Menopausal women are particularly at risk for obesity because their metabolism slows down, and they burn calories less efficiently."

According to Dr. Lark, many American women center their main meals around large steaks, chops, and oversize meat and cheese sandwiches.

"Large amounts of meat protein can increase the risk of osteoporosis," she says. "Meat protein is acidic. When a woman eats meat in excessive amounts, her body must buffer that acid load by leaching calcium from bone."

Dr. Lark recommends limiting or avoiding red meats, whole-milk dairy products, and saturated fats and oils. "Emphasize a diet high in whole grains, soy milk, beans, peas, green leafy vegetables, and fish high in omega-3s. These foods are very nutritious, low-fat, high-fiber, and are easy to digest."

healing diet

PROBLEM FOODS	GOOD FOODS
Alcohol	Bananas
Hot, spicy foods	Beans and legumes
Meat and other foods high in fat	Fish
Salt	Flax seed
	Oats and other whole grains
	Skim milk
	Soy products

BEST ADVICE: Eat a diet low in fat and high in whole grains, fruits, and vegetables. And ask your doctor to give you options for dealing with any unpleasant symptoms of menopause.

osteoporosis

Drink your milk! Remember how your parents used to hound you? No doubt they knew that milk helps build strong bones— better than just about any food. And building strong bones when you're young is one of the best ways of preventing osteoporosis later in life.

In Latin, the term osteoporosis literally means "porous bones." And that's a pretty accurate description of this condition. Look through a microscope at a healthy person's bones; they'll appear as a near-solid mass. But look at the magnified bones of someone with advanced osteoporosis, and you'll see something about as porous as a fishnet.

Osteoporosis is a common condition, affecting more than 24 million Americans, according to U.S. government figures. Four out of five of those who have this condition are women. The Duke University Medical Center in Durham, North Carolina, estimates that if you're a woman older than 50, your risk of developing osteoporosis is greater than your combined risk of developing breast, ovarian, or uterine cancer.

Bone Basics

Osteoporosis isn't caused by a virus. And it's not a genetic disease. This is a condition brought on by a variety of factors, many of them having to do with diet. In the years following menopause, women can lose up to a quarter of their bone mass. People born with thin bones also face a heightened risk, for the simple (if unfair) reason that they have less bone mass to begin with. Another major culprit: lack of exercise. When you jog, mow the lawn, or ride a bike, your bones—just like your muscles—literally grow stronger. Spend all your time slumped before a computer or TV, and the opposite happens.

Long-term use of steroid drugs such as prednisone can likewise increase your risk. But people who fail to eat a proper diet face the greatest risk of all, experts say.

Which brings us back to milk. Like other dairy products, milk is rich in calcium, the very stuff that makes up your bones. Calcium, the same mineral found in blackboard chalk, causes bones to be solid and hard. Take away the calcium, and humans would turn into land-roving jellyfish—no bones about it.

Bones constantly need calcium to patch and repair themselves and to replace old dead cells with new ones. Elsewhere in the body, calcium performs other vital tasks: It aids in blood clotting, helps nerves function smoothly, and it assists the heart and every other muscle.

Little wonder calcium is the most common mineral in your body. Fortunately, it's also plentiful in many of the foods we eat. Chalk one up to Mother Nature.

"Calcium's pretty cheap. You ought to be able to get enough of it," says Dr. C. Conrad Johnston Jr., M.D., an osteoporosis researcher at Indiana University School of Medicine in Indianapolis.

Just one glass of whole milk contains roughly 300 milligrams of calcium. Cheese, yogurt, and other dairy products are also calcium-rich. And you find the mineral in vegetables, soy foods, even breads. "The beauty about breads is that you eat quite a few servings of them," says Mona Calvo, Ph.D., a nutritionist with the Food and Drug Administration (FDA), who specializes in osteoporosis. Dr. Calvo starts counting off all the familiar bread group foods that form staples of the American diet—everything from pasta and hamburger rolls to crackers and tortillas. All of these contain some calcium and help boost your daily intake. "It all adds up," she says.

Investing in Precious Minerals

When you eat calcium-rich foods, it's a like putting money in the bank. That's because your bones—besides providing a framework that defines your basic shape and holds you together—function as a kind of calcium bank vault. Say your body needs a little extra calcium to keep your heart muscle running at a brisk clip during your morning walk. Or let's say your muscles have a lot of mending to do after the day you try in-line skating for the first time. No problem. Your bone bank stays open 24 hours a day. And your body can go in there and take whatever extra calcium it needs to get the job done.

Hopefully, any calcium your body withdraws from your bones today will be replaced with calcium contained in the foods you eat tomorrow. But suppose you're a picky eater? Day after day, month after month, you fail to replace the calcium that your body withdraws. That's a lot like draining a savings account. Your body keeps making withdrawals that aren't replaced. Your bones grow weaker and weaker. It's that simple.

Well, it's almost that simple. A couple of other factors come into play as well. As you age, your body grows less and less able to process the calcium you eat. After about age 30, your bones actually lose a tiny percentage (about .03 to .05 percent) of their mass each year.

With women, this bone loss greatly accelerates after they've gone through menopause, around age 50. That's because following menopause women produce far less of the hormone estrogen. And estrogen, when it's present, helps the body channel calcium efficiently to the bones. In males, the hormone testosterone performs a similar function.

In the years during and after menopause, a woman can lose up to 10 percent of the hardened shell portion of her bones (so-called cortical bone) and as much as 25 percent of the softer (trabecular) bone contained inside. After 10 years, bone loss continues at about 1 percent each year. The same rate occurs in men once they've reached their mid-60s.

As you age, you don't feel this bone loss. It takes place silently, painlessly. You may not even know it's happening without a doctor's exam. X-rays, the most common way of detecting osteoporosis, only reveal the disease when bones have deteriorated by up to 30 percent.

Weakened bones break easily, and some people find out that they have osteoporosis only after breaking a bone. Some people who have advanced osteoporosis have bones so weak that the slightest bump causes a break. Unfortunately, this advanced stage, complete with fragile, easily broken bones, happens a lot. According to the FDA, 1.5 million osteoporosis-related fractures occur annually. Complications from these bone fractures can cripple and even lead to death.

As osteoporosis progresses, women in particular can develop what's known as a dowager's hump. That's a curvature of the spine caused when individual vertebrae, weakened by osteoporosis, are literally crushed.

The best strategy for dealing with this crippling disease is prevention. And the good news is that you can do a great deal early on to keep osteoporosis at bay.

Eat Right from the Get-Go

The very best way of fending off osteoporosis is to eat right as a youngster. That brings us back to milk once again. "It's very important that you have an adequate amount of calcium as you're growing," says Dr. Johnston. No surprise, kids with rapidly growing bones need plenty of calcium. But Dr. Johnston goes a step further. He says the more calcium kids take in as they're growing, the better. An extra measure of calcium at this crucial time helps them build extra-strong bones that will offer them a measure of protection later in life.

In the late '80s Dr. Johnston set out to prove his theory with a simple experiment. He looked at identical twins. For each set of twins participating in the study, one twin (the control subject) ate a regular healthy diet. The other twin (the test subject) ate the same healthy diet, but also received a calcium supplement. Dr. Johnson used a supplement so he could precisely measure the amount of calcium his test subjects received. (Although calcium supplements are not harmful, Dr. Johnston recommends that kids get the calcium they need through regular foods, not supplements.)

After three years, Dr. Johnston found that those twins that received the extra calcium had developed a measurably heavier bone structure. They'd taken that extra calcium and stored it in their bones.

Think back to the bone bank analogy: All that calcium stored up within young bones is really a kind of investment for later in life—a time when menopause and plain old age cause bones to lose density. The more calcium deposited in the bone bank early on, the more will be available for withdrawal later.

Building Strong Bones

J ust how much calcium should kids receive? Most experts put the amount between 400 and 1,200 milligrams, depending on age.

A typical kid's diet can easily supply that 1,200 milligrams. How? Cereal with milk for breakfast, some cheese on that sandwich at lunch, a couple of glasses of milk, ice cream, or yogurt at some point during the day and you have it.

Two of the U.S. government's most important health organizations support the 400- to 1,200-milligram recommendation: The FDA and the National Institutes of Health (NIH). But you should be aware that the FDA and the NIH don't always see eye to eye about how much calcium people need. Prime example: recommendations for the 11- to 24-year-old age group. This is a crucial time in terms of bone building. First, kids enter adolescence and typically sprout up by awkward leaps and bounds, their bones growing apace. Then, during their late teens and early adult years, they reach their full height. Young people don't grow as much in their late teens and early twenties, but their bones do continue to harden.

The NIH considers this bone-building-and-hardening period crucial for protecting people from osteoporosis later. After all, you only get one chance to build a skeleton. That's why the NIH recommends that those in the 11-to-24-year-old group receive 1,500 milligrams of calcium per day. This is the exact same dosage the NIH recommends for older folks, who may have already developed osteoporosis.

Take a look at the chart on page 248. The FDA continues to recommend 1,200 milligrams of calcium daily for 11- to 24-year-olds. That puts the two groups just a 300-milligram glass of milk apart.

Whose recommendations should you follow? If you're fighting osteoporosis, or concerned about preventing osteoporosis, you should be aware that powerful groups like the National Osteoporosis Foundation, the Mayo Clinic, and the Duke University Medical Center stand behind the higher NIH estimates. And we'll stick with these same recommendations through the remainder of this section.

The NIH maintains that a calcium intake up to 2,000 milligrams a day is safe. Exceed 2,000 milligrams per day, however, and over the long haul you may risk such things as painful calcium deposits and kidney stones. These occur when your system stores more calcium than it can use.

Hooked on Pop

R ather than being concerned about getting too much calcium, say Drs. Johnston and Calvo, the majority of us need to be far more concerned about getting enough. This is a special concern when it comes to children. The Duke University Medical Center estimates that one-third of children younger than age five only receive about 75 percent of the recommended daily calcium they need. That tendency to get too little calcium continues as kids age, explains Dr. Calvo.

your calcium requirement
how much is enough?

The Federal Food and Drug Administration (FDA) and the National Institutes of Health (NIH) disagree on how much calcium a person needs during various stages of his or her life. Many groups, such as the National Osteoporosis Foundation and the Mayo Clinic, support the NIH guidelines, insisting the FDA's recommendations are too low, especially for people with a high risk of developing osteoporosis, such as postmenopausal women and men and women age 65 and older. The FDA, by the way, is the government group that determines the Recommended Dietary Allowance (RDA) for each vitamin and mineral. This chart shows at a glance what the RDA for each nutrient is, along with the NIH recommendation, which tends to be somewhat higher.

Age	RDA Milligrams Daily	NIH Recommendation Milligrams Daily
Birth to 6 months	400	400
6 to 12 months	600	600
1 to 5 years	800	800
6 to 10 years	1,200	800 to 1,200
11 to 21 years	1,200	1,200 to 1,500
Women, 25 to 50	800	1,000
Men, 25 to 65	800	1,000
Women, pregnant or lactating	1,200	1,200 to 1,500
Postmenopausal women on estrogen replacement therapy	800	1,000
Postmenopausal women not on estrogen replacement therapy	800	1,500
Men and women over 65	800	1,500

Source: The NIH Consensus Development Conference on Optimal Calcium Intake

Poor family eating habits take part of the blame, she says. And sometimes children go through phases of just not wanting to eat right. When it comes to milk, kids can really put up a lot of resistance. "There are a lot of kids who don't like the taste and texture," says Dr. Calvo.

Don't make the mistake of putting all the blame on the kids, Dr. Calvo insists. Milk, she explains, has a powerful rival for their affections—one that's part of the very backbone of kid culture: soft drinks. Include in this category all the diet and sweetened colas, the fruit-flavored drinks, trendy iced teas, and flavored waters. "They're all pretty void of nutrients," says Dr. Calvo.

And they're everywhere. There's no escaping the message. Sometimes it seems like soft drinks all pour out directly out of TV sets. Company logos appear on everything from kids' lunch boxes to T-shirts. Taken together, this advertising has a powerful effect, says Dr. Calvo. "You rarely see people order milk in a restaurant today," she notes. Instead, they order soft drinks. "Kids ought to be consuming something that's delivering nutrients," she says.

Overcoming the soft drink media blitz may be tough. "People would think it would be easier to change behavior than genetics, but having raised teenagers I'm not sure," says Dr. Johnston.

But, says Dr. Calvo, even kids who won't drink their milk can still get the calcium they need—and from foods young people like.

"Go to the freezer section of your grocery store," she advises. "Freezer pancakes and waffles can have 15 percent of the recommended daily intake for calcium. And it's rare that you get a kid that doesn't like cheese." And cheese, after all, figures into just about every kid-favorite dish: tacos, cheeseburgers, and, of course, pizza. Just one slice of pizza has 220 milligrams of calcium.

Diet Now, Pay Later

Alas, cheese, like other dairy products, has a well-known problem: fat content. A single slice of American cheese with a whopping

123 milligrams of calcium also contains a whopping 7 grams of fat. Eight ounces of ice cream, which contains 200 milligrams of calcium, also contains 14 grams of fat. There's no getting around it. That's a lot of fat.

This high fat content of all those delicious dairy foods is not exactly welcome news to people watching their weight. And who fears fat more than appearance-conscious teenage girls? asks Dr. Johnston. "When my daughter became a teenager, she went from milk to Diet Coke," he laments.

The danger, according to Dr. Johnston, is that females by age 16 or 17 have already gained their maximum bone growth. They've stopped laying in new bone. And if they cut back on calcium in their teen years, girls can actually begin losing bone mass.

That loss of bone mass can occur with amazing speed when teens—or anyone for that matter—go on crash diets. One 1997 study followed a group of women who crash-dieted on less than 1,000 calories per day. The researchers measured the women's bone density before and after the study. Within less than six months, researchers found that some of the women's bones had already declined by "significant amounts."

Skimming the Dairy Case

The key, say Drs. Calvo and Johnston, is convincing teens—or anyone concerned about their weight—to try out low-fat or nonfat dairy products. An 8-ounce serving of low-fat ice cream, for instance, contains just under 7 fat grams. That's half the fat of regular ice cream, yet

as good as milk

When it comes to calcium-rich foods, you just can't beat a good, tall glass of milk. Or can you? For a variety of reasons, not all kids (or adults for that matter) enjoy whole milk. Fortunately, there are plenty of alternatives. Here are several foods with calcium content equal to an 8-ounce glass of whole milk:

    1   cup 2 percent fat milk
    1   cup 2 percent fat chocolate milk
    8   ounces plain nonfat yogurt
    8   ounces plain low-fat yogurt
    8   ounces low-fat fruited yogurt
    8   ounces low-fat vanilla yogurt
  1½   ounces natural cheese
    2   ounces process American cheese

it still has more than 200 milligrams of calcium. A ½-cup serving of part skim mozzarella cheese, enough to top off half a pizza, holds a whopping 413 milligrams of calcium. But it has just 10 fat grams and 158 calories.

Here are some other low-fat tips for getting more calcium into your kids (and yourself):

🍎 **Pack in the powder.** To really boost calcium content, make powdered milk a staple in your kitchen, Dr. Calvo advises. Glass per glass, powdered milk nets you roughly half the 300 milligrams of calcium you receive from whole milk. But 150 milligrams of calcium is still worth going after, and you can use powdered milk to give you an extra calcium boost. Powdered milk works great as a thickener in soups, sauces, casseroles, meat loaf—any recipe that requires milk.

Here's how: When soup can directions call for 8 ounces of whole milk, use skim milk instead. (It contains the same amount of calcium as whole milk.) Then, stir in a tablespoon or two of powdered milk. "I add it all the time and don't tell people," Dr. Calvo admits. The powdered milk not only boosts the calcium content, it adds richness and flavor.

🍎 **Reach for the yogurt.** Yogurt's another great low-fat calcium source, says Dr. Calvo. Eight ounces of nonfat plain yogurt contains about 300 milligrams of calcium—again, the same as whole milk. But the yogurt weighs in at just 100 calories.

Add yogurt containers to your kids' lunch meals. (Be aware that if you're using the sweetened, fruit-flavored varieties, the calcium is still there, but the calories go up.) Use plain yogurt instead of mayonnaise in salad dressings and snack dips. Substitute yogurt for sour cream in Mexican dishes such as fajitas, and top off desserts like fruit, Jell-O, or pudding treats with your favorite flavored yogurts.

🍎 **Test your tolerances.** What if you don't do dairy? People who are lactose intolerant have trouble digesting the sugars contained in dairy products. They experience bloating after consuming dairy products that are high in lactose. Although more common in adults, this condition isn't limited to adults. "More kids have difficulty digesting milk than we realize," says Dr. Calvo.

Happily, people with lactose intolerance can still get plentiful portions of calcium. In some cases they can help their digestive system get used to dairy products. (For more information about dealing with this condition, see page 225). And some dairy products such as hard, aged cheeses have a lower amount of lactose (milk sugar) and may be tolerated by people who experience minor symptoms.

If you or your kids have this problem, try low-lactose and acidophilus milk and yogurt products and see if those are more easily digested.

Get some help from the drug store. If you have lactose intolerance, you might want to try Lactaid or other over-the-counter remedies available in drug stores. These are taken when you eat dairy products and can help you digest lactose and eliminate those unpleasant symptoms.

Know your best calcium sources. Even with the best of intentions, not everyone can eat dairy products. And not everyone likes them. The good news is that dairy products are not the only source of calcium. You can also get a good supply of calcium from bread and other calcium-enriched grain products; any fish with the bones left in (think canned sardines and salmon); broccoli, kale, bok choy, and other greens; seeds and nuts; and legumes (peas and beans). And don't forget that calcium-fortified orange juice that often sits close to milk in the dairy case.

Pay special attention if you're a vegetarian. Vegetarianism has become quite the trend—especially among teenage girls. Some vegetarians eat dairy products, and generally such a diet contains plenty of calcium, according to the FDA. But what about that strict group of vegan vegetarians who choose to omit all animal-based foods from their diets, including dairy? At least one study done in 1997 found that this strict dietary practice increases the risk of osteoporosis. Researchers from Taiwan looked at 258 Buddhist nuns who'd shunned meat for years. As a whole, the group showed abnormal bone loss in the neck and spine areas. The study's researchers recommended that vegan vegetarians take calcium supplements.

Learn to love tofu. One well-known meat substitute, tofu, is especially high in calcium. A chunk of this soy-based food about the size of a small steak contains 100 milligrams of calcium. Tofu makes a tasty addition to soups, salads, and rice dishes. Besides tofu, there are numerous other soy-based high-calcium products—from soy milk to soy cheeses.

The calcium in tofu and other soybean products comes in a form that appears to be easily absorbed and retained by the body. There's even evidence that certain compounds in soybeans may actually strengthen your bones. Researchers call these compounds isoflavones. One such isoflavone, daidzein, for example, is a close cousin to a drug widely used in Asia and Europe to treat osteoporosis. Another isoflavone, genistein, was found in one 1996 study to help inhibit the breakdown of bone in laboratory animals. The study found that after just one month, the animals that had been deprived of estrogen were still able to build up their back and thigh bones when fed a steady diet of soy foods.

Calcium for Adults

It's clear that children need their calcium in order to build strong bones. But what about adults? If your teenage years are a distant memory, is it too late for you to worry about getting enough calcium to keep your bones strong? The answer can be given in one word—no.

No matter what kind of skeleton you constructed as a youth, whether you're male or female, and no matter what kind of bones you're carrying around inside you now, your muscles still need a certain amount of calcium to do their thing. And if they don't have enough, they withdraw it from your bone bank. And if you can keep those withdrawals to a minimum, you can help protect your precious savings.

Whether you get your calcium from milk or soybeans, the need for this mineral is constant and ongoing. And women need more than men. Women who are pregnant need extra calcium for their babies. So do women who are breast-feeding. That's why the NIH maintains that women who are pregnant or who are breast-feeding need 1,500 milligrams of calcium daily. When

breast-feeding stops, the NIH lowers the amount to 1,000 milligrams.

The NIH returns to its 1,500-milligram per-day recommendation for women during the years following menopause. That's the time, you'll recall, when bone loss greatly accelerates.

Later in Life

The NIH maintains that both men and women age 65 and older need 1,500 milligrams of calcium per day. This is a reasonable amount of calcium—nothing a standard American diet can't supply. Problem is, older folks, like teenagers, don't always eat as they should. And lack of exercise or illness can cause loss of appetite.

For this reason, doctors sometimes recommend that people with poor eating habits take supplements in order to get the calcium they need. Calcium supplements come in many forms, and they're available over the counter in the vitamin section of food and drug stores. One of the cheapest, plain old Tums antacid, contains 200 milligrams of calcium or more per tablet.

If you suspect you're not getting enough calcium, it's a good idea to check with your doctor about whether you should take a calcium supplement and to get some advice on type and dosage. The amount of calcium in a supplement is clearly labeled on the bottle. Sometimes supplements such as antacids list calcium carbonate as the main ingredient. Calcium carbonate is made up of 40 percent elemental or pure calcium. So 750 milligrams of calcium carbonate will equal 300 milligrams of elemental calcium.

hope for a cure

Calcium supplements can actually slow bone loss, according to research published in the *New England Journal of Medicine*. That's good news, of course. But what if your skeleton has already deteriorated?

Some doctor-prescribed therapies take the next important step and can actually increase bone mass. Although prescription drugs are obviously not food, there is an important dietary component to this therapy that we'll get to in a minute.

Estrogen (hormone replacement therapy) is the most common medication that doctors prescribe for osteoporosis. Many women opt to take this hormone in the years during and after menopause to replace the estrogen their bodies no longer produce. Estrogen relieves some of the unwanted symptoms of menopause, such as mood swings and hot flashes. Researchers have determined that it also helps prevent bone loss, the same way a woman's own estrogen does. (There are a lot of pros and cons to hormone replacement therapy, so you should discuss it with your doctor to see if it is appropriate for you.)

Another drug, alendronate, may show even more promise than estrogen. After a three-year study, a group of women taking the drug experienced an increase of more than 8 percent in the density of their bones. By contrast, a similar group of women, who did not take the drug, showed a decrease in bone density. The group that took the drug also experienced half as many bone fractures.

A number of other drugs—calcitonin, residronate, and tiludronate—also show promise in reversing bone loss. Even flouride, the stuff found in toothpaste, has built up people's bones in studies. The jury is still out on which drug is best, and again, if you're a candidate for bone-protecting drugs, you'll want to discuss your options with your doctor.

Significantly, though, all these osteoporosis drugs work in tandem with calcium. They're not substitutes for the calcium that you get from foods (or supplements). The test group in the alendronate study, for example, also took 500 milligrams of calcium supplements each day. In one way or another the drugs all help bones hold onto the calcium they already contain and better absorb calcium from foods.

The bottom line here is that, even if you're taking hormone replacement therapy or some other drug to protect your bones, you still need to get adequate amounts of dietary calcium.

The Duke University Medical Center recommends taking supplements with meals or at some other regular time that's easy to remember. If you're taking 600 milligrams per day, it's better to divide the dosage in two, the group says. That is, take 300 milligrams with breakfast and the same amount with lunch.

Calcium's Natural Helpers

Like osteoporosis-fighting prescription drugs, certain common vitamins and minerals also help your body retain calcium from the foods you eat. Among them: magnesium, vitamin K, zinc, strontium, vitamin B6, vitamin C, silicon, copper, and boron.

In truth, you need only very small amounts of these vitamins and minerals in order for calcium to do its job. And all of these nutrients are provided in a normal balanced diet.

One vitamin, however, plays an especially important role in assisting calcium: vitamin D. Working in the small intestine, vitamin D absorbs calcium from the foods you eat so that it can pass that calcium on to your body. Without vitamin D, your body wouldn't be able to pick up any calcium at all. Few vitamins are more pleasant to take than vitamin D. To satisfy the daily requirement of 400 international units, just stand in the sun for 10 or 15 minutes a day.

Barring that, there are any number of foods that can help you get your minimum RDA. You'll find vitamin D in butter and eggs and in so-called fatty fish like herring, mackerel, and salmon. Most milk these days is fortified with vitamin D, as are most breakfast cereals.

Watch Those Calcium Robbers

Although some vitamins and minerals help calcium do its job, some foods and common substances can rob your system of this important mineral. Alcohol and nicotine both inhibit bone building, for instance. And too much salt can force your body to excrete calcium in urine.

In the past caffeine has been singled out as an osteoporosis risk factor. More recent studies have concluded that moderate amounts of caffeine present no risk. One study, for example, found that college-age women who drank one cup of coffee daily still had normal rates of bone growth. Another study tested women age 55 to 70 and found they experienced bone loss normal for their age, even after drinking three to four cups of coffee per day.

So, the latest word is that caffeine poses a problem only if you're a major league coffee addict, notes Dr. Johnston.

Dr. Calvo's advice to anyone concerned about caffeine and osteoporosis: Drink your coffee with milk.

In short, it's not the number of cups of coffee you have today or tomorrow that's important. Nor the meal you skip tomorrow or the alcohol you drank New Year's Eve.

What is important is the calcium you get on average, day after day, year after year.

Eating to fend off osteoporosis is a "lifelong adventure," explains Dr. Calvo. "So drink your milk, eat your yogurt, and have a piece of cheese."

healing diet

PROBLEM FOODS	GOOD FOODS
Salty foods	Breads
Alcoholic beverages	Foods fortified with vitamin D and calcium
	Milk and other dairy products
	Tofu and other soy products

BEST ADVICE: Make calcium-rich foods a part of your daily diet. If you smoke, quit.

256

overweight

Americans spend more than $30 billion every year to lose weight—make that to try to lose weight. But we just keep on getting fatter.

Some 32 million women and 26 million men are overweight—33.4 percent today compared to 25 percent two decades ago—according to the latest National Health and Nutrition Examination Survey. Obesity is also weighing more heavily on our children. One in every five kids is overweight, a 42 percent increase since 1980.

Fewer and fewer of us are looking good in a slinky bathing suit, but that's not the scary part, experts say. Former U.S. Surgeon General C. Everett Koop, M.D. , founder of Shape Up America!, notes: "After smoking, which causes an estimated 400,000 deaths annually, weight-related conditions are the second leading cause of death in the U.S., resulting in about 300,000 preventable deaths each year."

Countless research studies have established a link between a fatter body and a shorter life due to heart disease, stroke, cancer, diabetes, and other degenerative diseases. Unhealthy weight is also associated with disabling conditions like osteoarthritis and gout.

Why We're Gaining Weight

Our bodies are cleverly designed to store excess energy in the form of adipose tissues, or fat cells, to meet our ongoing energy needs without having to eat every couple of hours. "The accumulation of adiposities is due to an imbalance between energy intake and energy expenditure," explains obesity expert Ian Yip, M.D., associate professor of medicine and director of nutritional endocrinology at the UCLA Center for Human Nutrition. In other words, we're eating too much and moving around too little.

We each have 30 to 40 billion fat cells, collapsible thin-walled storage tanks that can swell to more than 10 times their original size. The more excess food we eat, the more our fat cells swell. This system was useful for ensuring survival in times when food was scarce; our bodies drew emergency energy from stored fat.

Nowadays, however, for most of us food is more than plentiful, including a plethora of high-calorie fast foods. Americans are eating 100 to 300 more calories a day than we were in the late 1970s, according to the Center for Science in the Public Interest.

What's more, says Dr. Yip, "the past 20 or 30 years have brought us more cars, computers, elevators, remote controls—you name it. Fewer of us have jobs that are physically demanding, and more than half of us report leading a couch potato lifestyle in our leisure time."

Other Factors Affecting Weight Gain

Why do some people seem to gain weight just by looking at a piece of pie while others can eat pie à la mode without gaining an ounce? Here's why:

Gender. Men have higher metabolisms and so burn more calories than women. Women are further challenged by pregnancy weight gain: Too much weight gained can be very hard to take off, studies show, but nursing one's baby helps. And women's metabolisms slow down during menopause.

Age. The older we are, the slower our metabolism, especially as we become more sedentary. Also, we don't respond as well to high-calorie meals, says nutrition expert Mary P. Clarke, Ph.D., R.D., professor of foods and nutrition at Kansas State University in Manhattan. "At least one study has shown that as we age, we tend to store calories as fat more easily. Our bodies just aren't as metabolically flexible."

Activity level. A sedentary lifestyle almost inevitably leads to a gradual but significant weight gain. It's a vicious cycle, explains William Evans, Ph.D., director of the Noll Physiological Research Center at Pennsylvania State University in University Park and co-author of *Biomarkers*. Physical inactivity leads to loss of muscle tissue and gain of fat, which lowers one's metabolism since muscle tissue burns more calories than fat. "In general, an inactive person can put on as much as a pound of fat a year after the age of 20," Dr. Evans says.

Heredity. People whose parents are obese are 25 to 35 percent more likely to be so, too, and other patterns seem to exist in families. One study, for instance, showed that identical twins who ate the same amount of extra calories gained the same amount of weight and in the same places in their bodies.

Modern genetic research is examining "fat genes" that may affect everything from appetite to fat storage. For instance, being closely studied is one gene that controls the production of lipoprotein lipase (LPL), an enzyme that helps store calories as fat.

Nonetheless, having "fat genes" doesn't mean you have to be overweight, says Rena White, M.D., director of the National Weight Control Registry, which tracks the success of people who have lost weight and kept it off. "Clearly, there are genetic factors in obesity," Dr. White says. "Over 70 percent of the people in our registry have at least one overweight parent, but they still succeeded in losing weight."

Do You Really Need to Lose?

Before you launch into a weight-loss regimen, consider this: Maybe you really would do well to lose weight— but maybe not. Many people, particularly women who aren't fat but just think they are, experts say, are trying to lose weight when they don't need to. There aren't any health benefits from shedding pounds you don't need to shed. How can you be sure you really need to lose weight?

Weight tables. Most of us gauge our weight by the bathroom scale and by weight tables—those charts showing that persons of a certain height should weigh within certain ranges. If you're more than 25 pounds above your range, you're probably too fat, say experts at the Mayo Clinic. But weight tables don't account for differences in body composition—proportions of muscle, fat, bone, and water.

"Obesity is an excess of body fat, not just body weight," says UCLA's Dr. Yip. "Most football players are overweight according to weight tables, but their weight is muscle, not fat." Along the same lines, Dr. Yip says, "not every 5'3" woman should weigh 115 pounds." Heavier weights with

good muscle tone can be just fine.

Body fat percentage. Checking how much of your weight is fat compared to muscle is a good measure of your weight status, according to the American Dietetic Association. Try this "pinch test" on the back of your upper arm: Using your thumb and forefinger, pinch a fold of skin. If the fold is more than an inch thick, you're probably too fat.

Body mass index (BMI). A calculation of body fat, a BMI of 19 to 25 is a "healthy weight target," according to the American Health Foundation. A BMI outside of this range (including a too-low BMI) makes one more prone to weight-related health problems. To calculate your own BMI:

Convert your pounds to kilograms (1 kilogram=2.2 pounds; so divide your weight in pounds by 2.2)

Convert your height to meters (1 meter=39.37 inches; so divide your height in inches by 39.37)

Calculate your BMI: Your weight in kilograms divided by your height in meters, squared

For example: For a 140-pound (63.6 kilograms), 5'6" (1.68 meters) woman: Her height squared is 1.68 X 1.68 = 2.82. Her BMI is 63.6 ÷ 2.82 = 22.55.

Body fat distribution. Where you store extra body fat is the most useful measure of overweight, some experts say. "Obesity should be defined in terms of waist-to-hip ratio," says obesity expert C. Wayne Callaway, M.D., associate clinical professor of medicine at George Washington University in Washington, D.C.

To calculate your waist-to-hip ratio, divide the number of inches around the most narrow part of your waistline by the measurement at the widest part of your hips. For example, a person with a 27-inch waist and 38-inch hips has a ratio of 0.71. A woman whose ratio is 0.8 or higher, and a man whose ratio is higher than 0.95, is at high risk of weight-related health problems.

Your body shape. Are you apple-shaped or pear-shaped? Research shows that extra fat around your waist resulting in an apple shape puts you at higher risk for heart disease, high blood pressure, stroke, and diabetes. Being pear-shaped however, doesn't appear to add health risk.

Healthy Weight Loss: Getting Started

Most of us can come up with plenty of reasons for losing weight, from fitting into a favorite pair of blue jeans to feeling better. Health reasons, however, should be number one on your list, weight-loss experts agree.

"Research shows that losing even 5 to 10 percent of excess weight can be greatly beneficial to health," says Dr. Clarke. This translates to as little as 7 pounds for a 5'2", 150-pound woman. "Modest weight loss,"

move that body

Adding exercise to lifestyle is the ideal way to manage your weight, says Barbara Moore, Ph.D., president and CEO of Shape Up America! "Physical activity is as critical as a good diet is for managing your weight," she says.

Aerobic exercise is one of the most efficient calorie-burners around. A brisk half-hour walk or swim can burn a hefty 300 calories. Strength-training exercise further aids weight loss by building muscle, metabolically active tissue that burns more calories even while you're sleeping.

An accumulated 30 minutes a day of moderate activity will do just fine.

"Many people think they need sweat running down their brow and to be out of breath in order to get health benefits," says James M. Rippe, M.D., a member of the Shape Up America! scientific advisory committee. "Physical activity shouldn't be a grim experience but a pleasant part of everyday life."

Make it fun. Walk the dog. Play ball with your kids. Learn a new sport.

Dr. Clarke says, "can reduce high blood pressure, lower cholesterol and triglyceride levels linked to heart disease, and return blood glucose levels to normal." (Blood glucose, or sugar, levels are related to diabetes.)

So you've decided that you really do need to lose weight? Here's what experts advise to get started:

🍎 **See your doctor.** If you think you need to lose more than 15 to 20 pounds, have any health problems, take medication on a regular basis, or have a family history of weight-related problems, see your doctor, advises Dr. Callaway. Your physician can help you decide the best approach to weight loss.

🍎 **Set a realistic goal.** "Try to reach a weight where you feel good," advises Dr. Clarke. "This isn't necessarily going to be what you weighed when you were 17, let alone what the emaciated models in fashion magazines look like they weigh."

Setting too-ambitious goals can set you up for frustration, says researcher Gary D. Foster, Ph.D., clinical director of the Weight and Eating Disorders Program at the University of Pennsylvania Medical Center in Philadelphia. Dr. Foster and his colleagues followed 60 overweight women through their weight-loss efforts and found that many of them expected as much as a one-third loss in body weight. Even while the women managed to lose an average of 35 pounds, 47 percent of the women said that they felt disappointed.

"If we keep our goals modest, we are more likely to achieve them," says Barbara Moore, Ph.D., president and CEO of Shape Up America! and former program consultant to Weight Watchers. "This helps us feel good about ourselves as well as providing the health benefits of weight loss."

🍎 **Go for gradual weight loss.** Dropping 1 to 2 pounds a week is ideal, experts agree. "Any more than that is probably temporary water loss or, worse yet, a reduction in muscle tissue," says Ellie Krieger, R.D., a nutritionist in private practice in New York. Weight lost gradually is also more easily kept off.

🍎 **Figure your calorie needs.** Calories are the amount of energy that different foods—protein, carbohydrates, and fat—supply.

To lose weight, you need to eat fewer calories than you burn. For a ballpark estimate of daily calories you need to lose 1 to 2 pounds of weight a week, multiply your current weight by 10. For a more precise calculation taking into account your gender, age, height, weight, and activity level, see a nutritionist or your doctor.

As a rule, women should consume no fewer than 1,200 calories a day to assure sufficient nutrients, and men should get no fewer than 1,400 calories, warns nutritionist Timi Gustafson, R.D., registered dietitian and co-founder of CyberDiet, an Internet nutrition counseling web site. Your doctor may advise going lower for brief, medically supervised amounts of time, but this is not something you should do on your own.

Eat for Good Health

Remember, you're losing weight to improve your health and feel good. So forget diets. From fruit juice fasts to high-protein, low-carbohydrate regimens, most diets are unrealistic, unhealthy, and don't even reward you with long-term weight loss.

A low-calorie diet doesn't supply all the nutrients you need, and it can mess up your metabolism, too, says Gustafson. "Your body is programmed to think you're going through a famine when you eat too few calories," she says. "What happens is your

helping your child lose weight

"The fact that one in every five children in America is overweight is of real concern," says obesity expert C. Wayne Callaway, M.D., associate clinical professor of medicine at George Washington University in Washington, D.C. Overweight in childhood is associated with heart disease, diabetes, and other problems later in life. An excess of fat cells developed as a child can also lead to a lifelong struggle with obesity. Some suggestions from experts:

Don't put your child on a diet. "Kids on a low-calorie diet will stop developing normally," warns Dr. Callaway. "At best, they'll start cheating, but then you've put them into the position of being duplicitous. Kids should be able to eat normally."
Follow the Food Guide Pyramid. A wide variety of nutritious foods is your best bet for retraining your child into healthy, satisfying eating habits.
Be sure your child gets enough calories. Energy demands for growing bodies, especially adolescents, are higher than for adults. Whereas a grown woman

may need 1,400 calories a day, a teenage girl may need 2,000 to 3,000. As long as a child is eating healthy food, calories consumed and calorie needs tend to balance out.
Make it a family affair. Don't single out your child. Healthy meals and snacks are for your whole family.
Encourage physical activity. Leisure time spent in front of a TV set instead of outside playing is one big factor in childhood obesity. Enroll your child in an after-school program. Better yet, get out of the house and play with your kids yourself.

metabolism slows down, which makes it even harder to lose weight."

Repeated dieting can lead to the "yo-yo syndrome," a frustrating pattern of losing weight then regaining it again and again.
🍎 **Follow the Food Guide Pyramid.** Established by the U.S. Department of Agriculture (USDA), the Food Guide Pyramid forms the basis of healthy eating for anyone and everyone, whether you're trying to lose weight or not. Daily guidelines include:

Bread, cereal, rice, and pasta: 6 to 11 servings
Vegetables: 3 to 5 servings
Fruit: 2 to 4 servings
Milk, yogurt, and cheese: 2 to 3 servings
Meat, poultry, fish, dry beans, eggs, and nuts: 2 to 3 servings
Fats, oils, and sweets: use sparingly

One look at this list may leave you wondering if you can really eat all the recommended foods and still lose weight. Absolutely yes, experts say.

"The key to losing weight is to eat from the low end of the serving ranges," says

eating out

Restaurants, especially of the fast-food variety, are notorious for huge portions and calorie-laden offerings. If you're like the typical American, eating out at fast-food restaurants two to three times a week and at regular restaurants a little less than once a week, you've got to make a plan if you're trying to lose weight. Experts advise:

Choose restaurants that let you choose. Instead of a "one-size-fits-all" place, find restaurants that let you make choices regarding everything from cooking methods to portion size.

Order broiled, baked, steamed, or poached items. Foods cooked by these methods are lower in fat.

Switch from burgers to a chicken or fish sandwich. This cuts fat and calories by up to one-third.

Pass on the bread and butter. Save your appetite and your calories for your entrée.

Split an entrée. Eat half a main course and a salad. Share other half with your dining partner or take leftovers home.

Order sauces on the side. Ask for gravy, salad dressing, and sauces on the side, then use them moderately.

At a salad bar, stick to salad. The greens and vegetables at a salad bar are great, but you counteract your calorie-cutting by adding cheese, lunch meats, or rich salad dressings. Stick to a little low-cal dressing or plain oil-and-vinegar.

Don't drink. One 5-ounce glass of wine contains 100 empty calories, and a 12-ounce beer has 150.

Gustafson. This adds up to about 1,600 calories a day, "which will leave you feeling full and satisfied," she says.

Eating a wide variety of foods from the Pyramid makes a healthy diet a long-term habit rather than a lose-weight-quick gimmick.

Watch your portions. What many Americans consider "normal" food portions are way out of whack, nutritionists say. Fast-food meals, from whopping hamburgers to bucket-size drinks, are calorie-laden disasters, says Dr. Clarke. But even low-fat foods can undermine weight loss if you eat too much of them.

"One portion of meat or poultry is 2 to 3 ounces, about the size of the palm of your hand, not the size of a paperback book," Gustafson says. "One portion of rice is a cup, not a heaping plate."

Eat foods that fit your life. A weight-loss program based on imported exotic foods available on Fridays only at a store in the next county might be interesting for awhile but won't last in the long run. Be practical: Consider your customary tastes and day-to-day lifestyle, advises nutritionist Krieger.

Then, perhaps once a week, add variety by trying something new.

"Have your basic shopping list, but once a week try a new item—something in season or something the store has on special," she suggests.

Cut Back on Fat

One of the easiest ways to cut calories is to cut the fat that abounds in everything from margarine to potato chips. Fat is the highest energy food source, providing 9 calories per gram compared to 4 grams for protein and carbohydrates. We require at least 15 percent but no more than 30 percent of calories from fat in our diets to maintain proper health. The average American gets considerably more than that.

Gustafson cites another reason cutting fat is especially effective for weight loss.

"If you eat more carbohydrates than you need, the excess is stored as glycogen in your muscles and liver, making it readily available as energy," she says. "But eat too much fatty food, and it's stored directly as fat cells."

The average American gets more than 80 grams of fat a day. Try these techniques to cut back to no more than 50 to 60 grams of fat for weight loss:

Change your meat, poultry, and fish habits. Eat less meat and more turkey, chicken, and fish. A 3-ounce portion of steak has 195 calories and 11 grams of fat, while skinless chicken has 160 calories and 6 grams of fat, and halibut has 95 calories and 1 gram of fat.

When you do choose meat, buy lean cuts such as loin and round cuts, and trim all visible fat. Broil, roast, bake, barbecue, or microwave meats to let fat drip away during cooking. In recipes such as lasagna or chili, cut meat in half and you won't even notice the difference, says Krieger.

Switch from processed meats like ham, bacon, hot dogs, sausages, bologna, and other luncheon meats to their reduced-fat or fat-free counterparts. Processed meats are the second leading source of fat (after ground beef) in Americans' diets.

Buy low-fat foods of all sorts. Skim milk has half the calories of whole milk and only a trace of fat. Try skim-milk-based cheeses, too. Look for fat-free yogurt and other dairy products. Switch from butter or stick margarine to reduced-fat tub margarine.

Low-fat or nonfat versions of your favorite salad dressings, mayonnaise, and other creamy condiments taste as good as the full-fat versions.

Prepare food low-fat. For cooking, use oil spray instead of bottled oil. And get creative with low-fat substitutes. For instance, prepare tuna salad with yogurt or low-fat cottage cheese and just a touch of mayonnaise. Or try plain fat-free sour cream in cold foods that call for sour cream. Plain low-fat yogurt works well in cooked recipes.

Spice it up. Fatty foods tend to taste good because we're genetically programmed that way as a survival mechanism for energy storage, says UCLA's Dr. Yip. He advises his patients to tantalize their tastebuds without fat by becoming adept with herbs and spices. Instead of deep-frying fish, for example, sprinkle it with lemon and a variety of herbs and broil it.

Fill Up on Fiber

Abundant in plant foods such as fruits, vegetables, and grains, fiber is not only good for you in all kinds of ways, but eating more fiber leaves less room in your stomach for fatty foods.

For good health, we should all eat 20 to 35 grams of fiber daily, but currently Americans average only about 11 grams. Follow the Food Guide Pyramid to include two to four servings of fruit, three to five servings of vegetables, and six to 11 servings of cereals, breads, rice, and pasta.

Add a little each day. Your digestive system could go gassy or get constipated should you suddenly go on a fiber-eating marathon. Instead, build up slowly over a period of weeks, and drink at least 8 to 12 cups of water and other fluids to keep everything running smoothly.

Switch to whole grain and whole wheat products. On the average, a slice of whole wheat bread has 2 to 3 grams of fiber, while white bread has virtually none. Whole grain pasta provides considerably more fiber than white flour pasta.

◖ **Add wheat bran to recipes.** For extra fiber plus better flavor and texture, add wheat bran cereal to muffin, cookie, bread, and casserole recipes.

◖ **Keep fruit and vegetables handy.** Remind yourself to eat two to three servings of fruit daily by keeping fresh fruit out in a bowl in your kitchen or carrying fruit as a snack in your purse or briefcase. Chop vegetables in advance—or buy a prechopped version—and keep them on hand for quick and easy snacks.

◖ **Play around with salads.** There's more to salad than iceberg lettuce. Experiment with a variety of vegetables to add interest and nutrients.

Slow Down on Sugar

Sugary foods are high in calories and often high in fat as well. Eating concentrated sweets can also play havoc with your blood glucose levels. A rapid rise followed by a rapid fall makes you crave even more sugar.

The sugar naturally present in complex carbohydrates such as bread, vegetables, and fruit isn't the problem. It's refined sugar, in foods like cake and candy, that you need to watch out for.

◖ **Cut back gradually.** Sweet tooth though you may have, you can train yourself to live without sugar, says nutritionist Krieger. Have a piece of fruit when the sugar urge strikes, she advises. "You may be uncomfortable at first," she says, "but after awhile, you'll get used to it. Sugary foods will start to taste way too sweet."

◖ **Switch off soft drinks.** The average American consumes 50 calorie-laden gallons of soda every year. Instead of a 12-ounce can of soda, containing 160 calories from 10 teaspoons of sugar, try switching to regular or flavored seltzer or a diet drink. Or try herbal teas.

🍎 **Bake with less sugar.** The sugar in most recipes for baked goods can be reduced by one-third and the cake or other items will still have a fine taste and texture.

Be Smart About a Lot of Little Things

Along with keeping the big picture in mind—calories, fiber, fat— there are a whole lot of smaller actions that taken together can add up over the weeks and months. Here are a number of additional ways to help you shed pounds.

🍎 **Watch those snacks.** Most of us consume about 20 percent of our daily calories in snacks, and that's just fine. Small between-meal snacks are great for boosting energy, and they can keep you from feeling famished when dinnertime finally rolls around. The trick is to eat healthy snacks. Buy snacks that say "low-fat" or "fat-free" on the label.

Check calorie content, too, as some low-fat snacks are high in calories. Good snack choices include rice cakes, fat-free yogurt, precut vegetables with fat-free dips, and air-popped popcorn seasoned with salt.

🍎 **Cut back on alcohol.** Alcohol is dense with non-nutritive calories. Just 5 ounces of wine contain a whopping 100 calories, and a 12-ounce beer has 150 calories. Even worse for weight loss, research shows that the relaxing effects of alcohol make some people more prone to overeating, especially high-calorie, fatty food.

🍎 **Eat smaller, more frequent meals.** Instead of eating two or three large meals a day, eating five or six smaller meals helps

keep body fat off, according to a study done at Tufts University. This encourages your body to convert food more readily into fuel for immediate energy instead of storing it as fat cells.

Make Friends with Your Appetite

Appetite control is a complex thing, says Dr. Clarke, involving both mind and body components. Everything from hormones to your emotional state seems to have an impact. "Many things are involved in helping you decide when it's time to eat and when you've had enough," says Dr. Clarke. "It's even harder for people who have undertaken strenuous dieting. By ignoring their body's signals, they put their systems out of whack." To help sort yourself out:

🍎 **Eat when you're hungry.** Try to pay attention to whether you're actually hungry (whether your stomach is grumbling) when you're about to eat. If so, go ahead and eat. If there's something else going on, address the situation instead of going straight for the comfort food.

🍎 **Eat slowly.** It takes about 20 minutes for your stomach to signal your brain that it's full. "If you're shoveling food into your mouth as fast as you can," says Gustafson, "you will eat beyond the point of satiety and fill up with food you don't even need."

Chew every bite of food thoroughly before you swallow. Put your fork down between bites.

🍎 **Keep a food diary.** A daily record of what and how much you eat, when you eat, what was happening at the time, and how you felt helps keep you wise to what you're eating and why. "A diary helps you become much more conscious of what you're doing and what you need to do to maintain your energy and a healthy weight," says Gustafson. It also clues you in to situations that trigger eating, from stress to boredom. You can then develop strategies for dealing with triggers, such as going for a long walk instead of wolfing down junk food.

Take It Easy on Yourself

As eager as you may be to change your life and shed pounds fast, trying to change everything at once can be overwhelming," says Krieger. "And this can paralyze you into not doing anything." Instead:

🍎 **Make three small changes a week.** "Decide, for instance, 'This week I'll have fruit as a snack instead of the usual chips, I'll switch from whole to 2 percent milk, and I'll eat a salad as a side dish instead of french fries,'" Krieger suggests. By incorporating change slowly, it's more likely to become a long-term habit.

🍎 **Treat yourself to your favorite foods.** There are no "bad" or "forbidden foods," weight-loss experts say. Go ahead and eat a favorite food once in awhile, but balance it out in your overall food plan. "If you really want a burger and fries for lunch with your friends," says Krieger, "go right ahead, but for dinner, stick to a big salad." Just make sure you don't have that kind of lunch every day.

🍎 **Forgive yourself.** If you really blew it, eating a day's worth of calories in an hour, don't give up. It's human nature to fall down once in awhile. Just pick yourself up and get back on track again.

healing diet

PROBLEM FOODS	GOOD FOODS
Alcohol	Foods high in fiber
Fatty foods	Fruits
Meat	Low-fat or skim milk and low-fat
Processed meats	dairy products
Sugary foods	Poultry
Whole milk and dairy products	Vegetables
	Whole grains

BEST ADVICE: Set realistic weight-loss goals: See your doctor if you plan on losing more than a few pounds. Don't lose more than 1 or 2 pounds a week.

parkinson's

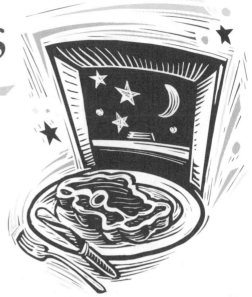

Meg Davis was 39 when she noticed that her left hand had become shaky. When the shakiness spread throughout her left arm, she went to her family doctor who recommended she see a neurologist. The neurologist did all kinds of tests, and everything came back normal. He couldn't diagnose anything. So Meg just dealt with it.

But the problem worsened—through difficulty walking, surgery, tremors so bad that her sleep was affected. It was time to see another neurologist. "I walked into his office, and he said to me, 'You look like you have Parkinson's disease,'" Meg recalls. After 12 years, her condition finally had been correctly diagnosed.

A Parkinson's Primer

Why wasn't Meg diagnosed earlier? Probably because Parkinson's disease doesn't commonly occur in young adults. It tends to target the elderly, usually showing up in persons older than 60. Furthermore, there is no lab test or brain scan that can definitively determine whether or not a person has this disease. It wouldn't have shown up on any of the tests that Meg's first neurologist performed. The best way to get an accurate diagnosis of Parkinson's disease, according to the American Parkinson Foundation, is to see a board-certified neurologist who specializes in movement disorders.

This disorder was named after London physician James Parkinson, who first described it in 1817. It begins when cells in an area of the brain called the substantia nigra (or black spot) start to die. These cells produce dopamine, a brain chemical that helps control muscle activity. At first, the lack of dopamine causes a tremor in one hand. As more cells die, less dopamine is produced, and a general slowness of movement develops on one side of the body. Eventually problems with balance and walking may occur. Other symptoms include foot drag, decreased facial expression, and difficulty with fine-motor tasks such as brushing teeth, buttoning clothes, and writing. Sometimes the effects flare up on the other side of the body.

Doctors don't know what causes Parkinson's and there's no cure, but the disease isn't fatal and can be controlled with medication. The primary drug used to treat Parkinson's is levodopa, or L-dopa (which combined with carbidopa is sold under the brand name Sinemet). Once in the brain, levodopa is converted to dopamine. As dopamine levels rise, the symptoms of

don't forget fiber

Besides affecting movement in your limbs, Parkinson's disease can slow down your bowels, causing constipation. If you're having trouble keeping things moving, make sure you're getting 20 to 35 grams of fiber daily. That should be simple if you're eating lots of fruits and vegetables.

Foods high in fiber include all dried fruits, pearled barley, all beans, lentils, blackberries, pears, raspberries, strawberries, brussels sprouts, broccoli, carrots, spinach, winter squash, and sweet potatoes.

Parkinson's disappear. Dopamine works until protein enters the picture.

The Role of Protein

All chemicals and nutrients must cross what's called the blood-brain barrier to enter the cells of your brain. Levodopa is no exception, and protein can get in its way. When you eat foods high in protein, your digestive system breaks them down into amino acids. Amino acids compete with L-dopa for the pathway that will bring them into the brain, thus slowing their entry, explains Jonathan Pincus, M.D., with the Department of Neurology at the Georgetown University Medical Center in Washington, D.C.

Individuals in the mild to moderate stages of Parkinson's disease, won't be affected, says Dr. Pincus. Their brains still produce and store some dopamine. But the 15 to 20 percent with severe Parkinson's

depend on levodopa to maintain normal muscular activity. And when not enough levodopa gets to the brain, normal muscular activity ceases. These individuals experience what's called an on-off response to the drug. They'll be symptom-free until levodopa is used up by their brain or is prevented from getting there in the first place. Some doctors try to treat this on-off response with drugs, but Dr. Pincus recommends the protein redistribution diet. You simply eat most of your protein in the evening when presumably the loss of mobility will be easier to tolerate. Reduced mobility begins about an hour after a high-protein meal and lasts for two to three hours. If you can't tolerate immobility during the evening, have supper just before bed so that you will be asleep when mobility is lost, says Dr. Pincus. (For information on a protein redistribution diet, see "Healing Diet" on page 269.)

The Value of Vitamin E

Experts have pondered the possibility that antioxidants (vitamins E and C and beta-carotene), which can protect various cells in the body from damage, might also prevent the degeneration of brain cells that causes Parkinson's. There's no evidence to show that taking supplements of any of these antioxidants will prevent or slow down Parkinson's disease, says Dr. Pincus. However, the Rotterdam study—research that examined the dietary habits of 5,342 individuals between the ages of 55 and 95— did suggest that eating foods high in vitamin E may have a protective effect. It can't hurt to include more foods rich in this antioxidant in your diet. Foods high in vitamin E include safflower oil, fortified cereal, wheat germ, soybeans, and cereal.

healing diet

The redistribution diet calls for limiting the amount of protein you eat before dinner to less than 10 grams. Until then you can consume as much as you want of the recommended foods. At dinner, go ahead and eat whatever you want.

PROBLEM FOODS

Stop after one serving of one of these low-protein foods:
Bread, English muffin, or bagel
Cereal (limit serving to provide no more than 2 to 3 grams of protein)
Corn or peas
Pasta
Popcorn
Potatoes, mashed with water, baked, broiled, or french-fried
Rice, white or brown

Avoid the following protein-packed foods until dinner:
All desserts: cake, cookies, pie, candy, ice cream, and frozen yogurt
All meats
All dairy products: milk, cheese, yogurt, and dressings and sauces made with milk or cream
Beans, peas, lentils
Eggs
Most prepared entrées: casseroles, soups, stews, chili, anything made with foods high in protein

GOOD FOODS

Beverages: coffee, tea, soda, fruit and vegetable juices, water
Condiments: oil, vinegar, margarine, butter, herbs, spices, salt, pepper, sugar, honey, jam, and nondairy creamer
Fruits, fresh, dried, or canned
Vegetables, except potatoes, corn, and peas

BEST ADVICE: If you have Parkinson's disease, you must be under the care of a physician. Discuss any dietary changes you wish to make with your doctor.

premenstrual syndrome

Are you confident, clear-headed, and physically fit throughout the month, then suddenly tearful, muddled, and uncoordinated the week before your period? At the same time, are you powerless to resist chocolate or doughnuts? Don't worry, you're not crazy, nor do your problems stem from a willpower shortage. Instead, you, along with up to 90 percent of women, might suffer from premenstrual syndrome (PMS).

The ABCs of PMS

The 10-day to two-week time span prior to the onset of a woman's period is defined as the premenstrual phase, and it is then that problems can develop. Medical researchers have found it difficult to isolate and define PMS, primarily because of its complexity. They've documented up to 150 different symptoms, from headaches, fatigue, forgetfulness, and mood swings to weight gain, breast tenderness, anxiety, and food cravings. A woman with PMS may have any one of the symptoms or a combination of symptoms. And the symptoms may vary in type and intensity each month.

The bit of good news in this murky picture is that the grin-and-bear-it approach to managing PMS that prevailed in the days when PMS was considered all in your head, has been replaced with a take-charge approach that begins with eating right. You'll need to consider both foods to avoid and foods to include in your diet.

Crave Control

Cravings for foods that are both sweet and creamy, such as ice cream, chocolate, and cookies, and for salty carbohydrates, such as potato chips and pretzels, are at an all-time high during PMS. Some women's daily sugar intake, for example, increases to 20 teaspoons or more. One out of every three women reports increased hunger and food cravings during the two weeks before her period and can consume as much as 87 percent more calories during this time.

What could be causing such a varied constellation of symptoms? The culprit could be serotonin, a neurotransmitter found in the brain, according to Judith Wurtman, Ph.D., research scientist in the Department of Brain and Cognitive Science at the Massachusetts Institute of Technology in Cambridge. Insufficient amounts of serotonin contribute to fatigue, mood swings that include anger and depression, poor concentration, spaciness, sleep disturbances, pain intolerance, food cravings, and other PMS-related symptoms.

Carbohydrate-rich foods, such as starches and sweets, are known to raise brain serotonin levels and just might improve mood. When comparing women who experience PMS symptoms with women who do not, Dr. Wurtman found that women with PMS increased their daily food intake by approximately 500 calories. Most of this increase came from carbohydrates. The carbohydrate cravings might have been an effort to self-medicate, since these women reported that they felt less depressed, tense, angry, confused, and sad, and more alert and calm after consuming carbohydrate-rich snacks.

Does this mean that you can turn to cookies, ice cream, potato chips, or other high-fat carbohydrates to solve your mood problems? Not necessarily. "The fat in these foods slows down digestion and interferes with the serotonin effect," says Dr. Wurtman.

👅 **Go for carbs, but avoid fat.** To maximize serotonin levels and help mood, a woman should eat a low-fat, carbohydrate-rich snack, such as honey on an English muffin, air-popped popcorn, or all-fruit jam on toast. And these should be eaten on an empty stomach.

👅 **Kiss chocolate, don't attack it.** Chocolate cravings are a different story. Chocolate is a seductive blend of sugar (which raises serotonin levels), caffeine (a nervous system stimulant), fat (which might alter morphinelike compounds in the brain called endorphins, which produce an immediate pleasure response), and a compound called phenylethylamine, which might stimulate the release of a hormone-like substance called dopamine that also affects mood.

Willpower is an unlikely defense against such a strong force, so a woman's best bet is to work with chocolate cravings. Choose small portions, such as a Hershey's Kiss or a Reese's Peanut Butter Cup, rather than grabbing an entire candy bar or ice cream sundae. And select low-fat (chocolate syrup instead of fudge topping as a dip for fresh fruit) and artificially sweetened options (such as hot cocoa mixes) whenever possible.

Using Food to Balance Hormones

An imbalance in the female hormones—estrogen and progesterone—may also be a contributing factor in PMS. Excess estrogen in the bloodstream may contribute to some PMS symptoms.

One way to lower these hormone levels is with fiber. According to a 1997 study from the American Health Foundation in Valhalla, New York, blood estrogen levels were lower during phases of the menstrual cycle in women who consume high-fiber diets compared to women who ate little fiber. A high-fiber diet enhances the body's ability to excrete excess estrogen and thus might help improve hormonal balance and PMS symptoms.

🍎 **Get more fiber.** Currently, women average only about 10 grams of fiber a day and should increase that to at least 25 grams. Increasing your fiber intake takes determination. To accomplish this feat, consume at least five fresh fruits or vegetables, several whole grains, and a serving of legumes every day.

🍎 **Learn to love soybeans.** Getting more fiber, however, is not the only means of dealing with excess estrogen. Soybeans and soy products contain estrogen-like compounds called phytoestrogens that help offset fluctuations in a woman's natural estrogen. Phytoestrogens act much like the female hormone, binding to the body's estrogen receptors and supplementing the effects of estrogen without the discomfort. But, how much is enough?

Preliminary evidence suggests that as little as 15 ounces of soy milk or 2 ounces of tofu daily might be all a woman needs to help balance her fluctuations in estrogen and curb PMS symptoms.

🍎 **Cut back on saturated fat.** The fats in meat and fatty dairy products help raise blood levels of estrogen. Substituting fillet of sole (or better yet, legumes and tofu) for filet mignon would help cut back on your saturated fat intake and might improve PMS symptoms. (The added benefit of switching to a low-fat diet is that it also lowers a woman's risk for hormone-related cancers, such as breast cancer.)

🍎 **Try safflower oil.** A special type of fat called linoleic acid, found in safflower oil, might help reduce PMS symptoms. Although poorly understood, it seems that linoleic acid might help regulate hormone-like compounds called prostaglandins that cause some of the abdominal bloating and breast discomfort associated with PMS. One or 2 tablespoons of safflower oil in the daily diet would supply enough linoleic acid to meet your body's needs, without jeopardizing your low-fat dietary goals.

Minerals Ease PMS

The vitamin-and-mineral-poor diets of some women might contribute to PMS. What's more, their symptoms often improve when these women switch from highly processed to balanced, nutrient-packed diets.

"Calcium and magnesium show real promise when it comes to preventing some symptoms of PMS," says James Penland, Ph.D., research psychologist with the USDA's Human Nutrition Research Center in Grand Forks, North Dakota.

🍎 **Try getting more calcium.** Women with PMS typically consume calcium-poor diets. In Dr. Penland's studies, increasing calcium intake to 1,600 milligrams (the equivalent of four to five servings of milk or other calcium-rich foods) reduced PMS symptoms, such as mood and concentration problems, pain, and water retention. Increasing calcium and vitamin D to optimal levels also might help lessen migraine headaches associated with PMS.

🍎 **Pay attention to magnesium.** Increasing your intake of magnesium-rich foods (nuts, wheat germ, bananas, and green leafy vegetables) also might reduce the frequency and severity of headaches associated with PMS.

"There is no need to take huge doses of these minerals," says Dr. Penland. "Just increasing dietary intake up to recommended levels often is enough to see an improvement in symptoms."

🍎 **Go for balance.** Dr. Penland and colleagues have investigated the role of other vitamins and minerals in PMS, but the results are inconclusive. In their study, low blood levels of iron, the B vitamins, and zinc were most common in women suffering from depression, mood swings, poor concentration, and breast pain. "These findings indicate that there might be an association between what a woman eats and PMS, especially with the trace mineral iron, but it is still too soon to make recommendations," says Dr. Penland.

However, since many women's diets fall short of optimal when it comes to these nutrients, it's a good idea to make sure that you're getting the recommended amounts of these nutrients in your diet. Iron and zinc are both found in the same foods—including extra-lean meats, oysters, cooked dried beans and peas, and dark green leafy vegetables. The B vitamins are found in minimally processed whole grains, low-fat milk products, beans, and vegetables.

Vitamins to the Rescue

Vitamin B6 is another controversial nutrient. Women who increase their intake of this B vitamin during the premenstrual phase often report that their moods improve and they are less prone to headaches, dizziness, vomiting, edema and bloating, breast discomfort, weight gain, and fatigue. However, medical research has not confirmed the vitamin B6-PMS link. In one study, vitamin B6 supplements (200 milligrams daily) had no effect whatsoever on PMS symptoms. In yet another study, women who took a placebo (a preparation they thought to be vitamin B6) also reported improvements in their PMS symptoms. This implies that the power of suggestion also seems to play a role in some cases of PMS.

If vitamin B6 is effective for some women, it is probably because at pharmacological doses (200 to 800 milligrams daily), the vitamin reduces blood estrogen levels or increases blood levels of the female hormone progesterone. Some researchers speculate that vitamin B6 helps in the manufacture and release of serotonin, which in turn regulates appetite, pain, sleep, and mood.

🍎 **Use caution with vitamin B6.** Even if the vitamin is effective, women should be cautious when self-medicating. Daily doses greater than 200 milligrams (the standard recommendation is 2 milligrams daily) have caused nerve damage in some people, so always consult a physician before taking doses of this vitamin above the RDA. Good food sources are brown rice, whole wheat, soybeans, bananas, beef, eggs, and peanuts.

🍎 **Consider vitamin E.** Vitamin E has shown promise in lessening some PMS symptoms. In some studies, daily doses of 150 to 600 international units (IUs) have reduced breast tenderness, bloating, and weight gain in some women with PMS. However, other studies show no effect, so the link between vitamin E and PMS remains speculative, leaving women in the dark as to whether or not to supplement.

🍎 **Discuss vitamins with your physician.** In general, it's best to get your nutrients from a balanced diet. If you'd like to try vitamin supplements to deal with the symptoms of PMS, it would be a good idea to get your doctor's recommendation about dosages.

Coffee, Wine, and PMS

Women with PMS tend to drink far fewer fluids than other women. But, while increasing fluid intake is important, the wrong kind might actually contribute to the problem. Coffee and other caffeinated beverages are a case in point. Women who consume caffeine-containing beverages, including coffee, tea, and colas, or even caffeine-containing medications, also might be more likely to experience PMS and suffer from mood swings, tiredness, irritability, headache, breast tenderness, and food cravings than are women who avoid caffeine.

🍎 **Ban caffeine.** Women with PMS should consider eliminating all caffeine from their diets to test whether it is contributing to their symptoms. Changes should be evaluated only after several months, since results may not show up immediately.

🍎 **Set limits on alcohol.** Women with PMS are also more likely than other women to drink more alcohol during the premenstrual phase. Although the increased alcohol intake might slightly reduce the pain and discomfort associated with PMS, it also aggravates mood swings and other emotional problems and should be avoided or limited to five drinks or less each week during the premenstrual phase. (One drink is the equivalent of a 6-ounce glass of wine, a 12-ounce can of beer, or one shot of hard liquor.)

A Diet for All Cycles

The only way you will know whether or not you have PMS is to keep a symptoms journal for three months, where you record your daily mood, health, and food intake. Any physical, emotional, or appetite changes during the 10 days prior to the onset of menstruation for at least two of the three months recorded serves as a red flag for PMS. From this information, you can try tailoring your diet to prevent or reduce symptoms.

Of course, diet is not the only factor to consider in dealing with PMS. It helps to avoid stress, which only amplifies PMS

the PMS-proof diet

Let's take a look at how eating to keep PMS at bay would translate into a typical daily diet. Here's a sample menu that incorporates the recommendations made in this section.

Breakfast:
1 cup oatmeal, cooked, topped with
    2 Tbsp. wheat germ
1 cup nonfat milk
1 slice whole wheat toast, topped with
    2 tsp. all-fruit jam
6 ounces orange juice

Midmorning Snack:
1 whole wheat tortilla, with
    1 Tbsp. peanut butter

Lunch:
Turkey sandwich:
    2 ounces turkey breast
    2 slices whole wheat bread
    1 leaf lettuce
    1 tsp. honey mustard or 2 tsp.
       cranberry chutney
1 cup carrot/raisin/apple
1 cup nonfat milk
¼ cantaloupe

Ice water with lemon

Afternoon Snack:
1 whole wheat bagel, topped with
    1 ounce fat-free cheese
1 cup carrot juice
Water

Dinner:
Tofu/vegetable stir-fry:
    1 cup tofu
    1 cup mixed vegetables
    1 to 2 Tbsp. safflower oil
Yogurt

The above diet supplies: 2,000 calories; protein, 20% of calories; carbohydrates, 59% of calories; refined sugar, 0%; fat, 21% of calories (47 grams); fiber, 35 grams; and 100 % or more of the Recommended Dietary Allowances for all vitamins and minerals.

symptoms. Instead, delegate work or treat yourself to a warm bath, a massage, a day off, or a walk in the country on the days when PMS symptoms are raging. Also, women who exercise daily are less prone to PMS symptoms, possibly because exercise helps balance the tidal wave of hormones, increases pleasurable endorphins, curbs hunger, and induces relaxation.

PMS might have come out of the closet, but it hasn't come out of the dark ages. There is still more to be learned about this syndrome before the final word is in on nutritional therapies. Keep in mind that the hormonal shifts and physical changes associated with PMS are part of a woman's natural monthly rhythm, and, therefore, should be viewed more as a time for awareness rather than as a disorder. In fact, in cultures where people honor the female cycle, PMS symptoms often are nonexistent.

However, for many women the monthly discomfort can be improved or remedied by a few simple changes in what they eat. In persistent or severe cases, consult a physician; hormone and/or drug therapy might be indicated.

healing diet

PROBLEM FOODS
Coffee and other beverages and foods
  that contain caffeine
High-fat foods
High-sugar foods

GOOD FOODS
Fiber-rich fruits and vegetables
Low-fat milk
Safflower oil
Yogurt

BEST ADVICE: Eat small, frequent meals and plan a carbohydrate-rich snack for your crave-prone time of the day. Limit your intake of processed sugars and satisfy chocolate cravings with small amounts of low-fat, sugar-free chocolate foods. Limit salt to minimize fluid retention.

Consider taking a well-balanced, moderate-dose vitamin and mineral supplement that contains 100 percent of the RDA for magnesium, iron, zinc, and the B-complex vitamins, and no more than 400 IU of vitamin E. (Some women report that a vitamin B6 supplement—50 to 150 milligrams—taken during the premenstrual phase improves their symptoms.)

Consult a physician if symptoms persist or intensify.

skin problems

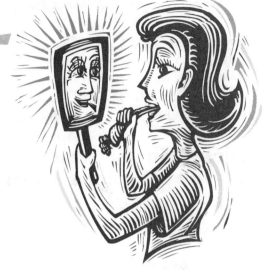

If it's true that beauty is only skin deep, then we're all gorgeous because our skin is very deep indeed. It's as deep as we are, in a sense, connecting with our innermost organs through a complex network of blood vessels, ducts, and glands. In fact, our skin can be a surprisingly accurate indicator of our overall health, as doctors prior to the advent of blood tests and X rays were obliged to learn.

Not only is our skin a highly informative organ, it's our largest, covering approximately 20 square feet and weighing about 7 pounds. It's also one of our more complex organs. It is not simply our body's shrink wrap. Rather, it's a highly intricate six-layered affair laced with millions of blood vessels, nerve fibers, muscle cells, connective tissue, hair follicles, oil and sweat glands, and receptors for sensing heat, cold, and pain.

And with this multitude of structures, not surprisingly, comes a multitude of duties: In addition to protecting us from the billions of microscopic invaders that would love access to our innards every day, our skin cools us with its sweat glands, keeps us warm with its rich vascular network, helps in the production of disease-fighting antibodies, and contributes to the making of vitamin D in conjunction with sunlight for the health of our bones.

What Can Go Wrong

Largely because of this wide range of duties, the skin also is vulnerable to a wide range of disorders, says Harvey Arbesman, M.D., clinical assistant professor in the Departments of Dermatology and Social and Preventive Medicine at the University at Buffalo in New York. The skin can fall prey to infection, inflammation, degeneration, congenital abnormalities, growths, lesions, and, of course, the pimples and blackheads that all too often blemish the adolescent years.

Can these conditions be controlled?

Many of them can, through proper hygiene, protection of the skin from the sun, and, yes, proper diet. "Because the skin and the body are, in fact, so intimately related, what's good nutritionally for the body in general tends to be good for the skin in particular," Dr. Arbesman says. "This means a diet rich in fruits and vegetables, high in fiber, and low in fat."

If that advice is beginning to sound like a broken record, so be it. "It's advice that really can't be stressed enough," Dr. Arbesman says. "So many of our major health problems today could be minimized significantly if we'd all just pay more attention to our diets." That said, let's take a closer look at the benefits of a healthy diet.

Less Cancer (and Maybe Wrinkles, Too)

Within the cells of your skin—and all your body's cells, for that matter—are highly unstable molecules called free radicals, created when cells use oxygen. Their instability is due to a shortage of an electron in their outer shell, a shortage that winds up being bad news for neighboring molecules because free radicals are forever seeking to rebalance themselves with an electron theft. "It's a long and involved molecular story," says Dr. Arbesman, "but what it boils down to is that free radicals can be very damaging to the cells of whatever tissue they populate, be it of the heart, the blood vessels, the lungs, or in this case the skin. The elasticity and hence smoothness of the skin can begin to break down under free-radical damage, age spots can form, and there can be increased risks of cancer."

Fruits and vegetables to the rescue. Most fruits and vegetables are rich in vitamins (C and beta-carotene) known as antioxidants, which research shows can help neutralize free radicals, thus preventing them from doing their harm. Other vitamins and minerals also have been found to blunt the effects of free radicals (vitamin E and the mineral selenium, for example).

Eat those fruits and veggies. Foods rich in antioxidants—potential skin-savers—should be included in your diet, Dr. Arbesman says. "People should try to include at least five servings of fruits and vegetables in their diets a day, especially citrus fruits high in vitamin C, and vegetables such as spinach, broccoli, carrots, kale, and winter squash."

Another advantage to a diet rich in antioxidants is that it may help reduce free radical damage caused by exposure to the sun, Dr. Arbesman adds. This damage includes wrinkles. "This doesn't mean forgoing a good sunblock when outdoors, or not wearing a hat or other protective clothing," says Dr. Arbesman, "but research does suggest that antioxidant vitamins may have a protective effect."

Less Fat for Healthier Skin

While you're stocking up at the produce counter, you might want to rethink your purchases in the meat and dairy aisles, Dr. Arbesman says. "We now have research to suggest that diets high in fat may increase risks for certain types of skin cancer." Why? Again, disorderly conduct from free radicals is suspected of playing a role. "We have evidence suggesting that sunlight may produce free radicals at a greater rate when greater amounts of fat are in the system," Dr. Arbesman says. "The process is called lipid peroxidation, and what it comes down to, really, is oxidation of fats within the body in a manner similar to that which, in the external world, turns fats and oils rancid."

Dr. Arbesman suggests limiting fat intake with that unappetizing scenario in mind.

🍎 **Cut fat.** Steer clear of fatty cuts of beef and pork, eschew the deep-fryer, and opt for dairy products sporting nonfat or low-fat labels. "This doesn't mean trying to avoid fat entirely, however," he says. "In limited amounts, the right kinds of fat—the monounsaturated type in olive oil, for example, and the fat in fish—can actually be quite healthful for the skin."

More Fish for Fewer "Scales"

Research shows that diets rich in fish oils may help minimize some of the flaking and itching caused by psoriasis, a skin disorder in which skin cells get produced approximately every three to four days instead of the normal rate of every 28 to 30. "We suspect the active components in fish oil are its omega-3 fatty acids, which may help reduce the inflammation associated with psoriasis," says Dr. Arbesman.

As encouraging as some of these studies have been, however, the results of others have been less so, Dr. Arbesman says, so it's clear that individual results can vary.

🍎 **Enjoy more fish.** Considering the other healthful benefits of fish for lowering cholesterol and reducing risks of heart attacks and stroke, however, including more

acne and the innocent candy bar

"Eat it today, wear it tomorrow." That's been a warning for kids with acne since the advent of the candy bar. But is it valid?

In most cases, no. "If you were to eat a greasy food with such abandon that you got some of it on your face, that might cause an adverse reaction by clogging the skin's pores, but otherwise there's no good research to show a connection between foods that are consumed and acne breakouts," says Douglas Kress, M.D., assistant professor of dermatology at the University of Pittsburgh School of Medicine.

A dietary connection does exist, however, with rosacea—a condition sometimes referred to as adult acne (although the conditions are not related) in which blood vessels become dilated in the area of the nose and cheeks. Blemishes resembling pimples can, in fact, appear. "Spicy foods, caffeine, and alcohol can exacerbate this condition in some people," Dr. Kress says.

fish in the diet can be a wise move to make, most nutritionists agree. Fish highest in omega-3 fatty acids are cold-water varieties such as salmon, mackerel, bluefin tuna, swordfish, herring, anchovies, sardines, and trout. Flaxseed oil is yet another good omega-3 source.

E Stands for Enforcer

As a final safeguard for the skin, some people may want to consider paying more attention to their intake of vitamin E, Dr. Arbesman says.

In addition to helping make other antioxidants more effective in neutralizing free radicals—and hence possibly helping to reduce risks of such degenerative illnesses as heart disease, cataracts, arthritis, and cancer—vitamin E has shown in laboratory studies that it can do an impressive job of arresting these molecular misfits even by itself.

Because most good sources of vitamin E (vegetable oils and nuts) tend also to be high in fat, however, upping your intake with the addition of a daily supplement can be a good idea, Dr. Arbesman says. (One good low-fat source of vitamin E is wheat germ, which supplies 39 percent of the RDA for vitamin E in just a ¼-cup, 110-calorie serving.)

The natural form of vitamin E, d-alpha tocopherol, taken in doses of between 100 and 400 international units a day, is what Dr. Arbesman recommends. Because vitamin E can thin the blood, however, supplementation may be dangerous for people already taking blood-thinning medications. Before taking supplemental vitamin E, people should always check first with their doctors, he says.

Diet and Eczema

People with eczema (clinically known as atopic dermatitis) should be glad to hear that diet, sometimes, can play a role in this agony of itches. "More and more, research is finding that outbreaks seem to be associated with the ingestion of certain foods in some people," Dr. Arbesman says. Foremost among these are milk and milk products, eggs, peanuts, wheat, and some varieties of fish and nuts, Dr. Arbesman says.

Research also suggests that the earlier in life one first experiences eczema, the greater the likelihood that food allergies play a role. If you experience outbreaks of eczema that seem to be connected with a particular food, discuss it with your doctor.

healing diet

PROBLEM FOODS	GOOD FOODS
Meat	Broccoli
Whole milk and dairy products	Carrots
	Citrus fruits
	Fish
	Kale
	Olive oil
	Spinach
	Wheat germ
	Winter squash

BEST ADVICE: Eat a varied diet rich in fruits and vegetables and low in fat.

stress

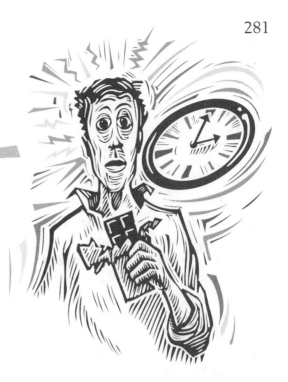

Does your typical day sound something like this? Your alarm goes off, and you push the snooze button a few times before jumping into the shower. You skip breakfast because you're already running late for a meeting, then you get stuck in a major traffic jam and miss the first 20 minutes of the meeting anyway.

At the end of your hectic day, you race from the office to the grocery store, then home to throw together a quick dinner and eat before collapsing into bed in exhaustion. You spend your weekends doing laundry, chores, and bills. You don't have much time for family or friends. Heck, you don't even have time to do something for yourself.

People all over America are struggling with endless demands on their time. They are stressed out. In this hectic, get-it-done-yesterday society, many people are stretched to the limit. Whether you realize it or not, the breakfast you didn't have this morning and the unhealthy dinner you threw together this evening contribute to your stress. Before we examine the relationship between stress and food, let's look at some facts about stress.

Stress, Close Up

Stress can come from anywhere—anger or frustration, an illness, the mere thought of April 15, deadlines at work, a big date, a new home, the birth of a child, shopping, the headlines in your newspaper. The stress of handling it all can make you anxious, cranky, and tired. Stress is exhausting. It also can make you sick. The less serious conditions that are stress-related are fatigue, headache, heartburn, indigestion, insomnia, and even hair loss.

But stress also undermines the immune system and can increase susceptibility to infections, heart disease, and cancer. Stress affects everything you do. According to Georgia Witkin, Ph.D., author of *The Truth About Women: Fighting the 14 Devastating Myths That Hold Women Back*, some behaviors that appear to be caused by low self-worth—overeating, not exercising, neglecting our own needs—are really caused by having too little time and too much stress.

In and of itself, stress is neither negative nor positive. It is our reaction to stress that affects our physical and emotional health. Although everyone experiences stress, not everyone handles it constructively. For instance, in addition to zapping your energy, stress depletes your time. You are then less likely to make yourself a salad for dinner and more likely to rip open a bag of corn chips while you sit on the couch and watch the evening news. You may think this is relaxing and that you're dealing with the stress of a crazy day, but you're not. You're really adding to your stress by not eating well. The healthier you are, the better you can handle stress. You need to have your body working at maximum capacity to deal with stress.

The bottom line in dealing with stress is to cope, to handle the stress in such a way that it doesn't harm you. Life is one stressful situation after another, and there's no way to remove stress from your life. And you shouldn't want to. It's stress that challenges you and makes you grow. Stress is what keeps us all going.

What should you do about stress? There are dozens of techniques for battling the negative effects of stress—everything from exercise and meditation to taking 15-minute mini-vacations from stress several times a day. The right diet can also help.

Eating Your Way to Stress Relief

A good diet will give you the strength you need and keep your immune system and nervous system in great shape. To understand why good nutritional habits are essential during periods of stress, it's important to recognize how the body responds to stress.

When faced with a huge dose of stress, the body relies on the digestive system. Epinephrine (adrenaline), the stress hormone, is released from the adrenal glands. This hormone travels through the body to increase blood pressure, heart rate, and breathing. Digestion shuts down, fats and sugars are released from stores in the body, and cholesterol levels rise.

The result of these hormonal changes is an aroused and tense state that prepares a person to meet danger. This is known as the fight-or-flight response. This response was needed back when cavemen had to react to physical danger. When the danger was no longer threatening, the body would return to normal.

Today, the body reacts to stress in the same way, but instead of running or fighting, you just get the stressed-out state. And you can stay in a state of tension unless you find ways to release it.

Food can affect stress in many ways. What you eat either can promote or relieve stress. It can also either help or hinder how the body handles the physical stress response. To build up your resistance to stress, try these eating tips:

🍎 **Don't skip meals.** Stress depletes you of energy. Many people really don't eat enough, either because they don't have time, or because they're trying to lose weight. Since food is essential for energy, these practices actually increase stress. When you skip meals, you don't tolerate stress as well because you lack energy.

🍎 **Eat for energy.** The first rule is to be consistent. "Eat at regular times each day, even if you're not hungry," advises Georgia Kostas, nutrition director at the Cooper Clinic in Dallas and author of *The Balancing Act Nutrition and Weight Guide*. "That way you'll head off hunger pangs that are bound to surface later." Kostas recommends spacing meals four to six hours apart and filling in with snacks when necessary.

Eat enough. If you know you have to expend an enormous amount of energy in the morning, say you have to deliver a report to a client, you've got to have a good breakfast. If you don't, you're asking for mood swings and fatigue in the early afternoon. Make your breakfast low in fat, focusing on complex carbohydrates. Some good suggestions are whole-grain cereal with low-fat milk or toast with yogurt or cheese for added protein. A breakfast full of sugar, such as a powdered doughnut or a cheese Danish, may give you a temporary boost but will leave you drained an hour later, just about the time you're ready to begin your presentation.

Do break for lunch. Eating lunch at your desk may sound like a good way to squeeze in some extra work, but it's better for your stress level to get away for a while. Eat separate from where you spend the rest of your stress-filled day. "Let coworkers know you don't want to talk about work or other stressful situations while you eat," says Charles B. Inlander, coauthor of *Stress: 63 Ways to Relieve Tension and Stay Healthy*. "A power lunch is okay once in a while, but don't make it a habit. It only adds to your stress level and interferes with your digestive process." Use your lunch break, even if it's only 30 minutes, to unwind.

Don't overeat. When people are under a great deal of stress, they tend to do things in excess, whether it's eating, drinking, or spending. If you're stressed out at work, you may find yourself stopping for ice cream on the way home. Giving in to the anxiety from stress makes you feel calm and in control. But this euphoria is only temporary.

A few days later there's guilt for the indulgent behavior, and that compounds the original stress. "Overeating and compulsive eating typically affect those who haven't learned to handle stress or how to express anxiety and tension orally," says Inlander. If you tend to overeat when feeling stressed, anticipate periods of high stress in your life and prepare for them. Don't bring snacks into your house. Stock up on fresh fruits, yogurt, rice cakes, and herbal tea.

Beware of lonely pasta. Can spaghetti really calm your nerves? Consuming a pure carbohydrate such as a bagel, a bowl of pasta, or rice with nothing else triggers an increase in the brain chemical serotonin. And serotonin makes you feel relaxed and calm at first. It also can make you feel sleepy and energy-starved later on. If you've ever had a big bowl of pasta at lunch, you are probably quite familiar with the energy cycle that follows. It helps to add some protein to your meal. Smear some cream cheese on your bagel, add some ground turkey to your pasta, or offset a bowl of pasta with a salad and grilled chicken.

Don't give in to sugar cravings. There isn't a person alive who hasn't at some point reached for a chocolate bar in the middle of a stress-packed afternoon. Some people, triggered by an onslaught of continual stress, go on sugar binges. They devour large quantities of sweets—a bag of cookies, a quart of ice cream—at a time. When you're feeling stressed, you're probably drawn to junk foods.

But let's face it. Chocolate and cookies won't make stress go away. Eating sweets may give you an initial boost of energy, but within an hour you're likely to feel even more sluggish, tense, and irritable. Sugary foods are digested quickly, producing a blood-sugar spike followed by an energy valley.

🍎 **Drink lots of fluids.** Dehydration causes fatigue and clouds your thinking. Try to have 2 quarts of fluid each day, either plain water or noncaffeinated beverages such as juice or herbal tea. If you work in an office all day, you should try to drink even more fluids. Dry, overheated, or highly air-conditioned buildings increase the rate at which the body loses water.

🍎 **Don't rely on coffee.** Many people turn to coffee, tea, or caffeinated soda for a quick pick-me-up. You feel more energetic at first, but after the effects wear off, you may feel even more tired and crave another energy boost. Too much caffeine also can make you edgy. Caffeine acts in the body like a shot of epinephrine, increasing the heart rate and blood pressure. In one North Carolina study researchers found higher amounts of the hormones related to stress in the subjects who drank coffee than in those who drank a noncaffeinated substitute (a placebo).

Because caffeine is a diuretic, it causes dehydration, which is fatiguing. Kostas recommends drinking no more than two cups of coffee or other caffeinated beverages per day. To counter the dehydration, drink a glass of water for every cup of coffee, tea, or soda you have.

🍎 **Don't use alcohol to relieve stress.** Many people drink when they're tense and uncomfortable. They reach for a glass of wine or some beer to unwind after a stressful day. Alcohol does give an immediate sense of stress relief, but once the buzz is gone, so is the good mood.

Alcohol also causes disrupted sleep, which makes stress even more likely to return. Alcohol deprives the body of nutrients from other foods. When alcohol is metabolized by the liver, it uses up niacin and thiamin, which means these B vitamins aren't available for other purposes. Alcohol also depletes your energy by dehydrating the body. Since alcohol is a diuretic, which increases the output of urine, it causes the loss of such water-soluble minerals as magnesium, potassium, and zinc. If you do drink, reserve your alcohol consumption for the weekends or special occasions. And for every glass of alcohol, drink a glass of water to prevent dehydration.

healing diet

PROBLEM FOODS	GOOD FOODS
Alcohol	Protein foods
Fatty foods	Whole grains
Sugary foods	

BEST ADVICE: Eat regularly and eat enough. Pay careful attention to eating a good, well-balanced diet when you're under a lot of stress.

urinary tract infection

You get the urge to go to the bathroom—again—even though you just went about an hour ago. And when you go, not much happens, except that it burns like crazy. This is the scenario of a pesky urinary tract infection (UTI), the most common problem that sends women of childbearing age to their physicians. Every year, UTIs account for more than 7 million visits to doctors' offices. Although UTIs do occur in men and children, this condition affects mostly women.

What's a UTI?

In a healthy bladder, urine is free of bacteria. However, bacteria from the rectal area may enter the urethra (the tube that leads from the outside of the body to the bladder) and travel the short distance up into the bladder. Normally, the bladder cleanses itself of bacteria. If for some reason it can't, the bacteria may cause an infection. About 80 to 90 percent of UTIs are caused by *Escherichia coli* (*E. coli*) bacteria, which are normally present in the rectum.

Urinary tract infection is the general term for a variety of conditions, such as cystitis (infection of the bladder) and urethritis (infection of the urethra).

Other conditions such as vaginitis and irritable bladder disorder may produce similar symptoms.

The urinary system is structured in a way that helps ward off infection. The ureters (the two tubes that carry urine from the kidneys to the bladder) and bladder normally prevent urine from backing up toward the kidneys. This ongoing flow of urine from the bladder helps wash bacteria out of the body.

Besides anatomy, immune defenses also prevent infection. And in men, the prostate gland produces secretions that slow bacterial growth. However, despite these safeguards, infections still occur.

A UTI commonly has the following symptoms:
- Frequent and urgent need to urinate
- Painful urination
- Cloudy urine
- Lower back or abdominal pain
- Blood in the urine

If you have these symptoms for more than 24 hours, contact your physician. Left untreated, a UTI can spread to the kidneys, causing a more serious condition called acute pyelonephritis. Symptoms of acute pyelonephritis include fever, chills, nausea, vomiting, difficult and painful urination, groin pain, and midback pain. If you have these symptoms, you should contact your physician immediately.

Who's at Risk?

Women are more than eight times as likely to get a UTI as men, according to the American Medical Women's Association. Part of the problem may be that bacteria have a shorter distance to travel in women than in men. In women, the urethra is about 1½ inches long. Compare this to men, whose urethras are about 8 inches in length. In addition, in women, the urethra is very close to the vagina and anus. This location makes it easier for bacteria to enter the urethra and then work their way up into the bladder.

Many women suffer from frequent UTIs. Nearly 20 percent of women who have a UTI will have another, and 30 percent of those will have yet another. Of the last group, 80 percent have recurrences.

Usually, the latest infection stems from a strain or type of bacteria that is different from the infection before it, indicating a separate infection. (Even when several UTIs in a row are due to *E. coli*, slight differences in the bacteria indicate distinct infections.)

Research funded by the National Institutes of Health (NIH) suggests that one factor behind recurrent UTIs may be the ability of bacteria to attach to cells lining the urinary tract.

The ABCs of UTIs

If you suspect a UTI, see your doctor. The first step he or she will take is to confirm a bacterial infection by reviewing your symptoms and having your urine tested. If a culture shows that there are bacteria in the urine, the doctor will prescribe a course of antibiotics. Be sure to take the entire dose. And if you feel discomfort or pain, be sure to ask about a urinary analgesic.

In the meantime, there are certain foods, vitamins, and beverages you can choose (and lose) in your diet to help ease symptoms.

Make water your best friend. "Drink large amounts of water to wash bacteria out of the urinary tract," advises John F. Bresette, M.D., chief of urology at Columbia Hospital for Women in New York City, and spokesperson for the National Women's Health Resource Center. "Drink eight to 10 glasses of water each day. Water will not contain any ingredients that can irritate the tract. And when your bladder is full, you will get a good contraction, which will empty the bladder completely."

Reach for cranberry juice. In one study, elderly women who drank 10 ounces a day of cranberry juice had less bacteria and white blood cells (which indicate infection) in their urine. "An acid environment in the urinary tract can inhibit bacterial growth," says Dr. Bresette. "Cranberry juice acidifies the urine."

"Cranberry juice contains compounds that prevent bacteria from sticking to the wall of the urinary tract," says Susan Lark, M.D., author of *The Estrogen Decision* and

factors that contribute to UTI

Gender. About 25 percent of women are estimated to have had at least one UTI in their lifetime. Compare this to men, with less than 1 percent (age 30 to 65 years) having had a UTI in their lifetime. An enlarged prostate gland also slows the flow of urine, raising the risk of infection.

Age. The occurrence of UTIs can increase after menopause when vaginal tissues become thinner and drier due to decreasing estrogen levels. This breakdown of vaginal tissues leaves them more delicate and more susceptible to irritation and injury. In men, from 5 to 15 percent of elderly men (more than 65 years old) have UTIs.

Sexual activity. There are bacteria in the vagina that help maintain a healthy environment. The more frequently young women have intercourse, the more likely they are to get UTIs.

Birth control methods. If a diaphragm is not fitted properly, it may put pressure on the bladder and increase the risk of infection. One study also found that spermicides selectively kill harmless bacteria and leave behind those that can irritate the urinary tract.

Lifestyle. If you don't drink enough water, your urine will be concentrated, and you will urinate less often. The longer you hold urine in your bladder, the more time bacteria have to multiply and gain a foothold, causing infection.

Pregnancy. About 4 percent of pregnant women develop a UTI. However, when a UTI does occur, it is more likely to travel to the kidneys. If left untreated, the infection can harm the fetus. Researchers suspect hormonal changes and shifts in the position of the urinary tract during pregnancy make it easier for bacteria to travel up the ureters to the kidneys.

Anatomy. Some women have an anatomical problem that makes them more susceptible to infections. Others are predisposed to UTIs because the cells covering the area of the vagina and urethra are more easily invaded by bacteria.

Genetics. If your mother or sister has UTIs, the chances are greater that you will have them.

Illness or disability. Any abnormality of the urinary tract that obstructs the flow of urine (a kidney stone, for example) sets the stage for an infection. Another common source of infection is catheters or tubes placed in the bladder. A person who cannot void, is unconscious, or is critically ill, often needs a catheter that stays in place for a long time.

In addition, people with diabetes have a higher risk of a UTI because of changes in their immune system. Any disorder that suppresses the immune system raises the risk of a urinary infection.

The Menopause Self-Help Book. She suggests using cranberry juice that is low in sugar. "Use only the tart, natural juice," she advises. "Drink one or two glasses each day. Don't drink more than this because the acidic juice may cause irritation."

lower your risk

Tired of contracting infection after infection? Although there is no proven way to prevent UTIs, following these tips will help keep these unpleasant infections at bay:

Drink up. Drink plenty of liquids to flush bacteria out of your system. Cranberry juice is especially helpful because it can prevent bacteria from gaining a foothold in your urinary tract in the first place.

Time it right. Drink water before and after sex so that you will urinate a good volume with a steady stream afterward. This will help eliminate any bacteria that may have entered.

Try yogurt. Yogurt with live acidophilus cultures (it will say that on the label) may help prevent urinary tract infections in some women, says Susan Lark, M.D.,

author of *The Estrogen Decision* and *The Menopause Self-Help Book*. "The live cultures help create an acid environment, which is healthier for the urinary tract," she says. "Taking supplements of acidophilus can also be helpful."

Opt for vitamin C. "Another easy way to create an environment that's acidic to bacteria is to take vitamin C supplements every day," notes Dr. Lark. "I recommend from 500 to 3,000 milligrams daily." Good sources of vitamin C are orange juice, red bell peppers, papaya, cranberry juice, strawberries, and kiwifruit.

Nix the java. Caffeinated foods and beverages, such as chocolate, coffee, tea, and colas, can irritate the urinary tract. Even some over-the-counter medications may contain caffeine.

Skip the irritants. Other common culprits that might increase discomfort include spicy foods, citrus fruits, tomatoes, and alcohol.

healing diet

PROBLEM FOODS	GOOD FOODS
Alcohol	Citrus fruit and other foods rich in vitamin C
Coffee and other foods containing caffeine	Cranberry juice
Spicy foods	Yogurt containing live cultures

BEST ADVICE: See your doctor for a diagnosis. If you're given antibiotics, make sure you take the whole course. Drink eight to 10 glasses of water a day.

healing recipes

<< There is no love sincerer than the love of food.
—George Bernard Shaw >>

Making a resolution to eat foods that boost good health is easy enough. But, let's face it, the food has to taste good, too. This bonus recipe section showcases ingredients a healthy body needs and also recognizes our love of good food. Sumptuous entrées, side dishes, desserts, breakfast recipes, and more are featured in this mini cookbook section for better health and healing.

beans and legumes

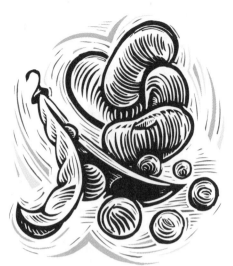

black bean corn salsa

Prep (salsa): 10 minutes **Stand:** 30 minutes
Prep (chips): 10 minutes **Bake:** 10 minutes (per batch)

This piquant good-for-you salsa scores high in flavor with a few stir-together ingredients. The baked chips are perfect partners for the dip. If you don't have time to make your own, look for baked tortilla chips next to regular chips at the supermarket.

½ of a 15-ounce can black beans, rinsed and drained
   (about ¾ cup)
⅔ cup corn relish
¼ cup thinly sliced radishes
1½ teaspoons lime juice
¼ teaspoon ground cumin
1 recipe Baked Tortilla Chips

1. In a bowl stir together the beans, relish, radishes, lime juice, and cumin. Let stand, covered, for 30 minutes.

2. Meanwhile, prepare Baked Tortilla Chips. Serve salsa with chips. Makes 12 appetizer servings.

Baked Tortilla Chips: Lightly spray eight 7-inch corn tortillas with nonstick spray coating. If desired, sprinkle lightly with onion powder. Cut each tortilla into 1-inch-wide strips. Spread strips in a single layer on a baking sheet. (You'll need to bake chips in batches.) Bake in a 350° oven for 10 to 12 minutes or until crisp.

Nutrition facts per serving: 89 calories, 1 g total fat (0 g saturated fat), 0 mg cholesterol, 141 mg sodium, 20 g carbohydrate, 1 g fiber, 2 g protein. Daily values: 0% vitamin A, 1% vitamin C, 0% calcium, 2% iron.

three–bean salad

Prep: 20 minutes **Chill:** 2 hours

1 9-ounce package frozen cut green beans
1 cup frozen whole kernel corn
1 15-ounce can black beans, rinsed and drained
3 medium carrots, chopped
1 8¾-ounce can garbanzo beans, rinsed and drained
1 medium red onion, thinly sliced
½ cup red wine vinegar
3 tablespoons orange juice
1 tablespoon snipped fresh cilantro or parsley
1 clove garlic, minced
¼ teaspoon ground turmeric
8 lettuce leaves

Black beans, garbanzo beans, and orange juice get high marks for immunity-boosting folate. This vinaigrette-dressed salad will appeal to your eye with colorful green beans, carrots, and corn.

1. In a medium covered saucepan cook the green beans and corn in a small amount of boiling water about 5 minutes or until crisp-tender. Drain in a colander. Rinse with cold water and drain again.

2. In a large bowl combine green bean mixture, black beans, carrots, garbanzo beans, and red onion.

3. For dressing, in a screw-top jar combine vinegar, orange juice, cilantro or parsley, garlic, and turmeric. Cover and shake well. Pour dressing over bean mixture; toss to coat. Cover and refrigerate for 2 to 24 hours, stirring occasionally. Serve on lettuce-lined plates. Makes 8 side-dish servings.

Nutrition facts per serving: 101 calories, 1 g total fat (0 g saturated fat), 0 mg cholesterol, 243 mg sodium, 21 g carbohydrate, 5 g fiber, 6 g protein. Daily values: 61% vitamin A, 15% vitamin C, 4% calcium, 11% iron.

garbanzo & barley salad

Prep: 25 minutes **Chill:** 4 hours

Barley and garbanzo beans team up for a great-tasting main-dish salad, perfect for lighter, summertime fare. The simple dressing—mint, lemon juice, and olive oil—adds a fresh, lively flavor, while cashews supply the crunch.

2 cups water
1 cup quick-cooking barley
½ of a 15-ounce can reduced-sodium garbanzo beans, drained and rinsed (about ¾ cup)
¼ cup shredded carrot
2 tablespoons snipped fresh parsley
1 tablespoon snipped fresh mint or 1 teaspoon dried mint, crushed
¼ cup lemon juice
1 tablespoon olive or salad oil
¼ teaspoon salt
¼ teaspoon pepper
¼ cup cashews or toasted sliced almonds
4 kale or lettuce leaves

1. In a medium saucepan bring water to boiling. Stir in barley. Return to boiling; reduce heat. Simmer, covered, for 10 to 12 minutes or until barley is tender. Drain in colander. Rinse with cold water; drain again. Transfer to a large bowl. Stir in garbanzo beans, carrot, parsley, and mint.

2. For dressing, in a screw-top jar combine the lemon juice, oil, salt, and pepper. Cover and shake well. Pour dressing over barley mixture; toss gently to coat. Cover and refrigerate for 4 to 24 hours, stirring once or twice.

3. To serve, stir the cashews or almonds into barley mixture. Spoon mixture onto kale- or lettuce-lined serving plates. Makes 4 main-dish servings.

Nutrition facts per serving: 298 calories, 9 g total fat (1 g saturated fat), 0 mg cholesterol, 250 mg sodium, 48 g carbohydrate, 6 g fiber, 9 g protein. Daily values: 18% vitamin A, 19% vitamin C, 1% calcium, 12% iron.

greek salad

Start to finish: 20 minutes

¼ cup lemon juice
2 tablespoons snipped fresh dill or 2 teaspoons dried dillweed
2 tablespoons olive oil
1½ teaspoons snipped fresh oregano or ½ teaspoon dried oregano, crushed
1 clove garlic, minced
⅛ teaspoon salt
⅛ teaspoon ground red pepper
1 15½-ounce can reduced-sodium red kidney beans, rinsed and drained
1 medium tomato, chopped
¼ cup sliced pitted Greek or ripe olives
6 cups torn romaine or mixed greens
½ of a medium cucumber, halved lengthwise and thinly sliced (about 1 cup)
½ of a small red onion, sliced and separated into rings
¼ cup crumbled feta cheese (1 ounce)

Craving a new type of bean salad for your next cookout? This updated bean salad boasts a Mediterranean flair. Dill, oregano, lemon juice, Greek olives, and feta add pizzazz to kidney bean salad.

1. In a medium bowl whisk together lemon juice, dill, oil, oregano, garlic, salt, and red pepper. Gently stir in kidney beans, tomato, and olives. Set aside.

2. In a large bowl toss together romaine or mixed greens, cucumber, and red onion. Arrange on 4 dinner plates. Top with the bean mixture. Sprinkle with feta cheese. Makes 4 main-dish servings.

Nutrition facts per serving: 246 calories, 12 g total fat (3 g saturated fat), 14 mg cholesterol, 298 mg sodium, 26 g carbohydrate, 8 g fiber, 11 g protein. Daily values: 27% vitamin A, 64% vitamin C, 13% calcium, 23% iron.

caribbean beans & rice

Prep: 15 minutes **Soak:** 1 hour **Cook:** 1 hour and 40 minutes

Bite into this heart-healthy dish for a taste of the Caribbean. The beans are loaded with cholesterol-lowering soluble fiber, while brown rice provides a good dose of magnesium, which helps control blood pressure.

1¼ cups dry red beans or red kidney beans
1 fresh jalapeño pepper
1 14½-ounce can reduced-sodium chicken broth
1 medium green sweet pepper, chopped
1 medium onion, chopped
1 tablespoon jerk seasoning
2 cloves garlic, minced
1¼ cups uncooked regular brown rice
1 8-ounce can pineapple tidbits (juice pack), drained
1 tablespoon snipped fresh cilantro or parsley
1 tablespoon frozen orange juice concentrate
1 14½-ounce can low-sodium stewed tomatoes, undrained

1. Rinse beans. In a large saucepan combine beans and 4 cups water. Bring to boiling; reduce heat. Simmer for 2 minutes. Remove from heat. Let stand, covered, for 1 hour. (Or, place beans and water in pan. Let soak, covered, overnight.)

2. Halve jalapeño pepper (wear plastic gloves). Remove stem, seeds, and membranes; finely chop. Drain and rinse beans. In the same pan combine beans, jalapeño pepper, broth, sweet pepper, onion, jerk seasoning, garlic, and ¾ cup water. Bring to boiling; reduce heat. Simmer, covered, for 1½ to 1¾ hours or until beans are tender.

3. Meanwhile, cook rice according to package directions, except omit any butter or salt. Keep warm. In a small bowl combine pineapple, cilantro or parsley, and juice concentrate; set aside. Stir tomatoes into cooked beans. Bring to boiling; reduce heat. Simmer, uncovered, about 10 minutes or until desired consistency. Spoon bean mixture over rice. Serve with pineapple mixture. Makes 5 main-dish servings.

Nutrition facts per serving: 393 calories, 2 g total fat (0 g saturated fat), 0 mg cholesterol, 387 mg sodium, 79 g carbohydrate, 8 g fiber, 15 g protein. Daily values: 12% vitamin A, 57% vitamin C, 6% calcium, 31% iron.

pinto bean burritos

Prep: 20 minutes **Bake:** 30 minutes

8 8-inch whole-wheat or regular flour tortillas
2 15-ounce cans pinto beans with jalapeño peppers,
   rinsed and drained
1 cup shredded reduced-fat Monterey Jack or cheddar
   cheese (4 ounces)
½ cup sliced green onions
   Nonstick spray coating
½ cup salsa
¼ cup light dairy sour cream
   Snipped fresh cilantro or parsley

These burritos make weeknight cooking a snap. Try flavored flour tortillas, such as spicy red pepper, tomato, or spinach, for an even better—and colorful— burrito. Can't find pinto beans with jalapeño peppers? Substitute regular pinto beans and stir in a finely chopped, seeded small jalapeño.

1. Stack tortillas and wrap tightly in foil. Heat in a 350° oven for 15 minutes to soften.

2. Meanwhile, mash beans slightly with back of a spoon. Place the beans, cheese, and green onions onto tortillas just below center. Fold over edge nearest filling, just until filling is covered. Fold in sides until they meet; roll up.

3. Spray a baking sheet with nonstick coating. Arrange the burritos, seam sides down, on prepared baking sheet. Bake in the 350° oven about 15 minutes or until heated through. Serve the burritos topped with salsa, sour cream, and cilantro or parsley. Makes 8 servings.

Nutrition facts per burrito: 263 calories, 6 g total fat (2 g saturated fat), 11 mg cholesterol, 677 mg sodium, 39 g carbohydrate, 5 g fiber, 14 g protein. Daily values: 6% vitamin A, 9% vitamin C, 15% calcium, 15% iron.

curried lentils & vegetables

Prep: 5 minutes **Cook:** 30 minutes

Hearty lentils can pinch hit for meat, just as beans do, but take much less time to cook than most bean varieties. Often used in East Indian dishes, lentils are a good source of iron.

⅔ cup lentils
1⅓ cups reduced-sodium chicken broth or vegetable broth
2 medium carrots, cut into thin bite-size strips
1 large onion, sliced
1 small zucchini or yellow summer squash, halved
    lengthwise and sliced
1 cup chopped, peeled Jerusalem artichokes or parsnips
1 cup cauliflower or broccoli flowerets
1 cup shredded cabbage
2 tablespoons dry sherry (optional)
2 teaspoons curry powder
1 clove garlic, minced
½ teaspoon salt-free seasoning blend
¼ teaspoon crushed red pepper

1. Rinse the lentils. In a large saucepan combine the lentils and broth. Bring to boiling; reduce heat. Simmer, covered, for 20 minutes.

2. Stir in the carrots, onion, squash, artichokes or parsnips, cauliflower or broccoli, cabbage, sherry (if desired), curry powder, garlic, seasoning blend, and red pepper. Return to boiling; reduce heat. Simmer, uncovered, for 10 to 15 minutes more or until the vegetables are tender. Makes 4 main-dish servings.

Nutrition facts per serving: 214 calories, 1 g total fat (0 g saturated fat), 0 mg cholesterol, 169 mg sodium, 41 g carbohydrate, 5 g fiber, 13 g protein. Daily values: 85% vitamin A, 64% vitamin C, 5% calcium, 38% iron.

north african bean stew

Prep: 15 minutes **Cook:** 25 minutes

4 cloves garlic, minced
1 tablespoon olive oil
2 teaspoons sweet paprika
½ teaspoon ground cumin
¼ teaspoon salt
¼ teaspoon ground allspice
¼ teaspoon ground ginger
1 14½-ounce can reduced-sodium chicken broth or
   vegetable broth
1 14½-ounce can low-sodium tomatoes, undrained and
   cut up
3 medium sweet potatoes, peeled and cubed
1 15-ounce can garbanzo beans, rinsed and drained
1 cup sliced fresh okra or frozen cut okra
1 recipe Turmeric Couscous
   Bottled hot pepper sauce

Sweet potatoes, which complement the various spices called for here, add a subtle sweetness to this hearty meatless stew. Sweet potatoes also burst with beta-carotene, an antioxidant that keeps your immune system healthy, reduces your risk for cancer, and protects against cataracts. They're quite impressive vegetables!

1. In a saucepan cook garlic in hot oil over medium heat for 15 seconds. Stir in paprika, cumin, salt, allspice, and ginger. Cook and stir over low heat for 1 minute. Stir in broth, tomatoes, and ¼ cup water. Stir in sweet potatoes and beans.

2. Bring to boiling; reduce heat. Simmer, covered, for 15 minutes. Stir in okra. Simmer, uncovered, for 10 to 12 minutes more or until vegetables are tender. Spoon over Turmeric Couscous. Serve with hot pepper sauce. Makes 4 main-dish servings.

Turmeric Couscous: In a medium saucepan combine 1 cup water, ¼ cup sliced green onions, and ⅛ teaspoon ground turmeric. Bring to boiling; remove from heat. Stir in ⅔ cup quick-cooking couscous. Let stand, covered, for 5 minutes.

Nutrition facts per serving: 381 calories, 6 g total fat (1 g saturated fat), 0 mg cholesterol, 821 mg sodium, 70 g carbohydrate, 14 g fiber, 13 g protein. Daily values: 209% vitamin A, 85% vitamin C, 11% calcium, 30% iron.

green soybean minestrone

Prep: 20 minutes **Cook:** 35 minutes

If your supermarket doesn't carry frozen green soybeans, look for these nutritional powerhouses at Asian food markets or health food stores. They provide a complete source of protein and serve up generous amounts of isoflavones and plant sterols that help fight heart disease and some types of cancer.

1 14½-ounce can reduced-sodium chicken broth or vegetable broth
1 14½-ounce can low-sodium tomatoes, undrained and cut up
1 cup tomato juice
1 large onion, chopped
1 medium carrot, finely chopped
1 clove garlic, minced
2 cups frozen green soybeans
1 cup frozen cut green beans or baby lima beans
2 ounces dried rotini pasta (about ⅔ cup)
1 medium yellow summer squash, halved lengthwise and sliced ¼ inch thick
1 tablespoon snipped fresh basil
1 teaspoon snipped fresh thyme
   Finely shredded Parmesan cheese (optional)

1. In a large saucepan combine 1 cup water, the broth, tomatoes, tomato juice, onion, carrot, garlic, and ¼ teaspoon pepper. Bring to boiling; reduce heat. Simmer, covered, for 20 minutes.

2. Stir in soybeans (if using), lima beans (if using), and pasta. Return to boiling; reduce heat. Simmer, covered, about 10 minutes more or until vegetables and pasta are nearly tender. Stir in green beans (if using), squash, basil, and thyme. Heat through. If desired, sprinkle each serving with Parmesan cheese. Makes 4 main-dish servings.

Nutrition facts per serving: 260 calories, 7 g total fat (1 g saturated fat), 0 mg cholesterol, 535 mg sodium, 37 g carbohydrate, 3 g fiber, 17 g protein. Daily values: 53% vitamin A, 70% vitamin C, 17% calcium, 29% iron.

soybean pilaf

Prep: 20 minutes **Cook:** 12 minutes

1   medium onion, chopped
2   cloves garlic, minced
1   tablespoon olive oil
1¼ cups orange juice
1   cup bulgur
1   cup frozen green soybeans or baby lima beans
¾   cup water
½   cup canned soybeans or small red beans, rinsed and
      drained
1   medium carrot, cut into thin bite-size strips
1   stalk celery, bias-sliced
⅓   cup dried tart cherries or raisins
¼   cup toasted wheat germ
2   oranges, peeled and sectioned

Soybeans are one of the best ways to get a significant amount of cancer-inhibiting, cholesterol-reducing, and osteoporosis-preventing isoflavones in your diet. This recipe uses green soybeans, which also are known as sweet beans or soybean kernels.

1. In a large saucepan cook onion and garlic in hot oil until onion is tender. Stir in orange juice, bulgur, frozen soybeans or lima beans, water, canned soybeans or red beans, carrot, and celery.

2. Bring to boiling; reduce heat. Simmer, covered, for 12 to 15 minutes or until soybeans are tender and liquid is absorbed. Stir in cherries or raisins and wheat germ. Serve with orange sections. Makes 4 main-dish servings.

Nutrition facts per serving: 404 calories, 10 g total fat (1 g saturated fat), 0 mg cholesterol, 74 mg sodium, 65 g carbohydrate, 12 g fiber, 19 g protein. Daily values: 52% vitamin A, 113% vitamin C, 11% calcium, 26% iron.

fruity tofu shakes

Start to finish: 10 minutes

If you've never tried tofu, this thick, fruity breakfast shake is a great start! Soy foods, like tofu, are tops in health benefits, providing cancer-fighting and heart-protecting phytochemicals, daidzein, and genistein.

1½ cups fresh or frozen fruit (strawberries, raspberries, peeled and cut-up peaches or mango, cut-up nectarines, or pitted dark sweet cherries)
1½ cups orange juice
1 10½-ounce package light tofu, cut up
2 tablespoons honey

1. Partially thaw the fruit, if frozen. In a blender container combine the fruit, orange juice, tofu, and honey. Cover and blend until nearly smooth. Pour into glasses. Makes three 1⅓-cup servings.

Nutrition facts per serving: 250 calories, 3 g total fat (0 g saturated fat), 0 mg cholesterol, 38 mg sodium, 51 g carbohydrate, 8 g fiber, 8 g protein. Daily values: 2% vitamin A, 168% vitamin C, 4% calcium, 12% iron.

pasta and grains

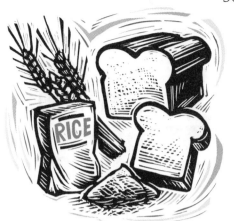

pasta with artichokes

Start to finish: 20 minutes

- 4 ounces dried fusilli pasta or fettuccine, broken
- 1 9-ounce package frozen artichoke hearts, thawed
- 2 medium red or green sweet peppers, chopped
- 1 small onion, finely chopped
- 2 cloves garlic, minced
- 1 tablespoon olive oil
- 1 medium tomato, seeded and chopped
- ¼ cup snipped fresh basil or 2 teaspoons dried basil, crushed
- 2 tablespoons grated Parmesan cheese

Infused with the flavors of olive oil and sweet basil, this pasta dish is simplicity at its best. The artichoke hearts, sweet peppers, and tomato dress up pasta—simply.

1. Cook pasta in boiling lightly salted water according to package directions. Drain. Return pasta to hot pan.

2. Meanwhile, in a large skillet cook and stir artichoke hearts, sweet peppers, onion, and garlic in hot oil over medium-high heat about 5 minutes or until vegetables are tender. Stir in tomato and basil; cook and stir about 2 minutes more or until mixture is heated through.

3. Add artichoke mixture to cooked pasta; toss gently to combine. Sprinkle each serving with Parmesan cheese. Makes 3 main-dish servings.

Nutrition facts per serving: 278 calories, 7 g total fat (2 g saturated fat), 3 mg cholesterol, 165 mg sodium, 46 g carbohydrate, 6 g fiber, 11 g protein. Daily values: 44% vitamin A, 171% vitamin C, 10% calcium, 21% iron.

pasta with swiss chard

Start to finish: 25 minutes

Bite into this red, white, and green wholesome main dish for a taste of Italy. Either Swiss chard or spinach provides a healthy serving of magnesium. This important mineral, needed for body-regulating enzymes, helps maintain healthy nerves, muscles, and bones.

12 ounces fresh Swiss chard or spinach
 8 ounces dried bow-tie or mostaccioli pasta
 4 cloves garlic, minced
 1 tablespoon olive oil
 ¾ cup light ricotta cheese
 ¼ cup light milk
 2 tablespoons snipped fresh basil or 2 teaspoons dried basil, crushed
 ¼ teaspoon salt
 ¼ teaspoon pepper
 ⅛ teaspoon ground nutmeg
 2 medium tomatoes, seeded and chopped
 ¼ cup finely shredded Parmesan cheese

1. Cut out and discard center ribs from Swiss chard or remove stems from spinach. Coarsely chop; set aside. Cook pasta according to package directions, except omit any oil or salt. Drain. Return pasta to hot pan.

2. Meanwhile, in a large skillet cook garlic in hot oil over medium heat for 15 seconds. Add Swiss chard or spinach. Cook over medium-low heat about 3 minutes or until Swiss chard or spinach wilts, stirring frequently. Stir in ricotta cheese, milk, basil, salt, pepper, and nutmeg. Cook and stir for 3 to 5 minutes more or until heated through.

3. Add Swiss chard mixture and tomatoes to cooked pasta; toss gently to combine. Sprinkle each serving with Parmesan. Makes 4 main-dish servings.

Nutrition facts per serving: 356 calories, 8 g total fat (1 g saturated fat), 14 mg cholesterol, 413 mg sodium, 54 g carbohydrate, 3 g fiber, 18 g protein. Daily values: 34% vitamin A, 45% vitamin C, 16% calcium, 29% iron.

penne with lemon asparagus

Start to finish: 30 minutes

8 ounces dried penne or mostaccioli pasta
1 14½-ounce can reduced-sodium chicken broth or
  vegetable broth
¾ teaspoon snipped fresh rosemary or ¼ teaspoon dried
  rosemary, crushed
¼ teaspoon pepper
1½ pounds fresh asparagus, trimmed and cut into 1-inch
  pieces (about 3½ cups), or two 9-ounce packages
  frozen cut asparagus
2 cups sliced fresh mushrooms
¼ cup dry white wine
1 teaspoon finely shredded lemon peel
2 tablespoons lemon juice
1 tablespoon cornstarch
¼ cup finely shredded Asiago cheese

A combo of rosemary, lemon, and asparagus flavors this elegant, light pasta dish. A sprinkling of shredded fresh Asiago adds a spirited finishing touch. If you like, add 8 ounces of peeled deveined cooked shrimp for a special entrée.

1. Cook pasta according to package directions, except omit any oil or salt. Drain. Return pasta to hot pan.

2. Meanwhile, in a large saucepan bring broth, rosemary, and pepper to boiling. Boil, uncovered, about 4 minutes or until mixture is reduced to about 1½ cups. Add asparagus and mushrooms. Simmer, uncovered, until asparagus is crisp-tender (allow 4 to 6 minutes for fresh asparagus or 3 to 4 minutes for frozen asparagus).

3. In a bowl stir together wine, lemon peel, lemon juice, and cornstarch; stir into asparagus mixture. Cook and stir until thickened. Cook and stir for 2 minutes more. Add asparagus mixture to cooked pasta; toss gently to coat. Sprinkle each serving with cheese. Makes 4 main-dish servings.

Nutrition facts per serving: 315 calories, 4 g total fat (0 g saturated fat), 5 mg cholesterol, 377 mg sodium, 55 g carbohydrate, 3 g fiber, 15 g protein. Daily values: 10% vitamin A, 63% vitamin C, 8% calcium, 24% iron.

304 pasta and grains

ravioli with sweet peppers

Start to finish: 20 minutes

This bright, fresh vegetable and pasta main dish scores high in flavor and nutrient value. Each serving provides more than half of your vitamin A and C needs, as well as quercetin and lycopene, important phyto-chemicals in the fight against cancer.

1 9-ounce package refrigerated light cheese ravioli
1 medium red sweet pepper, chopped
1 medium green sweet pepper, chopped
1 medium carrot, cut into thin bite-size strips
1 small onion, chopped
2 cloves garlic, minced
1 tablespoon olive oil
1 medium tomato, chopped
¼ cup reduced-sodium chicken broth or vegetable broth
3 tablespoons snipped fresh basil or 2 teaspoons dried
    basil, crushed, or 1 tablespoon snipped fresh tarragon
    or 1 teaspoon dried tarragon, crushed

1. Cook pasta according to package directions, except omit any oil or salt. Drain. Return pasta to hot pan.

2. Meanwhile, in a large skillet cook sweet peppers, carrot, onion, and garlic in hot oil over medium-high heat about 5 minutes or until vegetables are tender. Stir in tomato, broth, and basil or tarragon. Cook and stir about 2 minutes more or until heated through.

3. Add vegetable mixture to the cooked pasta; toss gently to combine. Makes 4 main-dish servings.

Nutrition facts per serving: 236 calories, 7 g total fat (2 g saturated fat), 43 mg cholesterol, 301 mg sodium, 33 g carbohydrate, 3 g fiber, 11 g protein. Daily values: 57% vitamin A, 86% vitamin C, 6% calcium, 8% iron.

herbed macaroni & cheese

Start to finish: 25 minutes

8 ounces dried elbow macaroni or rotini pasta
1 cup fat-free milk
1 tablespoon all-purpose flour
3 ounces reduced-fat cream cheese (Neufchâtel)
1 tablespoon snipped fresh basil or oregano or 1 teaspoon
  dried basil or oregano, crushed
¼ teaspoon pepper
5 slices light process American-flavored cheese
  product, torn
¼ cup sliced green onions
1 tablespoon grated Parmesan cheese
1 tablespoon toasted wheat germ

Old-fashioned macaroni and cheese can be part of a modern, healthy diet. This creamy version uses low-fat cheeses and fat-free milk to reduce the fat, while mustard and herbs boost the flavor and make it more updated than Mom's recipe.

1. Cook pasta according to package directions, except omit any oil or salt. Drain. Return pasta to hot pan.

2. Meanwhile, in a large saucepan gradually stir milk into flour. Add cream cheese, basil or oregano, and pepper. Cook and stir over medium heat until slightly thickened and bubbly. Cook and stir for 1 minute more. Remove from heat. Add torn American cheese, a little at a time, stirring until cheese melts. Stir in green onions.

3. Add cheese mixture to cooked pasta; toss gently to coat. Spoon into a serving dish. Sprinkle with Parmesan cheese and wheat germ. Makes 4 main-dish servings.

Nutrition facts per serving: 386 calories, 11 g total fat (6 g saturated fat), 33 mg cholesterol, 511 mg sodium, 51 g carbohydrate, 2 g fiber, 19 g protein. Daily values: 14% vitamin A, 3% vitamin C, 25% calcium, 17% iron.

couscous & feta salad

Prep: 25 minutes **Chill:** 4 hours

Fresh spinach and feta cheese mingle with couscous in a spicy Mediterranean salad that is easy, flavorful, and healthy. It provides a generous helping of folate, a B vitamin that lowers your risk of heart disease and stroke.

¼ cup dried tomatoes (not oil packed)
1½ cups water
2 cloves garlic, minced
1 cup quick-cooking couscous
½ of a medium cucumber, halved lengthwise and
    thinly sliced
2 green onions, sliced
⅓ cup red wine vinegar
2 tablespoons olive oil
2 teaspoons sugar
¼ teaspoon ground mustard
¼ teaspoon ground cumin
⅛ teaspoon ground red pepper
2 cups torn fresh spinach
¼ cup crumbled feta cheese (1 ounce)
¼ cup sliced almonds, toasted (optional)

1. In a small bowl combine dried tomatoes and enough warm water to cover. Let stand for 10 minutes. Drain and snip tomatoes; set aside.

2. Meanwhile, in a medium saucepan combine the 1½ cups water and garlic. Bring to boiling; remove from heat. Stir in couscous. Let stand, covered, for 5 minutes. Stir in cucumber and green onions. Transfer to a large bowl.

3. For dressing, in a small bowl whisk together vinegar, oil, sugar, mustard, cumin, and red pepper. Stir in drained tomatoes. Drizzle over couscous mixture; toss to coat. Cover; refrigerate for 4 to 24 hours. Before serving, stir couscous mixture. Stir in spinach and feta cheese. If desired, sprinkle each serving with almonds. Makes 4 main-dish servings.

Nutrition facts per serving: 282 calories, 9 g total fat (2 g saturated fat), 6 mg cholesterol, 181 mg sodium, 44 g carbohydrate, 8 g fiber, 9 g protein. Daily values: 22% vitamin A, 20% vitamin C, 7% calcium, 11% iron.

roasted vegetables & quinoa

Start to finish: 55 minutes

Nonstick spray coating
2 cups peeled and cubed butternut squash
4 plum tomatoes, cut into eighths
2 small onions, cut into thin wedges
1 tablespoon cooking or olive oil
1 tablespoon snipped fresh thyme or 1 teaspoon dried thyme, crushed
1½ teaspoons snipped fresh savory or ½ teaspoon dried savory, crushed
¼ teaspoon pepper
6 cloves garlic with skin
1½ cups quinoa
1 14½-ounce can reduced-sodium chicken broth or vegetable broth
1¼ cups water

Quinoa (KEEN-wah), called the "mother grain" by the ancient Incas, is a grain native to South America. It contains more protein than any other grain and is touted as the "supergrain of the future." Combined here with roasted butternut squash, plum tomatoes, garlic, and herbs, it's an irresistible main dish.

1. Line a 15×10×1-inch baking pan with foil; spray foil with nonstick coating. Spread squash, tomatoes, and onions on foil. Drizzle vegetables with oil; sprinkle with thyme, savory, and pepper. Place garlic cloves to one side of foil-lined pan. Bake in a 400° oven for 20 minutes. Remove garlic from pan; set aside to cool. Bake remaining vegetables for 15 to 20 minutes more or until tender.

2. Meanwhile, thoroughly rinse quinoa; drain. In a large saucepan combine broth and water. Bring to boiling. Stir in quinoa. Return to boiling; reduce heat. Simmer, covered, about 15 minutes or until quinoa is tender and liquid is absorbed. Squeeze softened garlic from each clove; discard skin. Stir garlic into quinoa. Add roasted vegetables to quinoa mixture; toss gently to combine. Makes 4 main-dish servings.

Nutrition facts per serving: 332 calories, 8 g total fat (1 g saturated fat), 0 mg cholesterol, 314 mg sodium, 57 g carbohydrate, 6 g fiber, 11 g protein. Daily values: 45% vitamin A, 37% vitamin C, 7% calcium, 46% iron.

millet–stuffed squash

Start to finish: 1 hour

Try fusion cooking at its best. Mild-flavored African millet combines with highly spiced Indian chutney to stuff the healthful, all-American acorn squash. Acorn squash contributes an abundance of beta-carotene to your diet.

2 acorn squash
2 tablespoons chutney
1¼ cups reduced-sodium chicken broth or vegetable broth
2 tablespoons sliced green onion
⅛ teaspoon pepper
½ cup millet
1 medium tomato, chopped
1 small apple, chopped

1. Halve squash; scoop out seeds. Place squash, cut sides down, in a large baking pan. Bake in a 350° oven about 45 minutes or until tender.

2. Meanwhile, cut up any large pieces of chutney. In a small saucepan stir together the chutney, broth, green onion, and pepper. Bring to boiling. Stir in the millet; reduce heat. Simmer, covered, for 15 to 20 minutes or until most of the liquid is absorbed. Stir in tomato and apple. Let stand, covered, for 5 minutes.

3. Fill the squash halves with the millet mixture. Bake, uncovered, about 10 minutes more or until heated through. Makes 4 main-dish servings.

Nutrition facts per serving: 216 calories, 2 g total fat (0 g saturated fat), 0 mg cholesterol, 213 mg sodium, 48 g carbohydrate, 9 g fiber, 5 g protein. Daily values: 136% vitamin A, 61% vitamin C, 7% calcium, 14% iron.

nutty brown rice patties

Prep: 35 minutes **Cook:** 48 minutes

½ cup uncooked regular brown rice
½ teaspoon instant vegetable or chicken bouillon granules
½ cup finely chopped onion
⅓ cup shredded carrot
1 clove garlic, minced, or ⅛ teaspoon garlic powder
1 teaspoon dried thyme, crushed
⅛ teaspoon pepper
2 beaten egg whites or ¼ cup refrigerated egg product
¼ cup finely chopped pecans, toasted
¼ cup fine dry bread crumbs
1 tablespoon cooking oil
⅓ cup fat-free dairy sour cream
2 tablespoons sliced green onion
1 small tomato, seeded and chopped

If you love burgers, this meatless version provides plenty of taste and texture with far less fat and cholesterol. Brown rice, the main ingredient, provides fiber to reduce your risk of cancer and helps to keep you slim and trim (fiber fills you up). Serve it for lunch topped with fat-free sour cream and fresh tomato.

1. In a medium saucepan cook the brown rice according to package directions, except omit any butter or salt. Transfer rice to a medium bowl; cool for 30 minutes. (Or, use 1½ cups leftover cooked brown rice.) In the same saucepan combine bouillon granules and ¼ cup water. Stir in the finely chopped onion, carrot, garlic, thyme, and pepper. Bring to boiling; reduce heat. Simmer, uncovered, for 4 to 5 minutes or until vegetables are very tender and liquid is evaporated.

2. Stir vegetable mixture, egg whites or egg product, pecans, and bread crumbs into cooked rice. With wet hands, shape into eight ½-inch-thick patties. In a large nonstick skillet heat 1½ teaspoons of the oil over medium-high heat. Add the 4 patties; cook about 2 minutes on each side or until golden. Remove and keep warm. Repeat with remaining oil and patties. To serve, mix sour cream and onion. Top patties with sour cream mixture and tomato. Makes 4 main-dish servings.

Nutrition facts per serving: 233 calories, 9 g total fat (1 g saturated fat), 0 mg cholesterol, 209 mg sodium, 31 g carbohydrate, 3 g fiber, 7 g protein. Daily values: 32% vitamin A, 9% vitamin C, 5% calcium, 7% iron.

tortellini soup

Prep: 15 minutes **Cook:** 43 minutes

Experiment on the wild side—with a little wild rice, that is. In this soup, the nutty flavor and chewy texture of wild rice, a long-grain marsh grass, lends contrast to the soft texture of tortellini pasta. Although it's more expensive than regular white rice, a little goes a long way. Be sure to wash wild rice thoroughly before using, as some dirt may still cling to the marsh-grown grass.

¼ cup uncooked wild rice
  Nonstick spray coating
1 large onion, chopped
1 stalk celery, thinly sliced
1 clove garlic, minced
6½ cups water
2 teaspoons instant vegetable bouillon granules
1 teaspoon dried oregano, crushed
½ teaspoon dried marjoram, crushed
⅛ teaspoon pepper
1 bay leaf
1 9-ounce package refrigerated cheese tortellini
2 cups chopped broccoli flowerets
2 tablespoons snipped dried tomatoes (not oil packed)

1. Rinse wild rice in a strainer under cold running water about 1 minute. Drain; set aside.

2. Spray an unheated large saucepan with nonstick coating. Heat saucepan over medium-high heat. Add the onion, celery, and garlic; cook, covered, for 3 to 4 minutes or until vegetables are crisp-tender, stirring once or twice. Carefully stir in wild rice, water, bouillon granules, oregano, marjoram, pepper, and bay leaf. Bring to boiling; reduce heat. Simmer, covered, about 35 minutes or until rice is nearly tender. Discard bay leaf.

3. Add tortellini, broccoli, and dried tomatoes to saucepan. Return to boiling; reduce heat. Cook, uncovered, for 5 to 6 minutes more or until tortellini and broccoli are just tender. Makes 4 main-dish servings.

Nutrition facts per serving: 268 calories, 5 g total fat (2 g saturated fat), 30 mg cholesterol, 737 mg sodium, 44 g carbohydrate, 2 g fiber, 13 g protein. Daily values: 7% vitamin A, 50% vitamin C, 13% calcium, 15% iron.

barley—vegetable salad

Prep: 25 minutes **Marinate:** 2 to 6 hours

½ cup quick-cooking barley
1 cup broccoli or cauliflower flowerets
1 cup fresh pea pods, strings removed and halved
    crosswise, or one 6-ounce package frozen pea pods,
    thawed and halved crosswise
1 medium red sweet pepper, cut into thin bite-size strips
½ cup chopped, seeded cucumber
¼ cup sliced green onions
2 tablespoons lime or lemon juice
2 tablespoons white wine vinegar
1 tablespoon olive or salad oil
2 teaspoons sugar
2 cloves garlic, minced
1 teaspoon dried thyme, crushed
¼ teaspoon crushed red pepper
¼ teaspoon black pepper

Rejoice in the summer sun with a backyard picnic featuring this chilly fresh vegetable and barley salad. One serving of this make-ahead salad provides 14 grams of fiber, more than half of your 25 gram goal for the entire day.

1. In a medium saucepan bring 1¼ cups water to boiling. Stir in barley; reduce heat. Simmer, covered, for 5 minutes. Stir in broccoli or cauliflower; cook, covered, for 5 minutes. If using, stir in fresh pea pods; cook, covered, about 1 minute more or until barley is tender. Drain in colander. Rinse with cold water; drain again. In a shallow glass dish combine barley mixture, thawed pea pods (if using), sweet pepper, cucumber, and green onions.

2. For dressing, in a screw-top jar combine lime or lemon juice, vinegar, oil, sugar, garlic, thyme, crushed red pepper, black pepper, and 2 tablespoons water. Cover and shake well. Pour over barley mixture; toss gently to coat. Cover and marinate in the refrigerator for 2 to 6 hours, stirring occasionally. Makes 8 side-dish servings.

Nutrition facts per serving: 84 calories, 2 g total fat (0 g saturated fat), 0 mg cholesterol, 12 mg sodium, 15 g carbohydrate, 14 g fiber, 3 g protein. Daily values: 6% vitamin A, 72% vitamin C, 2% calcium, 6% iron.

honey—nut granola

Prep: 10 minutes **Bake:** 30 minutes

Homemade granola wins hands-down over store-bought. For breakfast or a snack anytime, keep a batch on hand. Granola also tastes great spooned over fresh fruit or fat-free frozen yogurt.

Nonstick spray coating
3 cups regular rolled oats
½ cup toasted wheat germ
½ cup slivered almonds
⅓ cup honey
⅓ cup orange juice
¼ teaspoon ground cinnamon
Dash ground nutmeg
¾ cup finely snipped dried apricots or dried fruit bits
Vanilla or fruit-flavored fat-free yogurt

1. Spray a 15×10×1-inch baking pan with nonstick coating; set aside. In a large bowl stir together oats, wheat germ, and almonds. In a small saucepan combine honey, orange juice, cinnamon, and nutmeg. Bring to boiling, stirring occasionally. Pour over oat mixture; toss to coat.

2. Spread oat mixture evenly in prepared pan. Bake in a 325° oven for 25 minutes, stirring once. Stir in apricots or fruit bits. Bake for 5 to 10 minutes more or until oats are lightly browned. Remove from oven. Immediately turn out onto a large piece of foil to cool.

3. Store in an airtight container in the refrigerator for up to 2 weeks or in the freezer for up to 3 months.

4. For one serving, spoon one 6- or 8-ounce carton yogurt into a serving bowl. Top with ⅓ cup of the oat mixture. Makes 17 servings.

Nutrition facts per serving (includes 6 ounces of yogurt): 283 calories, 7 g total fat (2 g saturated fat), 9 mg cholesterol, 100 mg sodium, 48 g carbohydrate, 1 g fiber, 11 g protein. Daily values: 7% vitamin A, 6% vitamin C, 20% calcium, 9% iron.

ginger oatcakes

Prep: 20 minutes **Cook:** 4 minutes each

1½ cups fat-free milk
 ¾ cup quick-cooking or regular rolled oats
  3 slightly beaten egg whites
  1 slightly beaten egg
  2 tablespoons cooking oil
  2 tablespoons dark-colored corn syrup or molasses
  1 cup all-purpose flour
  2 tablespoons finely chopped crystallized ginger or
       ¼ to ½ teaspoon ground ginger
1½ teaspoons baking powder
 ¾ teaspoon ground cinnamon
 ¼ teaspoon baking soda
 ¼ teaspoon salt
     Fresh blueberries or sliced banana (optional)
     Orange marmalade or maple-flavored syrup (optional)

The secret to the wonderful flavor of these pancakes is the crystallized ginger and corn syrup stirred into the batter. Make this batter up to 2 days ahead and keep it in the refrigerator for a spur-of-the-moment breakfast.

1. In a medium saucepan heat milk over low heat just until hot, stirring occasionally. Stir in oats. Remove from heat; let stand for 5 minutes. Combine egg whites, egg, oil, and corn syrup or molasses; stir into oat mixture. In a medium bowl combine flour, ginger, baking powder, cinnamon, baking soda, and salt. Add oat mixture all at once to flour mixture; stir just until moistened. (Batter may be covered and stored in the refrigerator for up to 2 days.)

2. For each pancake, pour a scant ¼ cup batter into a hot, lightly greased heavy skillet. Cook over medium heat until golden brown, turning to second sides when pancakes have bubbly surfaces and edges are slightly dry. If desired, serve pancakes topped with blueberries or banana and marmalade or syrup. Makes 14 pancakes.

Nutrition facts per pancake: 94 calories, 3 g total fat (0 g saturated fat), 16 mg cholesterol, 132 mg sodium, 14 g carbohydrate, 1 g fiber, 4 g protein. Daily values: 2% vitamin A, 0% vitamin C, 6% calcium, 5% iron.

berry french toast

Prep: 20 minutes **Bake:** 11 minutes

Delicious! That's how our Better Homes and Gardens® Test Kitchen taste testers described this baked French toast. The orange-scented sauce is studded with plump, juicy berries of your choosing. It's a great way to begin the day.

Nonstick spray coating
¾ cup refrigerated or frozen egg product, thawed or 3 eggs
¾ cup fat-free milk
1 teaspoon finely shredded orange peel
½ teaspoon vanilla
¼ teaspoon ground nutmeg
8 1-inch-thick slices French bread
¼ cup frozen orange juice concentrate, thawed
1 tablespoon sugar
1 tablespoon cornstarch
1 cup water
3 cups fresh blueberries, raspberries, and/or sliced strawberries

1. Spray a large baking sheet with nonstick coating; set aside. In a shallow bowl combine egg product or eggs, milk, orange peel, vanilla, and nutmeg. Dip bread slices into egg mixture, coating both sides. Place on prepared baking sheet.

2. Bake in a 450° oven about 6 minutes or until bread is lightly browned. Turn bread over and bake for 5 to 8 minutes more or until golden.

3. Meanwhile, for sauce, in a medium saucepan combine orange juice concentrate, sugar, and cornstarch; stir in water. Cook and stir over medium heat until thickened and bubbly. Cook and stir for 2 minutes more. Remove from heat. Stir in berries. Serve the sauce with French toast. Makes 4 servings (2 slices per serving).

Nutrition facts per serving: 306 calories, 4 g total fat (1 g saturated fat), 1 mg cholesterol, 420 mg sodium, 56 g carbohydrate, 3 g fiber, 13 g protein.
Daily values: 14% vitamin A, 70% vitamin C, 11% calcium, 16% iron.

eggs and dairy

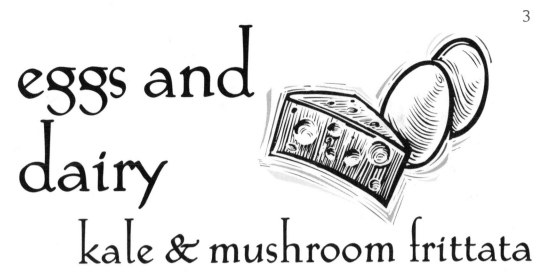

kale & mushroom frittata

Prep: 15 minutes **Bake:** 7 minutes

¼ cup reduced-sodium chicken broth or vegetable broth
2 cups shredded fresh kale or spinach
1 cup sliced fresh mushrooms
¼ cup chopped onion
5 egg whites
1 egg
½ teaspoon dried basil, crushed
¼ teaspoon dried thyme, crushed
⅛ teaspoon salt
⅛ teaspoon pepper
  Nonstick spray coating
¼ cup shredded reduced-fat Swiss or mozzarella cheese

A frittata is the Italian version of the French omelet. Instead of being flipped over onto itself as an omelet is, a frittata gets popped in the oven to finish cooking. Kale, herbs, and cheese flavor this frittata. Kale has a mild, cabbagelike flavor. Although best during the winter months, kale is available year-round.

1. In a medium saucepan bring broth to boiling. Stir in kale or spinach, mushrooms, and onion; reduce heat to medium. Cook, covered, for 9 to 12 minutes or until vegetables are tender; drain well.

2. Meanwhile, in a bowl combine egg whites, egg, basil, thyme, salt, and pepper. Spray an unheated ovenproof skillet with nonstick coating. Heat skillet over medium heat. Add kale mixture; pour egg mixture over kale mixture. Bake in a 350° oven for 6 to 8 minutes or until eggs are set. Sprinkle with cheese. Bake frittata for 1 to 2 minutes more. Makes 3 main-dish servings.

Nutrition facts per serving: 111 calories, 4 g total fat (2 g saturated fat), 76 mg cholesterol, 285 mg sodium, 7 g carbohydrate, 2 g fiber, 12 g protein. Daily values: 36% vitamin A, 32% vitamin C, 11% calcium, 8% iron.

enchilada skillet

Start to finish: 20 minutes

Here's an egg dish that is as good for dinner as it is for breakfast. Although the baked tortilla wedges take a short time to make, if you don't want to heat up the oven, use purchased baked tortillas instead.

 3 6-inch corn tortillas
 6 egg whites*
 5 eggs*
 ⅓ cup fat-free milk
 2 tablespoons sliced green onion
 ⅛ teaspoon garlic powder
    Nonstick spray coating
 ¼ cup shredded reduced-fat cheddar cheese (1 ounce)
 ¾ cup picante sauce
 ¼ cup fat-free dairy sour cream
 2 tablespoons sliced pitted ripe olives

1. Cut each tortilla into 8 wedges. Arrange wedges on a large baking sheet. Bake in a 350° oven for 5 to 10 minutes or until dry and crisp; set aside.

2. Meanwhile, in a medium bowl beat together egg whites, eggs, milk, green onion, and garlic powder. Spray an unheated large skillet with nonstick coating. Heat skillet over medium heat. Pour egg mixture into skillet. Cook, without stirring, until mixture begins to set on the bottom and around the edge. Using a spatula or large spoon, lift and fold the partially cooked eggs so the uncooked portion flows underneath. Continue cooking for 2 to 3 minutes or until eggs are cooked through, but are still glossy and moist. Sprinkle with cheddar cheese. Top each serving with picante sauce, sour cream, olives, and baked tortilla wedges. Makes 4 main-dish servings.

***Note:** You may substitute 2 cups refrigerated or frozen egg product, thawed, for the egg whites and eggs.

Nutrition facts per serving: 226 calories, 10 g total fat (3 g saturated fat), 272 mg cholesterol, 608 mg sodium, 17 g carbohydrate, 0 g fiber, 18 g protein. Daily values: 20% vitamin A, 14% vitamin C, 14% calcium, 10% iron.

tortilla casserole

Prep: 25 minutes **Bake:** 40 minutes

   Nonstick spray coating
1½ cups frozen whole kernel corn
  6 6-inch corn tortillas
  1 cup shredded reduced-fat mozzarella cheese (4 ounces)
½ cup sliced green onions
  1 4-ounce can diced green chili peppers, drained
¼ cup finely chopped red sweet pepper
  1 cup buttermilk
  2 egg whites*
  1 egg*
¼ teaspoon garlic salt
⅓ cup salsa

You don't need to shun using buttermilk because of its name. Buttermilk is made by adding a harmless bacteria to either fat-free or light milk, creating a tangy, slightly thickened milk. So, even though the name gives the impression of being high in fat, it's not. Serve this casserole for a brunch or simple evening meal. Pinto beans on the side or a fresh fruit salad completes the menu.

1. Spray a 2-quart square baking dish with nonstick coating. Cook corn according to package directions; drain well. Tear tortillas into bite-size pieces. Arrange half of the tortillas in baking dish. Top with half of the cheese, half of the corn, half of the green onions, half of the chili peppers, and half of the sweet pepper. Repeat the layers using the remaining tortillas, cheese, corn, green onions, chili peppers, and sweet pepper.

2. In a medium bowl beat together the buttermilk, egg whites, egg, and garlic salt. Pour over tortilla mixture. Bake in a 325° oven about 40 minutes or until a knife inserted near the center comes out clean. Let stand for 5 minutes before serving. To serve, cut into squares. Serve with salsa. Makes 4 main-dish servings.

*****Note:** You can substitute ½ cup refrigerated or frozen egg product, thawed, for the egg whites and whole egg.

Nutrition facts per serving: 260 calories, 7 g total fat (1 g saturated fat), 65 mg cholesterol, 600 mg sodium, 36 g carbohydrate, 0 g fiber, 18 g protein. Daily values: 13% vitamin A, 51% vitamin C, 15% calcium, 10% iron.

egg & potato casserole

Prep: 15 minutes **Bake:** 40 minutes

What a lifesaver! You can make this casserole up to 24 hours in advance to save you from spending a lot of time in the kitchen in the morning. Pull it from the refrigerator the next morning, bake it, and serve. We have also pared the fat to only 5 grams, which makes it a real lifesaver.

Nonstick spray coating
2 cups frozen loose-pack diced hash brown potatoes with onion and peppers
1 cup frozen cut broccoli or asparagus
⅓ cup finely chopped Canadian-style bacon or lean cooked ham (2 ounces)
⅓ cup evaporated fat-free milk
2 tablespoons all-purpose flour
2 8-ounce cartons refrigerated or frozen egg product, thawed
½ cup shredded reduced-fat cheddar cheese (2 ounces)
1 tablespoon snipped fresh basil or ½ teaspoon dried basil, crushed
¼ teaspoon black pepper
⅛ teaspoon salt

1. Spray a 2-quart square baking dish with nonstick coating. Arrange hash brown potatoes and broccoli or asparagus in bottom of baking dish; top with Canadian bacon or ham. Set aside. In a medium bowl gradually stir milk into flour. Stir in egg product, half of the cheese, the basil, black pepper, and salt. Pour egg mixture over vegetables.

2. Bake in a 350° oven for 40 to 45 minutes or until a knife inserted near center comes out clean. Sprinkle with remaining cheese. Let stand for 5 minutes. Makes 6 main-dish servings.

To make ahead: Assemble as above, but do not bake. Cover and refrigerate for 4 to 24 hours. To serve, remove cover and bake as above.

Nutrition facts per serving: 188 calories, 5 g total fat (2 g saturated fat), 11 mg cholesterol, 373 mg sodium, 18 g carbohydrate, 2 g fiber, 17 g protein. Daily values: 23% vitamin A, 25% vitamin C, 13% calcium, 17% iron.

pepper & broccoli omelet

Start to finish: 25 minutes

4 egg whites
2 tablespoons water
½ cup refrigerated or frozen egg product, thawed
1 tablespoon snipped fresh basil or 1 teaspoon dried basil, crushed
¼ teaspoon black pepper
⅛ teaspoon salt
1 tablespoon margarine or butter
1 cup broccoli flowerets, coarsely chopped
1 small red sweet pepper, chopped
3 tablespoons freshly grated Parmesan cheese

Get a super dose of immune-enhancing vitamin C from the bright-colored broccoli and red sweet pepper combination in this puffy baked omelet. Just one serving provides well over 100 percent of the RDA for vitamin C.

1. In a medium bowl beat egg whites until frothy. Add water; continue beating about 1½ minutes or until stiff peaks form (tips stand straight). Fold in egg product, basil, black pepper, and salt. In a 10-inch ovenproof skillet heat margarine or butter over medium-high heat until a drop of water sizzles. Pour in egg mixture, mounding slightly at sides. Reduce heat to low. Cook for 8 to 10 minutes or until puffed, set, and golden on bottom. Bake in a 325° oven for 8 to 10 minutes or until a knife inserted near center comes out clean.

2. Meanwhile, place a steamer basket in a medium saucepan. Add water to just below bottom of basket. Bring to boiling. Add broccoli and red pepper; reduce heat. Steam, covered, for 6 to 8 minutes or until vegetables are crisp-tender. Drain vegetables. Loosen sides of omelet with a metal spatula. Make a shallow cut slightly off-center across omelet. Top with the vegetables. Sprinkle with Parmesan cheese. Fold smaller side of omelet over vegetables and cheese. Cut in half crosswise. Makes 2 main-dish servings.

Nutrition facts per serving: 202 calories, 11 g total fat (2 g saturated fat), 8 mg cholesterol, 557 mg sodium, 6 g carbohydrate, 2 g fiber, 21 g protein. Daily values: 48% vitamin A, 140% vitamin C, 13% calcium, 13% iron.

broccoli–ricotta calzones

Prep: 25 minutes **Bake:** 12 minutes

Full of cheeses—ricotta, Parmesan, and mozzarella—these Italian turnovers won't blow your fat budget. Cheeses are available in lower fat versions making it easy to include them in a heart-healthy diet. Stoked with broccoli, these calzones (kal-ZOH-nays) are a meal in themselves. Simply add a fruit or mixed greens salad.

1 10-ounce package frozen chopped broccoli
⅓ cup chopped onion
¼ cup shredded carrot
1 clove garlic, minced
1¼ cups fat-free ricotta cheese
¾ cup shredded reduced-fat mozzarella cheese (3 ounces)
2 tablespoons grated Parmesan cheese
½ teaspoon dried Italian seasoning, crushed
⅛ teaspoon pepper
1 10-ounce package refrigerated pizza dough
1 tablespoon fat-free milk
   Nonstick spray coating
1 tablespoon grated Parmesan cheese

1. Cook broccoli, onion, carrot, and garlic according to the broccoli package directions; drain well.

2. In a large bowl stir together the broccoli mixture, ricotta cheese, mozzarella cheese, the 2 tablespoons Parmesan cheese, the Italian seasoning, and pepper. Unroll pizza dough. Roll or stretch dough into an 18×12-inch rectangle. Cut into six 6-inch squares. Divide broccoli mixture among squares. Brush edges of each square with milk. Lift one corner and stretch dough over to the opposite corner, making a triangle. With a fork, press edges of the dough well to seal.

3. Spray a baking sheet with nonstick coating. Arrange calzones on the baking sheet. Prick tops with a fork. Brush with milk. Sprinkle with the 1 tablespoon Parmesan cheese. Bake in a 425° oven for 12 to 15 minutes or until golden. Makes 6 main-dish servings.

Nutrition facts per serving: 195 calories, 5 g total fat (1 g saturated fat), 13 mg cholesterol, 325 mg sodium, 25 g carbohydrate, 2 g fiber, 16 g protein. Daily values: 32% vitamin A, 28% vitamin C, 14% calcium, 10% iron.

spinach—cheese tart

Prep: 25 minutes **Bake:** 10 minutes/20 minutes

1 recipe Pastry Shell
2 eggs
1 cup light ricotta cheese
½ cup crumbled semisoft goat cheese
¼ cup fat-free milk
½ cup chopped fresh spinach
¼ cup chopped, well drained, canned roasted red sweet
  peppers
2 teaspoons snipped fresh oregano or ¾ teaspoon dried
  oregano, crushed

1. Prepare Pastry Shell. Line pastry with a double thickness of heavy foil. Bake in a 450° oven for 10 to 12 minutes or until edge is golden. Remove from oven. Reduce oven temperature to 325°.

2. Meanwhile, in a medium bowl beat eggs slightly with an electric mixer. Add ricotta cheese, goat cheese, and milk. Beat until smooth. Stir in spinach, roasted peppers, and oregano. Pour mixture into pastry. Bake in the 325° oven about 20 minutes or until a knife inserted near the center comes out clean. Let stand for 5 minutes before serving. Makes 12 appetizer servings.

Pastry Shell: In a medium bowl stir together 1¼ cups all-purpose flour and ¼ teaspoon salt. In a 1-cup measure combine ¼ cup fat-free milk and 3 tablespoon olive oil. Add oil mixture all at once to flour mixture. Stir with a fork until dough forms a ball. On a lightly floured surface roll into a 12-inch circle. Transfer to a 9½- or 10-inch tart pan with a removable bottom, being careful not to stretch pastry. Trim pastry even with rim of pan. Do not prick.

Nutrition facts per serving: 140 calories, 8 g total fat (2 g saturated fat), 47 mg cholesterol, 137 mg sodium, 11 g carbohydrate, 0 g fiber, 6 g protein. Daily values: 8% vitamin A, 15% vitamin C, 4% calcium, 6% iron.

Here's a delectable savory appetizer tart to serve to guests. Light ricotta cheese makes up the bulk of the cheese used in the tart, keeping the fat low, while flavorful goat cheese, a higher fat cheese, is added in a smaller quantity. Fresh spinach, roasted sweet peppers, and oregano complement the goat cheese flavor.

3—mushroom garlic soup

Start to finish: 30 minutes

A mushroom trio—dried, button, and shiitake—lends this creamy garlic-flavored soup an earthy flair. We've added dry milk powder, increasing the calcium content by about 125 milligrams per serving. Calcium is important in helping prevent osteoporosis.

1 14½-ounce can vegetable or beef broth
⅓ cup dried mushrooms
¾ cup chopped onion
4 cloves garlic, minced
1 teaspoon butter or margarine
1 cup sliced fresh button mushrooms
1 cup sliced fresh shiitake mushrooms
1 tablespoon snipped fresh thyme or marjoram or
     1 teaspoon dried thyme or marjoram, crushed
⅛ teaspoon pepper
2¼ cups fat-free milk
⅓ cup nonfat dry milk powder
2 tablespoons cornstarch
1 medium carrot, shredded
1 tablespoon dry sherry (optional)

1. In a small saucepan bring broth to boiling. Add dried mushrooms; remove from heat. Let stand for 10 minutes. Drain, reserving broth. Chop mushrooms; set aside.

2. In a large saucepan cook onion and garlic in hot butter or margarine until tender. Carefully stir in reserved broth, chopped dried mushrooms, button mushrooms, shiitake mushrooms, dried thyme or marjoram (if using), and pepper. Bring to boiling; reduce heat. Simmer, covered, for 5 minutes.

3. Meanwhile, stir together the milk, milk powder, and cornstarch; stir into mixture in saucepan. Stir in carrot and, if using, fresh thyme or marjoram. Cook and stir until thickened and bubbly. Cook and stir for 2 minutes more. If desired, stir in sherry. Makes 3 main-dish servings.

Nutrition facts per 1½-cup serving: 193 calories, 3 g total fat (1 g saturated fat), 8 mg cholesterol, 719 mg sodium, 36 g carbohydrate, 3 g fiber, 12 g protein. Daily values: 70% vitamin A, 14% vitamin C, 28% calcium, 12% iron.

meat and poultry

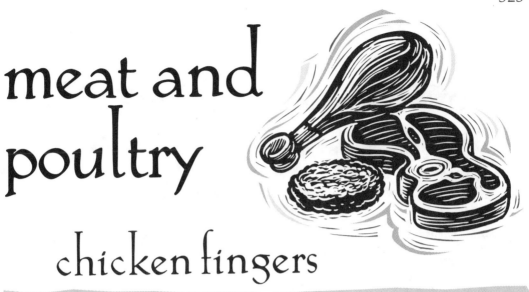

chicken fingers

Prep: 15 minutes **Bake:** 11 minutes

12 ounces skinless, boneless chicken breasts
 2 egg whites
 1 tablespoon honey
 2 cups cornflakes, crushed
 ¼ teaspoon pepper
 ¼ cup honey
 4 teaspoons prepared mustard or Dijon-style mustard
 ¼ teaspoon garlic powder

Got a craving for some crunchy chicken nuggets but shun the grease and fat? These chicken fingers are for you! The honey-mustard dipping sauce is the perfect partner to these baked chicken strips, a fat-skipping alternative to their fast-food cousins.

1. Rinse chicken; pat dry. Cut chicken into 3x¾-inch strips. In a small bowl combine egg whites and the 1 tablespoon honey. In a shallow bowl combine crushed cornflakes and pepper. Dip chicken strips into egg white mixture, then roll in crumb mixture to coat. Place in a single layer on an ungreased baking sheet.

2. Bake in a 450° oven for 11 to 13 minutes or until tender and no longer pink. Meanwhile, for sauce, in a small bowl stir together the ¼ cup honey, the mustard, and garlic powder. Serve with chicken. Makes 4 main-dish servings.

Nutrition facts per serving: 230 calories, 2 g total fat (1 g saturated fat), 45 mg cholesterol, 275 mg sodium, 31 g carbohydrate, 1 g fiber, 19 g protein. Daily values: 15% vitamin A, 10% vitamin C, 1% calcium, 10% iron.

oven–fried chicken

Prep: 15 minutes **Bake:** 45 minutes

Making healthy changes in your diet doesn't mean you have to give up favorite comfort foods. This easy, oven-prepared fried chicken keeps fat to a minimum. The drizzle of melted margarine or butter before baking provides the chicken with the deceiving richness of the pan-fried version.

2 whole medium chicken breasts (about 1½ pounds total), skinned and halved lengthwise
⅔ cup crushed low-fat crackers or onion-flavored crackers (about 40 crackers)
¼ teaspoon ground red pepper
1 egg white
1 tablespoon water
1 tablespoon margarine or butter, melted

1. Rinse chicken; pat dry. In a pie plate combine crushed crackers and red pepper. In a small bowl combine egg white and water.

2. Brush chicken with egg mixture. Sprinkle with crumb mixture; gently press crumbs onto chicken. Place in an ungreased shallow baking pan. Drizzle with the melted margarine or butter.

3. Bake in a 375° oven for 45 to 55 minutes or until tender and no longer pink. Makes 4 main-dish servings.

Nutrition facts per serving: 242 calories, 8 g total fat (1 g saturated fat), 73 mg cholesterol, 237 mg sodium, 11 g carbohydrate, 0 g fiber, 29 g protein. Daily values: 6% vitamin A, 0% vitamin C, 0% calcium, 4% iron.

lemongrass chicken

Start to finish: 30 minutes

2 stalks fresh lemongrass or 1 teaspoon finely shredded
   lemon peel
½ cup reduced-sodium chicken broth
2 teaspoons cornstarch
2 teaspoons rice vinegar or white wine vinegar
2 teaspoons light soy sauce
12 ounces skinless, boneless chicken breasts
   Nonstick spray coating
2 cloves garlic, minced
1 teaspoon grated fresh ginger
2 small zucchini, quartered lengthwise and sliced
6 green onions, cut into 1-inch pieces
2 teaspoons peanut or cooking oil
1 11-ounce can mandarin orange sections, drained
2 cups hot cooked rice

If you've never tasted lemongrass, try it in this delicious chicken recipe. Most often used in Thai cooking, lemongrass is considered an herb. It has long gray-green leaves and a green onionlike base. Remove any tough outer leaves, using only the inner, most tender portion of the stalk.

1. Peel off and discard heavy outer stalks of lemongrass; finely chop tender inner stalks. For sauce, stir together lemongrass or lemon peel, broth, cornstarch, vinegar, and soy sauce; set aside. Rinse chicken; pat dry. Cut chicken into 1-inch pieces.

2. Spray an unheated wok or large skillet with nonstick coating. Heat wok over medium heat. Add garlic and fresh ginger; stir-fry for 15 seconds. Add zucchini and green onions; stir-fry for 2 minutes. Remove vegetables from wok. Pour oil into wok. Add chicken; stir-fry for 3 to 4 minutes or until chicken is no longer pink. Push from center of wok. Stir sauce; pour into center of wok. Cook and stir until bubbly. Return vegetables to wok. Stir all ingredients together to coat with sauce. Cook and stir for 2 minutes more or until heated through. Gently stir in the oranges. Serve immediately with hot rice. Makes 4 main-dish servings.

Nutrition facts per serving: 286 calories, 6 g total fat (1 g saturated fat), 45 mg cholesterol, 216 mg sodium, 39 g carbohydrate, 1 g fiber, 20 g protein. Daily values: 5% vitamin A, 9% vitamin C, 2% calcium, 14% iron.

vegetable–stuffed chicken

Start to finish: 35 minutes

A simple Madeira wine sauce complements this elegant mushroom and cheese stuffed chicken. If you like a more earthy-flavored mushroom, use a wild mushroom, such as shiitake, chanterelle, or porcini.

Nonstick spray coating
1½ cups chopped fresh mushrooms
1 clove garlic, minced
2 tablespoons chopped roasted red sweet pepper
¼ teaspoon dried marjoram, crushed
4 medium skinless, boneless chicken breast halves
1½ ounces Gruyère cheese, cut into 4 slices
1 teaspoon olive oil
⅔ cup reduced-sodium chicken broth
⅓ cup Madeira wine or reduced-sodium chicken broth
2 teaspoons cornstarch
1 tablespoon snipped fresh parsley

1. For stuffing, spray an unheated large nonstick skillet with nonstick coating. Heat skillet over medium heat. Add mushrooms and garlic; cook until mushrooms are tender. Stir in roasted pepper and marjoram. Rinse chicken; pat dry. Cut a horizontal slit in the thickest portion of each chicken piece, forming a pocket. Place a slice of cheese and some of the stuffing in each pocket. Secure with wooden toothpicks.

2. In a large skillet cook chicken in hot oil over medium heat about 4 minutes or until browned, turning once. Pour broth and wine into skillet. Bring to boiling; reduce heat. Simmer, uncovered, about 8 minutes or until chicken is tender and no longer pink. Transfer chicken to a platter. Strain pan juices; measure juices. If necessary, return to skillet and boil gently until liquid is reduced to ¾ cup. Combine cornstarch and 1 tablespoon cold water; stir into liquid in skillet. Cook and stir until thickened and bubbly. Return chicken to skillet; cook for 2 minutes more. Remove toothpicks from chicken. Sprinkle with parsley. Makes 4 main-dish servings.

Nutrition facts per serving: 208 calories, 8 g total fat (3 g saturated fat), 71 mg cholesterol, 199 mg sodium, 4 g carbohydrate, 1 g fiber, 26 g protein. Daily values: 7% vitamin A, 25% vitamin C, 10% calcium, 9% iron.

chicken with apples & sage

Start to finish: 30 minutes

4 medium skinless, boneless chicken breast halves (about 1 pound total)
⅛ teaspoon salt
   Nonstick spray coating
1 cup apple juice
1 red or green sweet pepper, cut into 1-inch pieces
¼ cup chopped onion
1 clove garlic, minced
1½ teaspoons snipped fresh sage or ½ teaspoon dried sage, crushed
¼ teaspoon black pepper
1 tablespoon cornstarch
1 tablespoon cold water
2 medium red and/or green cooking apples, thinly sliced

Apple juice adds a pleasant sweetness to the sauce for this chicken dish. Serve it over hot cooked rice or wild rice for a satisfying meal. Steamed green beans or asparagus completes the menu.

1. Rinse chicken; pat dry. Sprinkle with salt. Spray an unheated large skillet with nonstick coating. Heat skillet over medium-high heat. Add chicken; cook for 8 to 10 minutes or until chicken is tender and no longer pink, turning once. Remove from skillet; keep warm.

2. Add apple juice, sweet pepper, onion, garlic, dried sage (if using), and black pepper to skillet. Bring to boiling; reduce heat. Simmer, covered, for 2 minutes. In a small bowl combine cornstarch and water; stir into skillet. Stir in apples. Cook and stir until thickened and bubbly. Cook and stir for 2 minutes more. If using, stir in fresh sage. Return chicken to skillet; heat through. Makes 4 main-dish servings.

Nutrition facts per serving: 203 calories, 4 g total fat (1 g saturated fat), 59 mg cholesterol, 123 mg sodium, 21 g carbohydrate, 2 g fiber, 22 g protein. Daily values: 14% vitamin A, 60% vitamin C, 2% calcium, 8% iron.

peppered pork

Prep: 15 minutes **Marinate:** 30 minutes **Broil:** 6 minutes

Through breeding and monitored feeding, pork now contains less fat and saturated fat. A wine and shallot sauce pairs well with the citrus and black pepper rub used on the pork.

    4 boneless pork loin chops, cut ¾ inch thick
    1 tablespoon whole black pepper, coarsely cracked
 1½ teaspoons finely shredded orange or lemon peel
    ½ cup dry red or white wine
    ½ cup sliced shallots or onion
    1 clove garlic, minced

1. Trim fat from pork. Combine pepper and orange or lemon peel. Rub evenly onto both sides of pork. Cover and marinate in refrigerator for 30 minutes to 2 hours.

2. Broil chops on the unheated rack of a broiler pan 3 to 4 inches from the heat for 6 to 8 minutes or until pork is slightly pink in center and juices run clear, turning once.

3. Meanwhile, in a small skillet bring wine to boiling. Add shallots or onion and garlic; reduce heat. Simmer, uncovered, for 5 minutes. Arrange pork on a serving platter; spoon shallot mixture over pork. Makes 4 main-dish servings.

Nutrition facts per serving: 143 calories, 6 g total fat (2 g saturated fat), 38 mg cholesterol, 52 mg sodium, 5 g carbohydrate, 0 g fiber, 13 g protein. Daily values: 25% vitamin A, 8% vitamin C, 1% calcium, 8% iron.

picture a portion

When you're trying to trim the fat, selecting the right portion size is half the battle. But it's not always easy, especially when you're eating away from home. These handy visual references can help:

● 3 ounces cooked meat, chicken, or fish = a deck of cards, a cassette tape, or the palm of a woman's hand
● 1 ounce cooked meat, chicken, or fish = a matchbox
● 1 ounce cheese = size of a thumb
● 2 tablespoons peanut butter, salad dressing, or mayonnaise = a golf ball

tomato–stuffed flank steak

Prep: 20 minutes **Cook:** 50 minutes

8 dried tomatoes (not oil packed)
1 1¼-pound beef flank steak
½ cup fine dry bread crumbs
¼ cup chopped onion
1 slightly beaten egg white
½ teaspoon dried basil, crushed
¼ teaspoon dried dillweed
¼ teaspoon pepper
  Nonstick spray coating
½ cup low-sodium tomato juice
2 cloves garlic, minced
1 tablespoon snipped fresh parsley
⅛ teaspoon salt

Iron from meat, poultry, or fish is more easily absorbed by your body than iron from plants. Vitamin C, found in tomatoes, also helps to absorb iron in meat and vegetables. Here, tomato juice and dried tomatoes provide the vitamin C to help mine the iron from flank steak.

1. In a small bowl combine dried tomatoes and enough warm water to cover. Let stand for 10 minutes. Drain and snip tomatoes; set aside. Trim fat from beef. Cover beef with plastic wrap. Pound lightly with a meat mallet to ¼-inch thickness. Remove wrap; set aside.

2. In a small bowl combine tomatoes, bread crumbs, onion, egg white, basil, dillweed, and pepper. Spread tomato mixture over beef. Roll up, jelly-roll style, starting from a narrow end; tie with kitchen string.

3. Spray an unheated large skillet with nonstick coating. Heat skillet over medium heat. Add beef; cook on all sides until brown. Add tomato juice and garlic. Bring to boiling; reduce heat. Simmer, uncovered, for 50 to 60 minutes or until tender. To serve, cut beef crosswise into 6 slices; arrange on a serving platter. Stir parsley and salt into pan juices; pass juices to spoon over beef. Makes 6 main-dish servings.

Nutrition facts per serving: 217 calories, 8 g total fat (3 g saturated fat), 44 mg cholesterol, 271 mg sodium, 14 g carbohydrate, 1 g fiber, 21 g protein. Daily values: 2% vitamin A, 13% vitamin C, 2% calcium, 15% iron.

sirloin with smoky sauce

Prep: 45 minutes **Marinate:** 2 hours **Grill:** 18 minutes

This simple sauce garners its smoky flavor from dried chipotle peppers, which are smoked jalapeños. A small amount of brown sugar adds a subtle sweetness to the sauce for a well-rounded hot-and-sweet flavor.

- 12 dried tomatoes halves (not oil packed)
- 1 to 3 dried chipotle peppers
- 1 cup dry red or white wine or 1 cup water plus
  ½ teaspoon instant beef bouillon granules
- 1 medium onion, chopped
- 1 tablespoon brown sugar
- 1 tablespoon lime or lemon juice
- 2 cloves garlic, quartered
- 12 ounces beef top sirloin steak, cut 1 inch thick

1. In a small bowl combine dried tomatoes, chipotle peppers, and enough boiling water to cover. Let stand for 30 minutes. Drain, reserving ¼ cup liquid. Cut up tomatoes. Halve chipotle peppers (wear plastic gloves). Remove stems, seeds, and membranes; cut up peppers.

2. For marinade, in a food processor bowl combine tomatoes, chipotle peppers, the ¼ cup liquid, wine or water plus bouillon granules, onion, brown sugar, lime or lemon juice, garlic, and ¼ teaspoon black pepper. Cover and process until nearly smooth. Trim fat from beef. Place beef in a plastic bag set in a shallow dish. Pour marinade over beef; close bag. Marinate in refrigerator for 2 to 8 hours, turning bag once.

3. Drain meat, reserving marinade. Grill beef on the rack of an uncovered grill directly over medium heat for 18 to 22 minutes for medium doneness, turning and brushing once with reserved marinade. (Or, broil beef on the unheated rack of a broiler pan 3 to 4 inches from the heat 18 to 22 minutes for medium doneness, turning and brushing once with marinade.) In a small saucepan heat remaining marinade to boiling; pass with meat. Makes 4 main-dish servings.

Nutrition facts per serving: 240 calories, 8 g total fat (3 g saturated fat), 57 mg cholesterol, 105 mg sodium, 12 g carbohydrate, 1 g fiber, 21 g protein. Daily values: 46% vitamin A, 17% vitamin C, 3% calcium, 20% iron.

fish and seafood

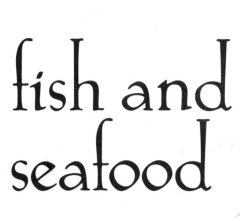
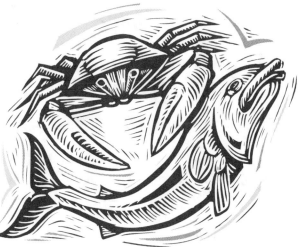

lemon & parmesan fish

Prep: 15 minutes **Bake:** 4 minutes

4 4-ounce fresh or frozen flounder, sole, or orange roughy
   fillets, ½ to 1 inch thick
   Nonstick spray coating
½ cup crushed cornflakes
1 tablespoon grated Parmesan cheese
1 tablespoon margarine or butter, melted
1 teaspoon finely shredded lemon peel
¼ teaspoon pepper
   Lemon wedges

1. Thaw fish, if frozen. Rinse fish; pat dry. Spray a
15×10×1-inch baking pan with nonstick coating. Place fish in
prepared pan, tucking under any thin edges.

2. In a small bowl combine crushed cornflakes, Parmesan
cheese, margarine or butter, lemon peel, and pepper. Sprinkle
crumb mixture on top of fish. Bake in a 450° oven until fish
flakes easily with a fork and crumbs are brown (allow 4 to
6 minutes per ½-inch thickness of fish). Serve with lemon
wedges. Makes 4 main-dish servings.

*Nutrition facts per serving: 158 calories, 5 g total fat (1 g saturated fat),
62 mg cholesterol, 221 mg sodium, 5 g carbohydrate, 0 g fiber, 22 g protein.
Daily values: 11% vitamin A, 6% vitamin C, 3% calcium, 4% iron.*

*Experts suggest eating
seafood two to three
times a week to take
advantage of its
excellent health benefits.
This recipe is so easy
that you can whip it up
on a busy weeknight.
Better yet, the crunchy
Parmesan crumb
topping on these oven-
baked fillets pleases kids
and adults alike.*

fish & fruit kabobs

Prep: 30 minutes **Grill:** 8 minutes

Pack sizzle into your summer by adding juicy ripe nectarines to firm-textured, mild-flavored fish. Broiled or grilled, just brush with the apple juice-rosemary-based mixture to lend the right touch of sweetness. Serve with hot cooked rice pilaf and grilled vegetables for a great meal.

1 pound fresh or frozen halibut steaks, cut 1 inch thick
4 nectarines, cut into 1½-inch pieces
2 medium zucchini, sliced ¾ inch thick
3 tablespoons apple or orange juice
1 tablespoon olive oil
1 teaspoon finely shredded lemon peel
1 tablespoon lemon juice
2 cloves garlic, minced
2 teaspoons snipped fresh rosemary or ½ teaspoon dried rosemary, crushed
¼ teaspoon salt
¼ teaspoon pepper
Nonstick spray coating

1. Thaw fish, if frozen. Remove skin and bones. Rinse fish; pat dry. Cut into 1-inch pieces. On 8 long metal skewers, alternately thread fish, nectarines, and zucchini.

2. In a small bowl combine apple or orange juice, oil, lemon peel, lemon juice, garlic, rosemary, salt, and pepper. Spray the unheated rack of an uncovered grill with nonstick coating. Brush kabobs with juice mixture.

3. Grill the kabobs directly over medium-high heat for 8 to 12 minutes or until the fish flakes easily with a fork, turning and brushing kabobs once with juice mixture. (Or, spray the unheated rack of a broiler pan with nonstick coating. Brush kabobs with juice mixture. Broil kabobs about 4 inches from the heat for 8 to 12 minutes, turning and brushing once with juice mixture.) Makes 4 main-dish servings.

Nutritional facts per serving: 240 calories, 7 g total fat (1 g saturated fat), 36 mg cholesterol, 197 mg sodium, 21 g carbohydrate, 3 g fiber, 25 g protein. Daily values: 16% vitamin A, 22% vitamin C, 6% calcium, 10% iron.

mustard jalapeño salmon

Prep: 10 minutes **Grill:** 4 minutes

4 5-ounce fresh or frozen salmon fillets, ½ to
   1 inch thick
1 teaspoon olive oil
2 tablespoons Dijon-style mustard
1 tablespoon honey
1 tablespoon bottled chopped red or green
   jalapeño pepper
⅛ teaspoon onion powder
⅛ teaspoon garlic powder
   Nonstick spray coating

This spicy glazed salmon not only is great tasting and simple, but it also provides your diet with omega-3 fatty acids—heart-saving fats found in salmon and other cold-water fish. These important fats help reduce the occurrence of hardening of the arteries and blocked blood vessels.

1. Thaw fish, if frozen. Rinse fish; pat dry. Brush with oil. For sauce, in a small bowl stir together mustard, honey, jalapeño pepper, onion powder, and garlic powder.

2. Spray the unheated rack of an uncovered grill with nonstick coating. Grill fish directly over medium heat until fish flakes easily with a fork (allow 4 to 6 minutes per ½-inch thickness of fish). Turn 1-inch-thick fillets once. Brush with sauce the last 5 minutes of cooking. (Or, spray the unheated rack of a broiler pan with nonstick coating. Broil fish about 4 inches from the heat. Allow 4 to 6 minutes per ½-inch thickness of fish. Turn 1-inch-thick fillets once during cooking time. Brush with sauce the last 5 minutes of cooking.) Makes 4 main-dish servings.

Nutrition facts per serving: 167 calories, 7 g total fat (1 g saturated fat), 25 mg cholesterol, 299 mg sodium, 5 g carbohydrate, 0 g fiber, 21 g protein. Daily values: 3% vitamin A, 2% vitamin C, 1% calcium, 6% iron.

tuna with mango sauce

Prep: 15 minutes **Grill:** 8 minutes

If you enjoy the sun-drenched Caribbean islands, this vitamin A-packed recipe is for you. It combines fiery hot habañero peppers, fresh ginger, and cool sweet mango. One serving provides more than 100 percent of your daily requirement of vitamin A.

4 5-ounce fresh or frozen tuna or halibut steaks, cut 1 inch thick
1 clove garlic, minced
¼ teaspoon salt
1 fresh habañero or jalapeño pepper
1 mango, peeled, seeded, and cut up (about 1 cup)
⅓ cup reduced-sodium chicken broth
1 tablespoon honey
3 thin slices fresh ginger
   Nonstick spray coating

1. Thaw fish, if frozen. Rinse fish; pat dry. Combine garlic and salt; rub evenly onto both sides of fish.

2. Halve pepper (wear plastic gloves). Remove stem, seeds, and membranes; chop pepper. For sauce, in a blender container or food processor bowl combine pepper, mango, chicken broth, honey, and ginger. Cover and blend or process until smooth. Pour into a small saucepan. Cook over low heat until heated through, stirring occasionally. Cover and keep warm.

3. Spray the unheated rack of an uncovered grill with nonstick coating. Grill fish directly over medium heat for 8 to 12 minutes or until fish flakes easily with a fork, turning once. (Or, spray the unheated rack of a broiler pan with nonstick coating. Broil fish about 4 inches from the heat for 8 to 12 minutes, turning once.) Serve sauce with fish. If desired, store any remaining sauce in refrigerator for up to 3 days. Makes 4 main-dish servings.

Nutrition facts per serving: 277 calories, 8 g total fat (2 g saturated fat), 59 mg cholesterol, 248 mg sodium, 14 g carbohydrate, 1 g fiber, 37 g protein. Daily values: 111% vitamin A, 43% vitamin C, 1% calcium, 11% iron.

linguine with scallops & asparagus

Start to finish: 25 minutes

12 ounces fresh or frozen sea scallops
 8 ounces dried linguine
 1 pound fresh asparagus, trimmed and cut into 1-inch
    pieces (about 2 cups)
 ½ cup sliced green onions
 2 cloves garlic, minced
 2 teaspoons olive oil
 1 pound ripe tomatoes, seeded and coarsely chopped
    (about 1⅓ cups)
 ½ teaspoon finely shredded orange peel
 ¼ cup orange juice
 3 tablespoons snipped fresh basil or 2 teaspoons dried
    basil, crushed
 ½ teaspoon cornstarch
 ¼ teaspoon salt

Sauté scallops with garlic and onion, then toss with fresh asparagus, pasta, and tomato sauce for a burst of flavor and a resplendent main dish. The fresh tomatoes provide plenty of lycopene, an antioxidant responsible for helping reduce the risk of cancer.

1. Thaw scallops, if frozen. Cut any large scallops in half. Rinse scallops; pat dry. Cook pasta according to package directions, omitting any oil or salt. Add asparagus to linguine the last 5 minutes of cooking. Drain. Return pasta to hot pan.

2. Meanwhile, in a large nonstick skillet cook green onions and garlic in hot oil over medium heat until tender. Add scallops; cook and stir for 2 to 3 minutes or until opaque. Remove scallops from skillet. Stir in ½ cup of the tomatoes, the orange peel, orange juice, dried basil (if using), cornstarch, and salt; cook and stir until slightly thickened. Cook and stir for 1 to 2 minutes more. Return scallops to skillet; heat through. Stir in the remaining tomatoes and, if using, fresh basil. Add scallop mixture to cooked pasta; toss gently to combine. Makes 4 main-dish servings.

Nutrition facts per serving: 351 calories, 5 g total fat (1 g saturated fat), 25 mg cholesterol, 275 mg sodium, 57 g carbohydrate, 4 g fiber, 22 g protein. Daily values: 15% vitamin A, 83% vitamin C, 8% calcium, 31% iron.

phytochemicals

Whatever term you may have heard regarding foods with disease preventative properties, such as phytochemicals, nutraceuticals, or functional foods, in this book we refer to them as phytochemicals. These foods have certain naturally occurring components that may play a beneficial role in optimum health. The following are examples of the foods and their specific health benefits:

Allylic sulfides: Chives, garlic, leeks, onion.
Benefits: Act as antibiotics and have antiviral potential, increase cancer resistance, help lower blood cholesterol and blood pressure.

Carotenes, carotenoids: Dark, green leafy vegetables; yellow and orange fruits and vegetables.
Benefits: May help reduce risk of heart disease, stroke, cataracts, macular degeneration of eyes, some types of cancers.

Flavonoids: Fruits, vegetables, red wine, tea.
Benefits: Antioxidants (page 26), antivirals, anti-inflammatories, antibacterials.

Glucosinolates, indoles: Broccoli, Brussels sprouts, cabbage, mustard greens.
Benefits: May help reduce risk of cancer.

Inositol hexaphosphates: Cereals, soybeans.
Benefits: Antioxidants.

Limonenes: Citrus fruits.
Benefits: Increase the enzymes that may help the body eliminate potential carcinogens.

Lycopenes: Tomatoes, tomato products.
Benefits: May reduce risk of prostate and cervical cancer.

Phytoestrogens: Fennel, legumes, linseed, soybeans, whole wheat.
Benefits: May help reduce menopausal symptoms, lower cholesterol, and reduce risk of prostate cancer.

Protease inhibitors: Legumes, seeds, soybeans.
Benefits: Inhibit growth of cancer cells.

citrus tuna pasta salad

Prep: 30 minutes **Chill:** 1 hour

6 ounces dried mafalda pasta or medium shell macaroni
1 9-ounce package frozen artichoke hearts, thawed
1 9¼-ounce can chunk white tuna (water pack), drained
    and broken into chunks
1 cup sliced fresh mushrooms
1 cup chopped yellow sweet pepper
¼ cup sliced pitted ripe olives
1 recipe Lemon Dressing
1 cup cherry tomatoes, halved
2 tablespoons finely shredded Parmesan cheese

Yellow sweet peppers, artichoke hearts, ripe olives, and a light lemon-herb dressing highlight this delicious pasta salad. Need a healthy potluck dish? Double the ingredients, chill the salad thoroughly, place in an airtight serving container and pack it in an insulated cooler along with lots of ice.

1. Cook pasta according to package directions, except omit any oil or salt. Add artichoke hearts to pasta the last 5 minutes of cooking. Drain in colander. Rinse with cold water; drain again. Halve any large artichoke hearts.

2. Transfer pasta mixture to a large bowl. Gently stir in tuna, mushrooms, sweet pepper, and olives. Prepare Lemon Dressing. Pour dressing over pasta mixture; toss to coat. Cover; refrigerate for at least 1 hour. Gently stir in tomatoes. Sprinkle with Parmesan cheese. Makes 4 main-dish servings.

Lemon Dressing: In a small bowl whisk together 1 teaspoon finely shredded lemon peel; 3 tablespoons lemon juice; 3 tablespoons rice vinegar or white wine vinegar; 2 tablespoons salad oil; 1 tablespoon snipped fresh thyme or basil or 1 teaspoon dried thyme or basil, crushed; 2 cloves garlic; ½ teaspoon sugar; and ¼ teaspoon black pepper.

Nutrition facts per serving: 389 calories, 11 g total fat (1 g saturated fat), 22 mg cholesterol, 369 mg sodium, 49 g carbohydrate, 5 g fiber, 27 g protein. Daily values: 7% vitamin A, 117% vitamin C, 8% calcium, 29% iron.

asparagus & shrimp salad

Start to finish: 30 minutes

Showcase fresh spring asparagus in this citrus and tarragon scented salad. Make everything ahead of time, then chill it for up to 2 hours. Ease preparation by using prewashed salad greens. At the last minute, toss it all together and serve.

1 pound fresh or frozen medium shrimp in shells
½ teaspoon finely shredded orange peel
2 tablespoons orange juice
1 pound fresh asparagus, trimmed and cut into 1-inch
    pieces (about 2 cups)
3 oranges
  Orange juice
1 tablespoon olive or salad oil
1 tablespoon white wine vinegar
1 clove garlic, minced
1 teaspoon snipped fresh tarragon
6 cups torn mixed greens
¼ cup sliced green onions

1. Thaw shrimp, if frozen. Peel, devein, and rinse shrimp. In a large saucepan bring 4 cups water to boiling. Add shrimp; reduce heat. Simmer, uncovered, for 1 to 3 minutes or until shrimp turn opaque. Drain in colander. Rinse with cold water; drain again. Transfer to a bowl. Add orange peel and the 2 tablespoons juice; toss gently to coat. In a covered medium saucepan cook asparagus in a small amount of boiling water for 4 to 6 minutes or until crisp-tender. Drain in colander. Rinse with cold water; drain again. Cover and refrigerate shrimp and asparagus for up to 2 hours.

2. Peel oranges. Working over a bowl, cut oranges into sections; reserve ⅓ cup of the juice. (If necessary, add additional orange juice to make ⅓ cup.) In a bowl whisk together the orange juice, oil, vinegar, garlic, tarragon, and ¼ teaspoon pepper. In a bowl combine shrimp, asparagus, orange sections, greens, and green onions. Pour dressing over all; toss gently to coat. Makes 4 main-dish servings.

Nutrition facts per serving: 180 calories, 5 g total fat (1 g saturated fat), 131 mg cholesterol, 162 mg sodium, 18 g carbohydrate, 5 g fiber, 19 g protein. Daily values: 21% vitamin A, 144% vitamin C, 8% calcium, 23% iron.

vegetables

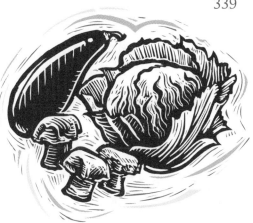

honey–glazed onions

Start to finish: 25 minutes

- 2 cups fresh or frozen small whole onions
- 2 tablespoons honey
- 2 tablespoons white wine vinegar
- 1 tablespoon fresh snipped basil or 1 teaspoon dried basil, crushed
- ¼ teaspoon ground sage

1. If using fresh onions, in a medium covered saucepan cook onions in boiling water for 8 to 10 minutes or just until tender; drain in colander. Cool slightly; peel. (Or, cook frozen onions according to package directions. Drain in colander.)

2. In the same saucepan combine honey, vinegar, basil, and sage. Add onions. Cook and stir until onions are glazed and heated through. Makes 4 side-dish servings.

Nutrition facts per serving: 78 calories, 0 g total fat (0 g saturated fat), 0 mg cholesterol, 4 mg sodium, 19 g carbohydrate, 2 g fiber, 1 g protein. Daily values: 0% vitamin A, 8% vitamin C, 2% calcium, 2% iron.

Just four ingredients make small whole onions grand enough for a very special meal. Onions contain naturally occurring allium, which have been linked with many health benefits including acting as a natural antibiotic and helping increase your cancer resistance.

citrus brussels sprouts

Prep: 15 minutes **Cook:** 10 minutes

Brussels sprouts pair up with sweet, mild carrots in a delicate orange sauce. Fresh Brussels sprouts are available between October and April. Look for firm, compact sprouts. Avoid larger sprouts, as their flavor is bitter. Smaller, vivid green sprouts taste sweeter.

2 cups fresh Brussels sprouts or one 10-ounce package frozen Brussels sprouts, thawed
3 medium carrots, quartered lengthwise and cut into 1-inch pieces
⅓ cup orange juice
1 teaspoon cornstarch
½ teaspoon sugar
¼ teaspoon salt
¼ teaspoon ground nutmeg (optional)

1. Halve Brussels sprouts. In a large covered saucepan cook Brussels sprouts and carrots in a small amount of boiling water for 10 to 12 minutes or until vegetables are crisp-tender. Drain in colander.

2. In the same saucepan combine orange juice, cornstarch, sugar, salt, and, if desired, nutmeg. Add Brussels sprouts and carrots. Cook and stir until thickened and bubbly. Cook and stir for 2 minutes more. Makes 4 side-dish servings.

Nutrition facts per sserving: 61 calories, 1 g total fat (0 g saturated fat), 0 mg cholesterol, 184 mg sodium, 14 g carbohydrate, 4 g fiber, 3 g protein. Daily values: 90% vitamin A, 100% vitamin C, 3% calcium, 8% iron.

don't be fat phobic

Don't try to forsake fat completely. Eating some fat is necessary for good health. Fat transports fat-soluble vitamins A, D, E, and K through the body and supplies essential fatty acids needed for growth, healthy skin, and production of body-regulating hormones.

Additionally, fat makes food flavorful and helps you feel satisfied longer after you eat than either pure protein or carbohydrates.

roasted ratatouille

Prep: 20 minutes **Roast:** 28 minutes

1 small zucchini or yellow summer squash, cubed (1 cup)
1 small eggplant, cubed (3½ cups)
1 medium yellow sweet pepper, cut into 1-inch strips
1 large onion, chopped (1 cup)
2 tablespoons snipped fresh Italian parsley or curly-leaf parsley
2 cloves garlic, minced
1 tablespoon olive oil
⅛ teaspoon salt
⅛ teaspoon black pepper
2 large tomatoes, chopped
1½ teaspoons lemon juice
   Focaccia, cut into wedges, or sliced French bread, toasted (optional)

Roasting vegetables in the oven at a high temperature brings out a robust flavor that can't be beat. Served as a side dish or spooned onto slices of bread, this blend of roasted vegetables is healthful as well as delicious.

1. In a greased 15×10×1-inch baking pan combine the zucchini or summer squash, eggplant, sweet pepper, onion, and parsley.

2. In a small bowl stir together garlic, olive oil, salt, and black pepper. Drizzle over vegetables and toss gently to coat.

3. Roast vegetables, uncovered, in a 450° oven about 20 minutes or until vegetables are tender and lightly browned, stirring once halfway through roasting. Stir in the tomatoes and lemon juice. Roast for 8 to 10 minutes more or until tomatoes are very soft and starting to juice out.

4. To serve, spoon vegetable mixture onto wedges of focaccia or toasted slices of French bread. Makes 4 side-dish servings.

Nutrition facts per serving (without focaccia or bread): 120 calories, 5 g total fat (1 g saturated fat), 2 mg cholesterol, 141 mg sodium, 18 g carbohydrate, 4 g fiber, 4 g protein. Daily values: 10% vitamin A, 189% vitamin C, 6% calcium, 7% iron.

spaghetti squash with tomatoes

Start to finish: 45 minutes

Spaghetti squash is known for what it doesn't have—a lot of fat, sodium, or calories. At just 45 calories per 1-cup serving, it's filling, but not fattening. Fresh herbs and tomatoes unite with the pale, tender spaghettilike squash, creating an ample side dish.

1 2½- to 3-pound spaghetti squash
1 small red or green sweet pepper, chopped
½ cup sliced green onions
2 tablespoons water
2 large tomatoes, chopped
2 tablespoons snipped fresh parsley
2 teaspoons snipped fresh dill or ½ teaspoon dried dillweed
2 teaspoons snipped fresh basil or ½ teaspoon dried basil, crushed
1 tablespoon grated Parmesan cheese

1. Halve squash lengthwise; scoop out seeds. Place squash halves, cut sides down, in a large baking dish. Bake in a 350° oven for 30 to 40 minutes or until tender.

2. Meanwhile, in a medium nonstick skillet combine sweet pepper, green onions, and water. Bring to boiling; reduce heat. Simmer, uncovered, for 2 minutes. Stir in tomatoes, parsley, dill, and basil. Simmer, uncovered, about 5 minutes more or until desired consistency.

3. Using two forks, remove stringy pulp from spaghetti squash and place on a serving platter. Spoon tomato mixture over squash; toss gently to combine. Sprinkle with Parmesan. Makes 6 side-dish servings.

Nutrition facts per serving: 66 calories, 1 g total fat (0 g saturated fat), 1 mg cholesterol, 52 mg sodium, 13 g carbohydrate, 3 g fiber, 2 g protein. Daily values: 15% vitamin A, 59% vitamin C, 5% calcium, 8% iron.

baked potato fries

Prep: 12 minutes **Bake:** 30 minutes

2 medium potatoes (12 ounces total)
2 teaspoons cooking oil
¼ teaspoon salt
¼ teaspoon paprika

Delight your family with homemade steak fries. No need to tell anyone there are just 2 grams of fat per serving. They'll love the crispy outsides with tender insides. You'll love avoiding messy, deep-fat frying.

1. Cut each potato lengthwise into 8 wedges. Place potato wedges in a plastic bag; add oil, salt, and paprika. Close bag and shake to coat.

2. Arrange the potato wedges in a single layer on a large ungreased baking sheet. Bake in a 425° oven for 30 to 35 minutes or until golden brown, turning once or twice. Makes 4 side-dish servings.

Nutrition facts per serving: 109 calories, 2 g total fat (0 g saturated fat), 0 mg cholesterol, 140 mg sodium, 20 g carbohydrate, 1 g fiber, 2 g protein. Daily values: 0% vitamin A, 21% vitamin C, 0% calcium, 7% iron.

Cheese Potato Fries: Prepare as directed above, except omit the salt and paprika. Add 1 tablespoon grated Parmesan cheese, ¼ teaspoon garlic powder, and ¼ teaspoon pepper to the potatoes along with the oil.

Nutrition facts per serving: 117 calories, 3 g total fat (1 g saturated fat), 1 mg cholesterol, 36 mg sodium, 21 g carbohydrate, 1 g fiber, 3 g protein. Daily values: 0% vitamin A, 21% vitamin C, 2% calcium, 7% iron.

Chili Fries: Prepare as directed above, except omit the paprika. Add 1 teaspoon chili powder; ¼ teaspoon dried oregano, crushed; and ⅛ teaspoon ground cumin to the potatoes along with the oil and salt.

Nutrition facts per serving: 111 calories, 2 g total fat (0 g saturated fat), 0 mg cholesterol, 147 mg sodium, 21 g carbohydrate, 1 g fiber, 2 g protein. Daily values: 2% vitamin A, 21% vitamin C, 1% calcium, 8% iron.

spicy spinach salad

Prep: 30 minutes

Spinach, a rich source of immune-boosting vitamin A, vitamin C, and folate, also contains magnesium, a mineral needed to protect your bones, heart, and arteries.

½ to 1 dried chipotle pepper or 1 canned whole green chili pepper
½ cup low-sodium tomato juice
2 tablespoons snipped fresh cilantro or parsley
1 tablespoon salad oil
1 teaspoon sugar
1 clove garlic, minced
¼ teaspoon salt-free seasoning blend
5 cups shredded fresh spinach
2 cups sliced fresh mushrooms
⅔ cup sliced red onion

1. If using dried chipotle pepper, in a small bowl combine the pepper and enough boiling water to cover. Let pepper stand for 20 minutes. Drain. Remove stem and seeds from chipotle or green chili pepper; finely chop.

2. For dressing, in a blender container or food processor bowl combine pepper, tomato juice, cilantro or parsley, oil, sugar, garlic, and seasoning blend. Cover and blend or process until nearly smooth.

3. In a large salad bowl combine spinach, mushrooms, and onion. Pour dressing over spinach mixture; toss gently to coat. Makes 5 to 6 side-dish servings.

Nutrition facts per serving: 62 calories, 3 g total fat (0 g saturated fat), 0 mg cholesterol, 49 mg sodium, 8 g carbohydrate, 3 g fiber, 3 g protein. Daily values: 39% vitamin A, 53% vitamin C, 5% calcium, 14% iron.

grilled vegetable burritos

Prep: 15 minutes **Grill:** 15 minutes

½ cup plain light yogurt or fat-free sour cream
1 small tomato, seeded and chopped
1 teaspoon snipped fresh oregano or ¼ teaspoon dried oregano, crushed
¼ teaspoon ground cumin
8 8-inch fat-free flour tortillas
1 small eggplant, halved lengthwise and cut into ½-inch-thick slices
1 medium zucchini, cut lengthwise into ¼-inch-thick slices
1 medium yellow summer squash, cut lengthwise into ¼-inch-thick slices
1 medium red sweet pepper, cut into ½-inch-wide strips
1 small red onion, cut into ½-inch-thick slices
1 tablespoon olive oil
1 teaspoon chili powder

When summer arrives and outdoor cooking beckons, grill some veggies for supper. A colorful combination of eggplant, red pepper, zucchini, yellow summer squash, and red onion fills the tortillas with panache. Top it all with herbed yogurt and fresh tomato for a sensational meatless meal.

1. In a small bowl stir together yogurt or sour cream, tomato, oregano, and cumin. Cover and refrigerate until serving time.

2. Stack tortillas and wrap tightly in a double thickness of foil; set aside. Brush vegetables lightly with oil; sprinkle with chili powder. Grill onion slices on the rack of an uncovered grill directly over medium heat for 5 minutes. Turn onion slices. Add remaining vegetables and tortilla package. Grill for 10 to 12 minutes more or until vegetables are tender, turning once. If some vegetables cook more quickly than others, remove and keep warm.

3. Divide the grilled vegetables among the tortillas. Top with some of the yogurt mixture, then roll up tortillas. Pass any remaining yogurt mixture. Makes 4 main-dish servings (2 burritos per serving).

Nutrition facts per serving: 308 calories, 4 g total fat (1 g saturated fat), 2 mg cholesterol, 712 mg sodium, 59 g carbohydrate, 5 g fiber, 7 g protein. Daily values: 20% vitamin A, 68% vitamin C, 6% calcium, 17% iron.

vegetable–stuffed chayote

Prep: 30 minutes **Bake:** 28 minutes

Add variety to your repertoire of vegetables with chayote (cha-YOH-teh). This pear-size squash tastes like a cross between an apple and cucumber and provides plenty of potassium. Filled with an herbed vegetable stuffing, it is hearty enough to be served as a meatless main dish.

2 medium chayote (8 ounces each)
1 cup sliced fresh mushrooms
1 small red sweet pepper, chopped
1 medium onion, chopped
1 clove garlic, minced
1 tablespoon margarine or butter
1½ cups soft whole-grain bread crumbs, toasted (2 slices)
½ cup finely shredded Parmesan cheese
1 slightly beaten egg
2 tablespoons snipped fresh cilantro or parsley
⅛ teaspoon salt
⅛ teaspoon black pepper
¼ teaspoon instant vegetable or chicken bouillon granules

1. Halve chayote lengthwise. In a saucepan cook chayote, covered, in enough boiling salted water to cover for 12 to 15 minutes or until tender; drain. When cool enough to handle, remove seeds. Scoop out and reserve pulp, leaving ¼-inch shells. Invert shells to drain. Chop pulp; drain. Squeeze pulp between paper towels to remove excess liquid.

2. For stuffing, in a large skillet cook mushrooms, sweet pepper, onion, and garlic in hot margarine or butter until tender. Remove from heat. Stir in chayote pulp, bread crumbs, ⅓ cup of the Parmesan cheese, the egg, cilantro or parsley, salt, and black pepper. Dissolve bouillon granules in ¼ cup water; stir into mushroom mixture. Spoon stuffing into shells. Place in a 2-quart square baking dish.

3. Bake, covered, in a 350° oven about 25 minutes or until heated through. Sprinkle with remaining Parmesan cheese. Bake, uncovered, for 3 minutes. Makes 4 main-dish servings.

Nutrition facts per serving: 175 calories, 9 g total fat (3 g saturated fat), 63 mg cholesterol, 428 mg sodium, 16 g carbohydrate, 4 g fiber, 10 g protein. Daily values: 28% vitamin A, 51% vitamin C, 29% calcium, 11% iron.

veggie whole wheat pizza

Prep: 30 minutes **Bake:** 20 minutes

3 cups cut-up fresh vegetables (sliced mushrooms; thin bite-size strips of zucchini, yellow summer squash, carrots, baby eggplant, onions, or sweet peppers; and/or small broccoli or cauliflower flowerets)

1 14½-ounce can Italian-style stewed tomatoes, undrained

1 6-ounce can low-sodium tomato paste

2 teaspoons red wine vinegar
Nonstick spray coating

1 16-ounce loaf frozen whole-wheat bread dough, thawed

1 15½-ounce can reduced-sodium red kidney beans, rinsed and drained

1½ cups shredded reduced-fat mozzarella or Monterey Jack cheese (6 ounces)

½ cup crumbled feta cheese or grated Parmesan cheese

2 tablespoons snipped fresh cilantro or parsley

Mama Mia—it's a pizza! It's not the traditional, fat-laden kind, but a whole wheat crust piled high with fresh, vividly colored veggies and low-fat cheeses. This healthful version of an Italian favorite provides generous amounts of vitamins and fiber.

1. Place a steamer basket in a medium saucepan. Add water to just below bottom of basket. Bring to boiling. Add vegetables; reduce heat. Steam, covered, for 2 to 5 minutes or until crisp-tender. Drain on paper towels.

2. For sauce, in a blender container combine tomatoes, tomato paste, and vinegar. Cover and blend until smooth.

3. Spray two 12-inch pizza pans with nonstick coating. Divide dough in half. Pat dough to 11-inch circles on prepared pans, building up edges slightly. Do not let rise. Bake in a 425° oven about 10 minutes or until browned. Remove from oven. Spread sauce over crusts to within ½ inch of edges. Layer with beans, cooked vegetables, and cheeses. Sprinkle with cilantro or parsley. Bake for 10 to 15 minutes more or until bubbly. Makes 8 main-dish servings.

Nutrition facts per serving: 331 calories, 9 g total fat (5 g saturated fat), 26 mg cholesterol, 513 mg sodium, 45 g carbohydrate, 5 g fiber, 18 g protein. Daily values: 58% vitamin A, 30% vitamin C, 28% calcium, 24% iron.

potato pancakes

Prep: 15 minutes **Cook:** 3 minutes (per batch)

If you love ham, eggs, and hash browns for breakfast, these potato pancakes are for you. Served with a spoonful of salsa, this entrée makes a satisfying breakfast or brunch. Just add whole wheat toast and fruit juice.

⅓ cup refrigerated or frozen egg product, thawed, or
    1 egg and 1 egg white
¼ cup all-purpose flour
2 tablespoons sliced green onion
⅛ teaspoon pepper
3 medium potatoes, peeled and shredded (about 2 cups)
½ cup finely chopped lean cooked ham (2 ounces)
1 tablespoon margarine or butter
½ cup salsa

1. In a large bowl combine egg product, flour, green onion, and pepper. Stir in potatoes and ham. In a large skillet melt 1½ teaspoons of the margarine or butter over medium heat.

2. For each pancake, pour about ¼ cup batter into skillet, spreading into a 3-inch circle. Cook for 1½ to 2 minutes on each side or until lightly browned, turning to second sides when pancakes have bubbly surfaces and edges are slightly dry. Keep warm. Repeat with remaining margarine and batter. Serve pancakes with salsa. Makes 4 main-dish servings.

Nutrition facts per serving: 195 calories, 5 g total fat (1 g saturated fat), 4 mg cholesterol, 348 mg sodium, 30 g carbohydrate, 2 g fiber, 9 g protein. Daily values: 12% vitamin A, 36% vitamin C, 2% calcium, 10% iron.

nutrition myth buster

MYTH: Starchy foods such as bread, potatoes, and pasta are fattening.

FACT: Not so! The real culprits are the calorie-dense fatty ingredients and toppings we pair them with—oil, butter, margarine, cheese, and rich sauces, to name just a few. Eating too much of any food can cause weight gain. But, keep in mind that, ounce for ounce, fats pack more than twice the calories of starches.

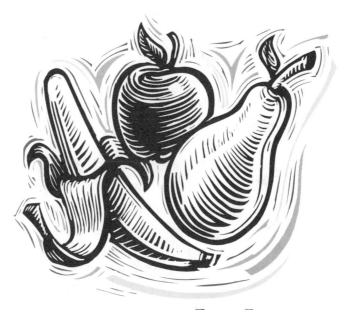

fruits

jicama—berry salad

Prep: 20 minutes

Romaine and/or white kale leaves
2   cups sliced strawberries
1   cup peeled jicama cut into thin bite-size strips
3   tablespoons white wine vinegar
3   tablespoons orange juice
2   medium shallots, finely chopped
1   tablespoon snipped fresh mint or 1 teaspoon dried
       mint, crushed
1   tablespoon olive or salad oil
    Dash salt-free seasoning blend

Low in fat and calories, fruits and vegetables are nutrition bargains. This salad combines the familiar strawberry with the less familiar jicama. Jicama, a root vegetable, adds a slightly sweet flavor and crisp texture to the freshness of this vitamin C-loaded salad.

1. Line 4 salad plates with romaine and/or kale leaves. Arrange strawberries and jicama on greens.

2. For dressing, in a screw-top jar combine vinegar, orange juice, shallots, mint, oil, and seasoning blend. Cover and shake well. Drizzle dressing over salads. Makes 4 side-dish servings.

Nutrition facts per serving: 80 calories, 4 g total fat (0 g saturated fat), 0 mg cholesterol, 4 mg sodium, 11 g carbohydrate, 3 g fiber, 2 g protein. Daily values: 14% vitamin A, 115% vitamin C, 2% calcium, 8% iron.

exotic fruit salad

Prep: 25 minutes **Chill:** 2 hours

Bite into a heavenly combination of fruits—strawberries, cantaloupe, kiwifruit, and papaya. An aromatic blend of lime juice, honey, and five-spice powder lightly dresses every succulent piece of fruit.

1 medium papaya or mango, peeled, seeded, and cut into bite-size pieces (1 cup)
1 cup cubed cantaloupe or honeydew melon
1 cup sliced strawberries
½ teaspoon finely shredded lime peel
3 tablespoons lime juice
1 tablespoon honey
⅛ teaspoon five-spice powder
2 kiwifruit, peeled, halved lengthwise, and sliced

1. In a large salad bowl combine papaya or mango, cantaloupe or honeydew melon, and strawberries.

2. For dressing, in a small bowl stir together lime peel, lime juice, honey, and five-spice powder. Pour dressing over fruit; toss gently to coat. Cover and refrigerate for up to 2 hours. Before serving, stir in kiwifruit. Makes 4 side-dish servings.

Nutrition facts per serving: 89 calories, 1 g total fat (0 g saturated fat), 0 mg cholesterol, 6 mg sodium, 21 g carbohydrate, 1 g fiber, 1 g protein. Daily values: 20% vitamin A, 177% vitamin C, 3% calcium, 3% iron.

pear salad with tofu dressing

Start to finish: 30 minutes

½ of a 10½-ounce package light tofu, cut into cubes
2 tablespoons water or milk
4 teaspoons lemon juice
2 teaspoons olive oil
1 teaspoon Dijon-style mustard
1 teaspoon Worcestershire sauce
1 teaspoon reduced-sodium soy sauce
¼ teaspoon sugar
¼ teaspoon pepper
1 clove garlic, minced
2 tablespoons grated Parmesan cheese
6 cups torn fresh spinach or mixed greens
1 medium pear, thinly sliced
1 stalk celery, sliced
½ cup seedless red grapes, halved
½ cup slivered almonds, toasted

Salad dressings like this one are a tasty way to start working more soy foods into your diet. Tofu, made from soybeans, is a gold mine of phytochemicals. They help lessen your risk of cancer, reduce symptoms of menopause, and lower cholesterol levels.

1. For dressing, place tofu, water or milk, lemon juice, oil, mustard, Worcestershire sauce, soy sauce, sugar, pepper, and garlic in a blender container. Cover and blend until smooth. Add Parmesan cheese; cover and blend until combined.

2. In a large salad bowl combine spinach or mixed greens, pear, celery, grapes, and almonds. Pour dressing over spinach mixture; toss gently to coat. Makes 4 main-dish servings.

Nutrition facts per serving: 171 calories, 9 g total fat (2 g saturated fat), 2 mg cholesterol, 240 mg sodium, 18 g carbohydrate, 5 g fiber, 9 g protein. Daily values: 57% vitamin A, 55% vitamin C, 14% calcium, 22% iron.

pears in red wine sauce

Prep: 15 minutes **Cook:** 18 minutes

Pears always are an elegant dessert—especially when paired with a sweetened wine sauce. Moderate amounts of red or white wine may help lower the risk for heart disease. It's thought that wine may boost the body's ability to dissolve blood clots and lower the amount of "bad" cholesterol formed.

4 medium pears, peeled, halved lengthwise, and cored
1 tablespoon lemon juice
1½ cups dry red wine
¼ cup sugar
3 strips orange peel
¼ cup orange juice
2 inches stick cinnamon
1 tablespoon finely shredded orange peel

1. Brush cut sides of pears with lemon juice. In a large skillet combine the wine, sugar, orange-peel strips, orange juice, and cinnamon. Bring to boiling. Carefully add pears; reduce heat. Simmer, covered, for 10 to 15 minutes or until pears are tender, turning once. Using a slotted spoon, transfer pears to 4 dessert dishes.

2. Return wine mixture to boiling. Boil, uncovered, about 8 minutes or until liquid is reduced to about 1 cup. Remove orange-peel strips and cinnamon; discard. Spoon wine mixture over pears. Sprinkle with the shredded orange peel. Makes 4 servings.

Nutrition facts per serving: 219 calories, 1 g total fat (0 g saturated fat), 0 mg cholesterol, 57 mg sodium, 41 g carbohydrate, 5 g fiber, 1 g protein. Daily values: 0% vitamin A, 30% vitamin C, 2% calcium, 5% iron.

apple–plum crostata

Prep: 25 minutes **Bake:** 40 minutes **Cool:** 30 minutes

1 recipe Pie Crust
3 tablespoons sugar
4 teaspoons cornstarch
1 teaspoon finely shredded lemon peel
¾ teaspoon ground cinnamon
2 medium cooking apples, thinly sliced
3 medium plums, sliced (about 2 cups)
1 teaspoon sugar

The reduced-fat crust for this tart is a cross between a biscuit and pastry. Best of all, it's easy—no tedious crimped edges. Simply fold the excess dough over the top of the fruit filling to make a wide, fuss-free crust. The recipe also can be used for your other favorite single-crust pies.

1. Prepare Pie Crust. In a large bowl stir together the 3 tablespoons sugar, the cornstarch, lemon peel, and cinnamon. Add apples and plums; toss gently to coat. Spread fruit mixture in pastry-lined pie plate. Lift excess dough up and over fruit. Sprinkle top edge of dough with the 1 teaspoon sugar.

2. Bake in a 375° oven for 20 minutes. Cover loosely with foil. Bake about 20 minutes more or until apples are tender. Cool on a wire rack for at least 30 minutes. Makes 8 servings.

Pie Crust: In a medium bowl stir together 1 cup all-purpose flour, 4 teaspoons sugar, 1 teaspoon baking powder, ⅛ teaspoon baking soda, and ⅛ teaspoon salt. Cut in 2 tablespoons butter or margarine until pieces are pea-size. Make a well in the center. Add ⅓ cup buttermilk all at once; stir just until moistened. If mixture seems dry, add 1 tablespoon water, tossing gently to moisten. Turn dough out onto a lightly floured surface. Quickly knead by gently folding and pressing dough for 5 or 6 strokes, or until it holds together. Roll into a 12-inch circle. Transfer to a lightly greased 9-inch pie plate, allowing excess to extend over edge.

Nutrition facts per serving: 146 calories, 3 g total fat (2 g saturated fat), 8 mg cholesterol, 139 mg sodium, 28 g carbohydrate, 2 g fiber, 2 g protein. Daily values: 3% vitamin A, 7% vitamin C, 5% calcium, 6% iron.

praline baked apples

Prep: 15 minutes **Bake:** 30 minutes

Apples win kudos as both a favorite harvest-time fruit and a great source of fiber (especially from the skin). The nut and cinnamon-sugar topping bakes up to crunchy golden brown.

½ cup apple juice
⅛ teaspoon ground cinnamon
4 small red cooking apples
¼ cup coarsely chopped pecans or walnuts
¼ cup packed brown sugar
⅛ teaspoon ground cinnamon
  Vanilla low-fat yogurt or low-fat ice cream (optional)

1. In a small bowl combine apple juice and ⅛ teaspoon cinnamon. Divide mixture among four 6-ounce custard cups. Core apples; remove peel from the top one-third of each apple. Cut apples into eighths, cutting to, but not completely through, the bottoms. Place apples in prepared cups.

2. Place custard cups in a shallow baking pan. In a small bowl combine pecans or walnuts, brown sugar, and ⅛ teaspoon cinnamon; sprinkle over apples. Bake, covered, in a 350° oven for 30 to 40 minutes or until apples are tender.

3. If desired, top each serving with a dollop of low-fat yogurt or ice cream. Makes 4 servings.

Nutrition facts per serving: 183 calories, 5 g total fat (0 g saturated fat), 0 mg cholesterol, 5 mg sodium, 37 g carbohydrate, 4 g fiber, 1 g protein. Daily values: 0% vitamin A, 13% vitamin C, 2% calcium, 5% iron.

frozen fruit yogurt

Prep: 20 minutes **Freeze:** 30 minutes **Ripen:** 4 hours

2 ripe medium bananas, cut into chunks
1 15-ounce can unpeeled apricot halves in light syrup, drained
½ cup apricot nectar or orange juice
¼ cup light-colored corn syrup
2 16-ounce cartons vanilla low-fat yogurt
½ cup light milk

Think dessert can't be good for you? Think again. Calcium and potassium in this frozen yogurt help control your blood pressure, while apricots lend cancer-fighting beta-carotene. This frozen concoction is refreshing on a hot day.

1. In a blender container combine bananas, apricots, and orange juice or apricot nectar. Cover and blend until smooth. Add corn syrup. Cover and blend until syrup is dissolved. In a large bowl combine banana mixture, yogurt, and milk.

2. Freeze mixture in a 2-quart ice-cream freezer according to the manufacturer's directions. Makes twelve ½-cup servings.

Nutrition facts per serving: 138 calories, 2 g total fat (1 g saturated fat), 4 mg cholesterol, 55 mg sodium, 29 g carbohydrate, 1 g fiber, 4 g protein. Daily values: 7% vitamin A, 14% vitamin C, 10% calcium, 3% iron.

a double dose of goodness

Satisfy your sweet tooth with delicious, nutritious snacks and desserts. Carrot-pineapple muffins, zucchini-nut bread, apple-cranberry crisp, and oatmeal-raisin cookies are sweetly satisfying and loaded with good nutrition, too. Additionally, look for desserts, such as the ones in this section, that include fruit as their main ingredient.

mango mousse

Prep: 20 minutes **Freeze:** 45 minutes **Chill:** 4 hours

This light and creamy mousse is a satisfying snack or dessert. Mangoes are the star ingredients, making this mousse rich in three antioxidants—beta-carotene, vitamin C, and vitamin E. All three work together to neutralize naturally occurring free radicals in your body.

2 ripe mangoes, peeled, seeded, and chopped
1 envelope unflavored gelatin
2 tablespoons sugar
2 teaspoons lemon juice
1 8-ounce container frozen light whipped dessert topping, thawed

1. Place mangoes in a food processor bowl or blender container. Cover and process or blend until smooth. Add enough water to make 2 cups total. Transfer the 2 cups mango mixture to a medium saucepan. Bring to boiling.

2. Meanwhile, in a large bowl stir together gelatin and sugar. Pour mango mixture over gelatin mixture; stir until gelatin dissolves. Stir in lemon juice. Cover and freeze for 45 to 60 minutes or until mixture mounds, stirring occasionally. Beat chilled mango mixture with an electric mixer for 2 to 3 minutes or until thick and light. Fold in whipped topping.

3. Spoon or pipe mango mixture into 6 dessert dishes or parfait glasses. Cover; refrigerate until set. Makes 6 servings.

Nutrition facts per serving: 149 calories, 5 g total fat (0 g saturated fat), 1 mg cholesterol, 31 mg sodium, 25 g carbohydrate, 2 g fiber, 1 g protein. Daily values: 31% vitamin A, 34% vitamin C, 2% calcium, 1% iron.

recipe index

general index

a

Acidophilus milk, 228

Acne, 279

Additives, 44–45, 84

African Americans
diabetes in, 124
hypertension in, 187, 189
salt sensitivity in, 191

Age
cholesterol level linked to, 196
at menopause, 235
weight gain linked to, 257

Aging
anti-aging diet, 66–68
anti-aging supplements, 62, 63
antioxidants linked to, 60–62
calorie intake and life span, 65
and fat, 62–65
and nutritional needs, 59–60
physiological changes of, 58–59
and vitamin B12 requirements, 75
and water intake, 66

Alcohol
calories in, 36, 265
and colds, 103
and depression, 121
energy-zapping effects of, 284
as headache trigger, 168
and heartburn, 185
and hypertension, 191
during menopause, 242
in moderation, 35–36
and PMS, 274
during pregnancy, 35
wine and macular degeneration, 232

Alendronate, 253

Allergies, food
diagnosing, 154–155
food reactions that aren't, 157
as not-so-common problem, 152–154
prevention of, 156, 158
symptoms of, 154
tips for coping with, 155–156

American Dietetic Association's Hot Line, 12

Amines, 168–169

Anaphylactic shock, 153

Anemia
B vitamins for, 75–76
versus iron deficiency, 70
iron-rich foods for, 73, 74
symptoms of, 69
in women, 71–72

Antioxidants
as anti-aging vitamins, 60–62
defined, 26
and diabetes, 129
for eye health, 231
for heart disease prevention, 178, 180
and osteoarthritis, 79
for skin protection, 278

Appetite control, 265–266

Apples
as cancer-fighting food, 90–91
as part of low-cholesterol diet, 198

Arthritis
excess weight linked to, 77–78
rheumatoid, 78–81
types of, 78
vegetarian diet for, 81–82
vitamin C for, 79
vitamin D for, 78–79

Aspartame, 44, 170

Asthma
coffee for, 85
and food allergies, 84–85
heartburn linked to, 85
problem foods, 86
symptoms of, 83

Atherosclerosis, 172

b

Bacteria
as cause of foodborne illness, 42
on skin, 203
on teeth, 113–114

Baking soda, 34

Bananas
for high blood pressure, 190
during menopause, 240

Barbecued food, 93

Beano, 90, 149

Beans
as cancer-fighting food, 90
as gas-causing food, 149

Beer, 35–36

Beta-carotene. See also Vitamin A
as anti-aging antioxidant, 60
as cancer-fighting antioxidant, 88, 89
defined, 26
sources of, 91
for vision protection, 230–231

Black tea, 91

Blood pressure
basics, 187–188
DASH diet for lowering, 188–189
and sodium, 33, 191–192
tips for lowering, 189–191

Body Mass Index, 22–23, 258

Body shape, 259

Bones, calcium for, 244–245, 247. See also Osteoporosis

Breast cancer
and alcohol, 11, 36
soy foods as protection against, 90
vegetables for prevention of, 89–90

Breasts, fibrocystic
and caffeine, 145
and fats, 143–144
fiber for, 144
food-hormone connection in, 142–143
good foods for, 146–147
phytoestrogens for, 145–146

Butter
versus margarine, 12, 64, 176
saturated fat in, 29, 195, 198

B vitamins
aging and intake of, 59–60
B6, 75–76, 146, 179
B12, 75, 179, 211
folic acid, 59, 75, 80, 211
for heart health, 59, 179
niacin (B3), 211
for prevention of anemia, 75–76
for sleep quality, 211

C

Caffeine
and depression, 121
and fibrocystic breasts, 145
as insomnia instigator,
209–210
in kids' foods, 32
during menopause, 241
as a natural laxative, 111
and osteoporosis, 254
and PMS, 271, 274
Caffeine withdrawal headaches,
167–168
Calcium
for adults, 252
for children, 246–249
in dairy products, 30
and kidney stones, 222
for menopausal women, 240
as natural sedative, 210
and osteoporosis, 10,
244–255
for prevention of PMS
symptoms, 272–273
Recommended Dietary
Allowance (RDA), 248
for rheumatoid arthritis,
79–80
robbers, 254–255
supplements, 246, 252,
253, 254
in tofu, 251
vitamin D as helper of, 254
Calories
in alcohol, 36, 265
defined, 260
moderate activities for
burning, 23–24
and serving size, 25
Campylobacter, 42
Cancer
antioxidants for prevention
of, 61, 88, 278
breast, 11, 36, 62, 89
colon, 27
foods that promote, 92–94
foods that protect against,
88–92
and free radicals, 87–88
skin, 92, 278–279
Canned goods
shopping for, 45–46
storage of, 50

Carbohydrates
daily calories of, 27
defined, 38
and depression, 119
and heart disease, 177
sugars, 31–33
Carotenoids
beta-carotene, 26, 60, 88, 89,
91, 230–231
as cancer-fighting food,
88, 91
lycopene, 91, 178, 180
as vision protection, 230–231
Celiac disease
cause and cure for, 95–97
forbidden foods list for, 96
gluten-dodging strategies for,
97–99
symptoms of, 95
Cereal
as beneficial grains, 25
as diabetes-fighting food, 128
fiber in, 108
as no-cholesterol snack, 199
Charcoal-broiled food, 93
Cheese
and dental caries, 115
for lactose-intolerant
individuals, 228
Chicken soup for colds, 103
Children
allergy prevention in,
156, 158
asthma in, 83
calcium for, 246–249
cholesterol levels in, 197
diabetes in, 123, 128
fiber for, 31
food allergies in, 152–154
and food safety, 40
heart disease prevention in,
196, 197
hyperactivity in, 31–32
iron needs in, 71, 72
milk-allergic babies, 156,
158, 212
obesity in, 256, 261
school lunches for, 52
tooth decay in, 116
Chili peppers, 102
Chocolate
cravings and PMS, 270, 271
and dental caries, 115

as headache trigger, 169–170
as poor stress reliever, 283
Cholesterol
defined, 29, 194
diabetes and intake of, 126
diet's effect on, 174–175
low-density lipoprotein,
172–173, 194–195
measurement, 194
types of, 194–195
Chromium, 129
Chronic Fatigue Syndrome
(CFS), 135
Citrus fruits as triggers for
asthma, 84
Cleanliness, 50–53
Cluster headaches, 164–165
Clyospora, 39, 42
Coffee
for asthma attacks, 85
and depression, 121
as energy-zapper, 284
with milk, 254
as a natural laxative, 111
and PMS, 274
Colds
facts about, 100–101
foods for fighting, 102–103
herbs for, 104
prevention of, 101–102
vitamin C for, 101
Colon cancer and insoluble
fiber, 27
Constipation
causes of, 105–106
fiber for, 106–111
Cooking
with food safety in mind,
53–55
low-cholesterol meal
preparation, 200
Cooking spray, nonstick, 199
Copper, 75–76
for immune system
function, 207
Crash dieting
and colds, 102
as gallstone instigator,
160, 163
Crucifers, 89–90
Culinary repertoire, 18–19
Cutting boards, 53

metric cooking hints

By making a few conversions, cooks in Australia, Canada, and the United Kingdom can use the recipes in *Better Homes and Gardens®Food for Health & Healing* with confidence. The charts on this page provide a guide for converting measurements from the U.S. customary system, which is used throughout this book, to the imperial and metric systems. There also is a conversion table for oven temperatures to accommodate the differences in oven calibrations.

Product Differences: Most of the ingredients called for in the recipes in this book are available in English-speaking countries. However, some are known by different names. Here are some common American ingredients and their possible counterparts:
● Sugar is granulated or castor sugar.
● Powdered sugar is icing sugar.
● All-purpose flour is plain household flour or white flour. When self-rising flour is used in place of all-purpose flour in a recipe that calls for leavening, omit the leavening agent (baking soda or baking powder) and salt.
● Light-colored corn syrup is golden syrup.
● Cornstarch is cornflour.
● Baking soda is bicarbonate of soda.
● Vanilla is vanilla essence.
● Green, red, or yellow sweet peppers are capsicums.
● Golden raisins are sultanas.

Volume and Weight: Americans traditionally use cup measures for liquid and solid ingredients. The chart, below, shows the approximate imperial and metric equivalents. If you are accustomed to weighing solid ingredients, the following approximate equivalents will be helpful.
● 1 cup butter, castor sugar, or rice = 8 ounces = about 250 grams
● 1 cup flour = 4 ounces = about 125 grams
● 1 cup icing sugar = 5 ounces = about 150 grams
  Spoon measures are used for smaller amounts of ingredients. Although the size of the tablespoon varies slightly in different countries, for practical purposes and for recipes in this book, a straight substitution is all that's necessary.
  Measurements made using cups or spoons always should be level unless stated otherwise.

equivalents: U.S. = Australia/U.K.

⅛ teaspoon = 0.5 ml
¼ teaspoon = 1 ml
½ teaspoon = 2 ml
1 teaspoon = 5 ml
1 tablespoon = 1 tablespoon
¼ cup = 2 tablespoons = 2 fluid ounces = 60 ml
⅓ cup = ¼ cup = 3 fluid ounces = 90 ml
½ cup = ⅓ cup = 4 fluid ounces = 120 ml
⅔ cup = ½ cup = 5 fluid ounces = 150 ml
¾ cup = ⅔ cup = 6 fluid ounces = 180 ml
1 cup = ¾ cup = 8 fluid ounces = 240 ml
1¼ cups = 1 cup
2 cups = 1 pint
1 quart = 1 liter
½ inch =1.27 cm
1 inch = 2.54 cm

continued

baking pan sizes

American	Metric
8×1½-inch round baking pan	20×4-cm cake tin
9×1½-inch round baking pan	23×3.5-cm cake tin
11×7×1½-inch baking pan	28×18×4-cm baking tin
13×9×2-inch baking pan	30×20×3-cm baking tin
2-quart rectangular baking dish	30×20×3-cm baking tin
15×10×1-inch baking pan	30×25×2-cm baking tin (Swiss roll tin)
9-inch pie plate	22×4- or 23×4-cm pie plate
7- or 8-inch springform pan	18- or 20-cm springform or loose-bottom cake tin
9×5×3-inch loaf pan	23×13×7-cm or 2-pound narrow loaf tin or pâté tin
1½-quart casserole	1.5-liter casserole
2-quart casserole	2-liter casserole

oven temperature equivalents

Fahrenheit Setting	Celsius Setting*	Gas Setting
300°F (slow)	150°C	Gas Mark 2
325°F (moderately slow)	160°C	Gas Mark 3
350°F (moderate)	180°C	Gas Mark 4
375°F (moderately hot)	190°C	Gas Mark 5
400°F	200°C	Gas Mark 6 (hot)
425°F	220°C	Gas Mark 7
450°F	230°C	Gas Mark 8 (very hot)
Broil		Grill

*Electric and gas ovens may be calibrated using Celsius. However, for an electric oven, increase the Celsius setting 10 to 20 degrees when cooking above 160°C. For convection or forced-air ovens (gas or electric), lower the temperature setting 10°C when cooking at all heat levels.